MW00380928

Board Stiff Too

Board Stiff Too

Preparing for the Anesthesia Orals

Second Edition

Christopher J. Gallagher, M.D.
Staff Anesthesiologist, Florida Gulf to Bay
Anesthesiology, Tampa General Hospital,
Tampa, Florida

Steven E. Hill, M.D.
Assistant Professor of Anesthesiology,
Duke University Medical Center,
Durham, North Carolina

David A. Lubarsky, M.D., M.B.A.
Associate Professor and Vice Chairman
of Anesthesiology, Duke University Medical
Center, Durham, North Carolina

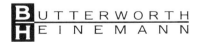

An Imprint of Elsevier

Boston   Oxford   Auckland   Johannesburg   Melbourne   New Delhi

Copyright © 2001 by Butterworth–Heinemann

 A member of the Reed Elsevier group

All rights reserved.

No part of this publication may be reproduced, stored in a retrieval system, or transmitted in any form or by any means, electronic, mechanical, photocopying, recording, or otherwise, without the prior written permission of the publisher.

Permissions may be sought directly from Elsevier's Health Sciences Rights Department in Philadelphia, USA: phone: (+1)215-238-7869, fax: (+1)215-238-2239, email: healthpermissions@elsevier.com. You may also complete your request on-line via the Elsevier Science homepage (http://www.elsevier.com), by selecting 'Customer Support' and then 'Obtaining Permissions'.

Every effort has been made to ensure that the drug dosage schedules within this text are accurate and conform to standards accepted at time of publication. However, as treatment recommendations vary in the light of continuing research and clinical experience, the reader is advised to verify drug dosage schedules herein with information found on product information sheets. This is especially true in cases of new or infrequently used drugs.

Recognizing the importance of preserving what has been written, Butterworth–Heinemann prints its books on acid-free paper whenever possible.

 Butterworth–Heinemann supports the efforts of American Forests and the Global ReLeaf program in its campaign for the betterment of trees, forests, and our environment.

Library of Congress Cataloging-in-Publication Data

Gallagher, Christopher J.
  Board stiff too : preparing for the anesthesia orals / Christopher J. Gallagher, Steven E. Hill, David A. Lubarsky.—2nd ed.
    p. ; cm.
  Rev. ed. of: Preparing for the anesthesia orals : board stiff / Christopher J. Gallagher, David A. Lubarsky. Boston : Butterworths, c1990.
  Includes bibliographical references and index.
  ISBN 0-7506-7157-2 (alk. paper)
  1. Anesthesia—Examinations, questions, etc.   I. Title: Preparing for the anesthesia orals.   II. Hill, Steven E.   III. Lubarsky, David A.   IV. Title.
  [DNLM: 1. Anesthesia—Examination Questions. 2. Anesthesiology—education. WO 218.2 G162b 2001]
  RD82.3 .G35 2001
  617.9'6'076—dc21

                                                                    00-041390

British Library Cataloguing-in-Publication Data
A catalogue record for this book is available from the British Library.

The publisher offers special discounts on bulk orders of this book.
For information, please contact:

Manager of Special Sales
Butterworth–Heinemann
225 Wildwood Avenue
Woburn, MA 01801-2041
Tel: 781-904-2500
Fax: 781-904-2620

For information on all Butterworth–Heinemann publications available, contact our World Wide Web home page at: http://www.bh.com

10 9 8 7 6 5 4
Printed in the United States of America

Contents

Preface to the Second Edition

"DRECK!"
"Wouldn't use this to line the bottom of a parakeet cage!
It's an insult to both parakeet and cage!"
"The trees that gave their lives for this book all died in vain."

Chris sat back and looked through the reviews of *Board Stiff: Preparing for the Anesthesia Orals.* Ah, to relive that past glory. Thems were the days.

Behind him, a curtain billowed. A breeze from the toxic waste dump wafted in through the window. Bills PAST DUE, old Lotto tickets, and pink slips blew off the Formica kitchen table. Chris reached for them, missed, shrugged them off as no loss, then kept going in one swift motion to the bag of fried pork rinds. With his other hand, he turned up the volume on his remote. On the TV, two women tore each other's hair out.

Jerry Springer's "Too Hot for Television III" played out the timeless drama of love affairs gone awry.

Footsteps crunched on the gravel walkway. The door banged.

"I know you're in there, Dr. Gallagher! I can hear your TV!" the proprietor of Fragrant Zephyrs Trailer Courts shouted. "Now I got people I gotta pay, and I can't do that 'til you pay me! Now I have my check by Monday or you're out, you hear me?"

The women on the Jerry Springer video increased their volume. After a few minutes, the footsteps on the gravel crunched away.

Chris picked up his phone, a plastic mockup of a Macintosh laryngoscope, and dialed the operator.

"I'd like to place a collect call."

"That's right, collect, to Dr. David Lubarsky."

The phone rang in David Lubarsky's office. His telephone, a mockup of a Miller laryngoscope.

Noticing his assistant was nowhere to be found, David found himself actually answering his own phone. In a somewhat annoyed tone, he said "Yes?"

"Will you accept a collect call from a Mister…" the operator started.

"That's DOCTOR, lady!" Chris protested.

"Will you accept a collect call from a…Doctor Gallagher?" the operator asked.

"Hey Dave, remember me?"

"Operator," David said, "I'll accept the call." He drummed his fingers on his desk. "So, Chris, looks like private practice is treating you right. Are you calling from prison? Is this the one phone call you get from the jail?"

Chris washed down his fried pork rinds with a gulp of JOLT!® Cola. "Very funny; they never convicted me that time. That's not what this is about anyway. What say we write a second edition of *Board Stiff*?"

David's eyebrows went up. "What would possess us to write a second edition of *Board Stiff*?"

Chris looked around at his bills PAST DUE.

"Uh, Dave, it's not so much a question of *possess* us, it's more a question of getting *repossessed*, if you follow my meaning," Chris explained.

"Oh," David caught it. "Well if we're going to do this, we'd better get some young blood on this. Someone closer to the exam."

"You mean dragoon some new assistant professor into doing all the work?" Chris asked.

"You understand the academic world to a T," David said.

"Then take all the credit and all the money?" Chris pressed.

"Sounds like a plan to me," David said. "His name is Steve Hill. He just took the test so he'll know all the latest."

"Done," Chris said. "Uh, one last thing." Chris looked around at the empty pizza boxes, the beer-can pyramid decorations. "Do you think we can squeeze an advance out of the publisher?"

C.J.G.
S.E.H.
D.A.L.

Preface to the First Edition

In the beginning there was half the big syringe, all the small syringe. Then came fentanyl, somatosensory evoked potentials, halothane hepatitis, and a host of other afflictions to vex the spirit of the average oral board examinee. Where to turn? The literature? Go ahead, open the last 17 volumes of *Anesthesiology*. Do you really care what happens to slices of salamander fetal hippocampus when exposed to the latest benzodiazepine antagonist? Are you about to try to disprove the findings yourself? Wrong, bucko. The questions that bother you are much more mundane—and more important.

Soon you'll be staring down the glare of two examiners who have forgotten more in the last 15 minutes than you've learned in your whole wretched lifetime. They aren't concerned with what happens in the achondroplastic dwarf on phenelzine who just aspirated a peanut and has had no IV access ever since a 99% burn. They want to know whether you'll cancel a generic case for a generically high blood pressure. Try to find the answer! Look long and hard. Read all the textbooks. Direct answers are hard to find!

Devoid of any national renown, the two of us have taken it on ourselves to distill the essence of the oral boards into a small, portable study guide. Academicians in the field of anesthesiology may cringe at the thought that this book is even associated with their discipline—the authors are the types you see at a meeting, not presenting abstracts, but hanging out at the pool demanding piña coladas for breakfast.

We have invented a large variety of oral board scenarios and present them step by step. To develop these questions, we culled information from scores of examinees. We talked to many who passed and a few who flunked. From the recurrent themes that appeared year after year, we invented questions similar to those encountered on the oral boards.

- No examiners were approached about specific questions.
- No examiners were connected in any way to the production of this book.
- These questions are meant to resemble oral board questions. Any verbatim reproduction of an actual board question is coincidental.

We have not annotated every fact in this book. We did that for three reasons. First, this is a review, a guide book. If you need a ton of references, then consult the heavily referenced textbooks. Second, most people in their last few weeks of preparation for the boards don't look up a lot of original articles. Third[1], when[2-4] you're[5] reading (Rumpelstiltskin, 1856) through[ibid.] a[4,6,7,8] review (Jumpinjehosephrat, 1977), the flow gets a little choppy if every other word is coated with superscripts and references.

This book will provide you with answers to those tough "there's no right answer" questions. Maybe not *the* answer, but an answer you can defend. We stick our necks out on a variety of complex and controversial questions. We discuss difficult cases where you must balance the anesthetic considerations for two or more organ systems concomitantly. We show you how to make a rational decision that you should be able to defend. Making rational decisions that you can defend should get you through the boards.

Good luck!

C.J.G.
D.A.L.

The Road Up Ahead

Lasciate ogni speranza,voi ch'intrate.
—Dante, *The Inferno*

(Abandon all hope ye who enter here.)

Oh, the Oral Boards for Anesthesiology aren't so bad. No need to abandon all hope. *Board Stiff Too* stands ready to help you through the big day. Here's how.

PART I: DRIVING SCHOOL

Tips for taking the test. The authors have worked with hundreds of test takers over the past decade. Certain methods of test preparation consistently work. Certain methods consistently fail. Learn the methods that work. (Hint: Practice aloud. Practice aloud early. Practice aloud often.)

PART II: MECHANIC'S MANUAL

A brief review of the major subjects that will appear on the test: pulmonary, cardiac, airway, trauma, renal, OB, peds, pain, regional, liver, equipment, fluids, and obesity. Each area is examined with the Anesthesia Oral Examination in mind, that is, what are the preop, intraop, and postop implications? Get in the "test mode" of thinking. See how to defend different answers.

PART III: TEST TRACK

Practice questions and practice exams—the meat of the book and the meat of your own preparation. You will receive two flavors of tests. The first batch of questions comes from Chris's kitchen. Chris sold his soul to private practice so his answers have a "real world" seasoning to them. David and Steve prepared the second batch of questions. As David and

Steve both reside in the pulsating nerve center of academe, their answers have an "academic world" piquancy.

This dual viewpoint serves the same function as diversifying your portfolio. You don't want all of Chris's prejudices, and you don't want all of David's and Steve's prejudices. Take all the answers given with a grain of salt. Disagree with them, come up with your own answers. Come up with better answers!

WHAT PROVED MOST USEFUL FROM THE FIRST EDITION OF *BOARD STIFF*?

The single review chapter that readers found most useful was "Vital Signs Are Vital." Every test taker had to explain some alteration in the vital signs, and the list from "Vital Signs Are Vital" helped.

All readers found the practice exams useful. And a decade's worth of readers all agreed with our constant nagging to "Practice aloud, practice aloud, practice aloud." You are holding a *written* book but you are preparing for an *oral* exam, so do the obvious: practice *saying* your answers.

WHAT HAS CHANGED SINCE *BOARD STIFF*?

The more things change, the more things stay the same. At the time of the first edition, the test consisted of two clinical scenes, each with preop, intraop, and postop questions. Now, the test consists of two clinical scenes, one with intraop and postop questions, the other with preop and intraop questions. Both exams emphasize the intraop portion of the exam. So, although divided up, you will still need to know the preop, intraop, and postop implications of everything.

The biggest educational change has been the explosion of the cyberworld. A wealth of online resources now offers the test taker more opportunities to look up material and to practice the exam. Today's test taker can "practice aloud" online with a friend, look up the latest Malignant Hyperthermia recommendations, go into a chat room with other anesthesiologists (Gasnet), look up emedicine.com for an online anesthesia textbook, or access an expert panel of subspecialty anesthesiologists on anesthesiaweb.com. All from the comfort of his or her own PC. Great stuff, this is.

THE FUNNIEST THING WE HEARD IN 10 YEARS OF *BOARD STIFF*-RELATED COMMENTS?

One brutally honest fellow may have hit upon a great truth when he said, "Face it, nothing you read does you any good anyway, but at least

Board Stiff is funny. So as long as you're killing time before the test, you might as well read something funny."

We hope you will find *Board Stiff Too* useful. Questions? Comments? Complaints? Threats? Please, let us know. Board Stiff, Inc. is a work in progress, and we are always eager to field your input on how to improve.

Board Stiff Too

Driving School

TIPS FOR TAKING THE TEST

In the not too distant future you will find yourself in a hotel room. In that room, there will be three things vital to your passing the anesthesia oral board examination:

1. The oral board examiners
2. The oral board exam
3. You

Driving School will give you insight into the first two components—the examiners and the test. How is the test given? Why is the test important? What motivates the examiners? What are the examiners looking for in a Board Certified Anesthesiologist? This information should help you relax a little. It's easier to go into a test knowing what's coming.

Driving School will give you insight into the most important element in the room—you. You, the test taker.

Over the past 10 years, the authors have prepared for the exam themselves, and have helped hundreds of others prepare for the exam. What method of test preparation works for you? What method of test preparation fails for you?

Driving School will reveal what works for you, so that *you* can walk out of that hotel room with a smile on your face.

Chapters 1–6 will look at the individual aspects of test preparation. Chapter 7 will tie it all together.

1 | Ten Little Indians

Ten little Indian boys went out to dine; one choked his little self and then there were nine.

Nine little Indian boys sat up very late; one overslept himself and then there were eight.

Eight little Indian boys traveling in Devon; one said he'd stay there and then there were seven.

Seven little Indian boys chopping up sticks; one chopped himself in halves and then there were six.

Six little Indian boys playing with a hive; a bumblebee stung one and then there were five.

Five little Indian boys going in for law; one got in Chancery and then there were four.

Four little Indian boys going out to sea; a red herring swallowed one and then there were three.

Three little Indian boys walking in the Zoo; a big bear hugged one and then there were two.

Two little Indian boys sitting in the sun; one got frizzled up and then there was one.

One little Indian boy left all alone; he went and hanged himself and then there were none.

Agatha Christie's murder masterpiece *Ten Little Indians* (the original title was *Then There Were None*) takes place on an island. Ten guests, all with murderous skeletons in their closets, are invited by an unknown host to attend a weekend party. One by one, the guests are murdered, each according to the nursery rhyme "Ten Little Indians."

For example, the first guest is poisoned at dinner, which corresponds to the nursery rhyme line, "one choked his little self."

The second guest is smothered with a pillow in his bed, which corresponds to the nursery rhyme line, "one overslept himself." And so it goes down the list.

As people die, one by one, suspicion among the surviving guests rises to a fever pitch. One of the remaining guests *has* to be the murderer! Imagine if you were one of the last two survivors? Your opposite, the other surviving guest, *must* be the murderer. And there you are, all alone on the island, with only you, a murderer, and eight dead bodies.

(That's way worse than taking your Boards could ever be!) Agatha Christie, master of the murder genre, keeps you hanging right up to the last page.

Will we keep *you* hanging? Will you have to hold your breath right up to the last paragraph of *Board Stiff Too* to see how to prepare for your Oral Board Examination?

No.

We will tell you right now, at the *beginning* of the book. You may want to read the next section, "The Trick," and put this book back on the shelf. You can do all your test preparation on your own at no cost. (That might be the best advice you'll get in this whole book.)

THE TRICK

To get good at playing tennis, you should play tennis.
To get good at swimming, you should swim.
To get good at speaking French, you should speak French.
To get good at the Oral Board Examination, you should practice
    taking oral board examinations.

Did you catch it?

Practice taking oral board exams. Practice aloud, starting today, now, this minute.

Practice aloud, even if that means talking to yourself, your dog, or a sympathetic wall or tree. Practice aloud early and often. Have your partners quiz you if you are in practice. Have your attendings quiz you if you are in residence. Give practice exams to other people, and listen to how they explain themselves *aloud*. Keep practicing always remembering the golden rule: IF I CAN'T EXPLAIN IT ALOUD THEN I DON'T KNOW IT. IF IT DOESN'T SOUND RIGHT ALOUD, THEN KEEP PRACTICING UNTIL IT DOES SOUND RIGHT ALOUD. Explain *aloud* what you do every day. Explain your next case *aloud*. Explain how you would handle a stat C-Section *aloud*, a trauma case *aloud*, anaphylactic shock *aloud*. Practice aloud, aloud, aloud. Make the words. Say the words. Move your mouth. Be like the Tin Man when they oiled his jaw.

At this point, you have gutted the most important lesson out of this book. If you want to slip the book back on the shelf, look around the medical bookstore with a guilty expression, and slip out to the parking lot, be our guest. Enjoy pizza and beer with the money you saved. Hoist a cold one in our honor. Good luck and God bless.

And when you pass the exam and finally have time to read non-anesthetic stuff, read *Ten Little Indians*. The ending will blow you away.

2 | Who, What, Where, When, Why

Journalists since time immemorial have asked the questions: Who, What, Where, and When? To these, we add Why?

WHO?

Who are the oral board examiners? Who are the people that will be facing you in that hotel room?

Some oral board examiners are academics; some are private practice anesthesiologists. They are a dedicated lot, true guardians of the faith. Consider what they go through; before consideration for oral examiner status, they have to design questions for the written boards. They do these exams on their own time, often using up their vacation or professional leave time. Reimbursement? Chump change. It's got to be a labor of love; it sure ain't a labor for money.

Fun? During the exams the examiners are almost in prison, able only to hang out with other examiners. Any "fraternization" with the examinees and they are hung up by their thumbs with piano wires.

So why do they do it? Believe it or not, to keep the specialty strong, to keep us tight as a profession. To understand this, look at the flip side of the issue. What would it mean to be board certified in anesthesiology if you walked into an exam, sat down in the exam room, shook hands with two other anesthesiologists, stated your hat size, and walked out with a passing grade? Nothing. That's what board certification would mean. Nothing. There would be no standard of excellence, no yardstick. How would that sit with the surgeons who pass a rigorous test to get their board certification? How would that sit with the OB-GYN docs, the internists, the cardiologists, all of whom work hard to pass their specialty tests? *How would that sit with the patients?*

So, these board examiners, this merry band of hard workers, are doing us the ultimate favor. They are keeping our specialty credible.

WHAT?

What are the examiners looking for?

Specifics will follow (the actual format), but for now, look at the question in the broad sense. What would *you* look for if *you* were an examiner? Before you give the label "Expert in the Field of Anesthesiology" to someone, you would expect that anesthesiologist to know about any aspect pertaining to perioperative management of a patient, would you not?

Preoperative

Is the patient ready for an elective procedure? Should anything else be done diagnostically or therapeutically before surgery? Is the patient an emergency? Even if an emergency, should anything else be done diagnostically or therapeutically before the operation? Economics are a reality now, do you really need to delay the case or order the million dollar workup? How do you explain risk to a patient, a family? What if a parent wants to come to the OR?

Name it. Think of anything, anything at all that can occur in the time before the case starts. It is all fair game. Why? Because the label of board certification, the label "Expert in the Field of Anesthesiology" means you can handle whatever comes up.

Intraoperative

(Of note, this area is the most heavily weighted in the exam.)
Again, what is fair game? Anything that happens in the OR is fair game—lines, monitors, machines, induction, vital signs, bleeding, coding. If it can happen in the OR, it can appear on the exam. You must know the induction of an 18-year-old marine with a twisted knee, a 75-year-old brought from the cath lab in full arrest, and anything else you can imagine. The rhythm can be sinus, V-tach, or flat line. You have to know what to do.

Alternatives. Why do a spinal? Why not a general? You induced with propofol, why not breathe down with sevoflurane? You try an arm block; it doesn't work, now what? Patient refuses an IV; what will you do in these cases? An "Expert in the Field of Anesthesiology" would know what to do, and, out loud, be able to defend his or her answer in a logical manner.

Disasters. Can a venous air embolism occur intraop? Myocardial ischemia? Failed intubation? Catastrophic bleeding? Sure. Is it reasonable for an examiner to ask you to explain your way through such disasters? Sure.

Postoperative

An "Expert in the Field of Anesthesiology" should be able to manage what in the postoperative period? *Anything.* That's the definition of an expert. That's the definition of a board certified anesthesiologist.

Laryngospasm? Oliguria? ARDS? Lost tooth? Inadequate pain relief? Respiratory arrest? Put yourself in the examiners' position. Of course you would expect an expert to know how to manage these problems.

That is the "What" of the exam. Anything at all that can happen to a patient under your care.

WHY?

Why bother getting board certified? Can't you practice without it? Don't plenty of people get by just fine without their boards? Yes, so far, but more and more, insurance companies, hospital privilege committees, and individual anesthesia groups are making board certification a necessity. No doubt, if you are board certified, you are better off.

WHEN?

Twice a year, in spring and fall.

A question we often get is, "Should I take the oral exam as soon as possible after the written exam?" Yes, yes, a thousand times yes. Take that exam while the stuff is fresh. Don't hold off on the vain hope that you will have "more time to prepare." That "more time" never comes. It's human nature to put off studying, and it's human nature to forget stuff as time passes. So just jump into the flames as soon as possible.

Hospitals have time limits, too. For example, a hospital may say you have 5 years from the end of your residence to become board certified. So if you hold off and hold off, then fail your exam, you may get in trouble with hospital privileges. If, in contrast, you take the test right away, then even if you flunk, you'll have time to take the test again.

If you fail, when can you test again? The next time it comes around, in about 6 months.

How many times can you take the exam? If you fail three times, you have to go back and retake the writtens. If you fail six times, then you have to do another year of residence to become eligible again. That means quite a hit in the wallet, if you think about going back to a resident's salary.

WHERE?

The exam is always at some nice resort. Of course, the resort's amenities are usually lost on the freaking-out test takers. Some people choose to stay at a nearby hotel to escape the supercharged atmosphere. Other examinees fly in just for the day. Better make sure you get to the right place on time if you do that. Taking this exam isn't like missing a flight. You can't just say, "Sorry, can you fit me in the next slot?"

That is the journalist's view of the boards—the who, what, where, when, and why. Now back to you. What is your best study material? What should you read? How can you get knowledge?

3 | With All Thy Getting Get Knowledge

Saint Thomas More described Utopia as the ideal world. If an oral board candidate were to prepare for an exam in this Utopia, the scheme would run something like this:

> Time: Years ahead of the exam, the candidate would say, "Hark! Those distant drums, yea verily they represent the sound of the approaching oral board examination! I shall now, this minute, steel myself to the task at hand and start reading, practicing aloud, and dedicate my every minute to prepare for this exam; this watershed event in my life. Not a grain of sand shall fall through the hourglass 'ere I begin my preparation."
> Study Schedule: Every day, month after month, year after year, the Utopian preparation continues. Read, study, practice aloud, practice exams without end from dozens of different examiners.
> Books Read: Miller, the magnum opus version. Then on to Barash's *Clinical Anesthesia*, then Stoelting's *Anesthesia and Co-Existing Diseases*, then a little poolside reading—Dorsch and Dorsch's *Understanding Anesthesia Equipment*. For fun, on vacation, the perfect oral board candidate brings along a waterproofed edition of the *Mass General Handbook* to read on his windsurf board.

To round out his reading, this most perfect of anesthesia students zips through the *ASA Refresher Course* book, the discussion section of each article in *Anesthesiology*, *Anesthesia and Analgesia*, and the British and Canadian journals of anaesthesia. (He laughs to himself how funny they spell "anaesthesia.") In the bathroom he has a copy of Snow's *On the Inhalation of Ether* in the magazine rack next to the commode.

Does he or she waste time in the car going to work? Heaven forfend! Enter Audio Digest, the bimonthly, one-hour cassette produced by the California Medical Association. Well-edited, clinically relevant, understandable, these tapes tell our hero or heroine the latest thinking on obstetric anesthesia, the difficult airway, pain management, and every other topic in anesthesia. And yes, Audio Digest comes with little quizzes to hammer home the important points.

> Study Atmosphere: In Utopia, the work, call, and personal schedule always leave plenty of time for uninterrupted study in a quiet atmosphere after a good night's sleep. A computer provides instant access to the website (www.AnesthesiaWeb.com) where Dr. Lubarsky is the chair of the editorial board. The computer also links to cyberchat rooms like Gasnet where tough questions are batted around.

A few centuries after Saint Thomas More, another term entered the lexicon, Realpolitik, the world as it really is rather than the way it should be. Let us examine a Realpolitik study plan.

> Time: "Oh good golly Miss Molly! Look at that calendar. The oral board exam is next week and I haven't read a damned thing!"
> Study Schedule: You ask your boss for a little time off to study for the exam. Boss says, "Are you talking to me? Is this some kind of joke? Does this hospital look like a study hall to you, or maybe you think we can pay the bills by sitting around all day doing nothing. Now get back into your room and be lucky I don't rip your head off."
> Books Read: Uh…
> Study Atmosphere: Junior has colic. The washing machine just leaked all over the hardwood floor. Another person at work quit, so your call schedule just got worse. The next-door neighbor's teenager is starting a rock band and they practice a lot.

Sound familiar? No mere mortal can do the Utopian test preparation. Most of us tend towards the Realpolitik end of the spectrum. Here's a time-tested way to maximize what study time you do have.

1. Your READING is best directed by HOW DO YOU DO ON A PRACTICE ORAL EXAM.
2. Baby Miller (or Miller Lite) has a ton of information. Go through Baby Miller slowly. Better to go through Baby Miller twice than Big Miller just partway through.
3. The crème de la crème of reading is the "Anesthetic Considerations" section of Stoelting's *Anesthesia and Co-Existing Disease.* If I had blown off everything and only had time to read one thing, I would read this.
4. Try taping yourself with a dictaphone or Walkman. (It's like filming your golf swing and studying the motions.) Over time, you will hear yourself improve.

5. *Audio Digest*. Fills in "down time" in the car or while out exercising. These tapes ask *and answer* the very questions likely to appear on the exam. They're a little expensive, but most anesthesia libraries in teaching programs should have them. Or you can share the cost with someone else taking the test.

6. *ASA Refresher Course*. The little chapters (4 or 5 pages, most of them) fit into a "real world" pattern of studying. Case delayed for 15 minutes? Whip out the Refresher Course and read a chapter. A few minutes' reading before you go to sleep at night? Time enough for one little ASA Refresher course.

7. Invisible reading. You're in a case, not much is happening. In your mind's eye, *make* something happen. Practice explaining what you would do if, say, the patient's pressure went through the roof, or through the floor. Imagine V-tach, A-fib, accidental extubation, imagine anything! Then explain, as if talking to another person, what you would do. Pick the worst case scenario and talk your way through it, only silently. Does your patient have a history of CAD? What about working through an intraoperative MI—how would it appear on your monitors; how would you respond?

     This silent reading, this "imagined oral boards" can provide you with a hundred examinations' worth of practice tests, a thousand. And you always have time for this studying, after all, you're in the operating room all day. Make your OR time study time.

8. Weekly conferences. Any residency has some kind of weekly meeting. Any group has some Q/A meetings. Make these meetings your own, personal, tailor-made oral board preparation course. Ask your attendings or colleagues, "Who should get a muscle biopsy for MH? What platelet count would you 'allow' for an epidural?" Listen how your colleagues explain their answers. Then give your own explanations. Can you answer, out loud, the questions that come up at these meetings? If you make every meeting a mini practice board, you should be in fine shape when the actual test comes along. Of note, many people fresh out of residency took and passed the oral boards with no "extra" preparation whatsoever. Universally, they told the authors that their weekly departmental meetings played a key role in their success. "Each week we saw an oral board exam, after years of that, the actual board exam was a snap."

9. *Mass General Handbook*. Great source for info like maximum doses of local anesthetics. Gives bullet explanations of mechanism of action of, say, bretylium. (Maybe you use bretylium rarely; you should still know something about it.) The *Mass General Handbook* has the distinct advantage of being portable so you can take it poolside.

10. Other board review books. The original *Board Stiff* generated a whole slough of *Board Stiff* knockoffs. To wit:

    What to Say on the Oral Boards
    What Not to Say on the Oral Boards
    What You Should Say on the Oral Boards
    What You Should Not Say on the Oral Boards

    The list goes on. Are these *Board Stiff* copycats any good? Yes! They ask questions. They make you think. That's good preparation.

11. Review courses such as Osler. You get out of them what you put into them. If you feel that you are going to some spa that will magically make you pass the exam, you're wrong. If you go there ready to roll up your sleeves, take a lot of practice exams, watch a lot of practice exams, and work your tail off, you will get a lot out of them. Are these review courses worth the money? Only you can answer that. If you can prepare yourself with self-study, practice exams with attendings or friends, then you need not attend such a course.

    If you're in solo practice, have little contact with colleagues, or if you have a house full of kids and just cannot find study time to yourself, or if your personality is such that you need to "go somewhere" to study, then these review courses may be for you. Are most people satisfied with these review course meetings? Yes.

Dr. Lubarsky even has a little cottage industry where he personally tutors a few students before each exam (even academics have to do something to earn $$).

Books, review courses, audiotape, self-taping, invisible reading—no matter what your method, remember the prime directive:

PRACTICE ALOUD, REMEMBER, THESE ARE *ORAL* BOARDS. IT'S WHAT YOU *SAY*, NOT WHAT YOU READ, THAT WILL MAKE FOR A PASSING GRADE.

There, now that we've cleared the deck, it should be smooth sailing through calm seas.

4 | God Himself Could Not Sink This Ship

The shipbuilder had thought of everything, even building watertight compartments in case the ship had a collision with, say, an iceberg. No idle boast, then, when the shipbuilder bragged, "God Himself could not sink this ship."

> "Iceberg dead ahead!"
> "Hard a port!"
> Scrape.
> Blub.

So much for unbridled confidence.

Shipbuilders learned from the failure of the Titanic. You too, can learn from failure. In particular, you can learn from those who attempted to take the oral boards, and sank beneath the waves. Here's what 10 years of observing oral board shipwrecks have taught.

1. Failure to prepare for the test.

    "I read a lot, but I never got around to taking a real, live practice oral exam."

    "Yeah, I did some practice orals…well, I did *a* practice oral…I lied, I never did a practice exam. I never practiced aloud."

    "I didn't want to look stupid in front of someone by practicing. So instead, I looked stupid in front of the official oral board examiners."

    "I wasn't ready to practice; I needed to do some more reading. I mean, isn't it important to know that frog legs bathed in electrolytes and coriander solutions require a higher dose of relaxant?"

    "It would have been an imposition to ask someone to give me a practice oral exam. Now, I'll have to impose on them to give me time off to take the exam again."

Lesson Learned: Since you have passed the written exam, you already *know* enough facts to pass the oral exam. You just have to string those facts together in a coherent fashion. So string them together in a practice exam. And do one right away, early on, today, this minute. Find some way, any way, to practice your answers in some kind of oral exam format. Can't find someone to do it in person? Do an exam over the phone. Do one over the Internet with a friend. Find a way. That "I never got around to taking a practice exam" is the A, number one, recurrent theme for failure. Follow the motto of the Nike Corporation: "Just do it!" Worried about looking dumb? Who cares? It's just a practice exam. Better to look dumb early on and have time to improve. If you wait until it's too late, you'll look dumb in front of the people who give out the grades. If you wait until that late, there will be no more room in the lifeboats.

2. Getting rattled early on and never getting back on track.

"They asked me to draw a line isolation monitor. I floundered and floundered, wouldn't admit I didn't know. Then, for the rest of the test, I kept thinking back to that damned line isolation monitor."

"It was a peds question. I said something wrong, then, later on, during a different part of the exam, I realized my mistake. I said, 'Wait, I would have done a rapid sequence before!'"

Lesson Learned: Cut your losses and move on. If you don't know, say you don't know or make your best guess and move along. A mistake or two or a few admissions of "I don't know" won't sink you. Getting flustered, rattled, and so preoccupied that you can't focus on the rest of the exam, now *that* will sink you. If the examiners persist in questioning you on a subject you really don't know, just ask politely to move on.

Of course, some questions you can bail out of and others you can't. For example, you can ask them to move on if you don't remember the pKa of bupivacaine. You can ask them to move on if you can't put together a stick model of amiodarone. But you can't ask them to move on after you couldn't intubate the patient.

3. Trying to cater to the examiner.

"I had Dr. X, you know, the big expert on regional, so I did a cholecystectomy with a combination celiac plexus, intrapleural, and intercostal block, with a Ketamine enema for sedation."

"I had Dr. Y, the big neuroanesthesia guru. When they asked me how I'd do a C-section for a patient with a placenta previa, I kept talking about cerebral protection and the blood brain barrier. Everything I said was neuro, neuro, neuro. I forgot the regular stuff, like, how to handle the tremendous blood loss that can accompany a placenta previa. I neglected to mention that I would put in two big IVs and I would have blood in the room, checked and ready to go."

"I had Dr. Z, the expert in blah, blah, blah. So instead of saying what I normally do, I bent myself in knots to convince Dr. Z that I, too, am an expert in blah, blah, blah."

Lesson Learned: Cool it. It doesn't matter who your examiners are or what they are "experts" in. The examiners will ask you questions about anesthesia, pure and simple. Answer the questions the way you normally would. Tailor the response to the question, not the questioner. A regular old anesthetic is often the right answer, after all, no need to do some super-complicated, ultra-weird technique you're completely unfamiliar with. You wouldn't do that in real life, would you? This above all else, to thine own self be true. Remember, these examiners aren't idiots. Try to bullshit them and they can tear you to pieces. (Think Rottweilers with no patience for stupid games.)

4. Getting mad.

"I'm doing a perfectly safe anesthetic, then the examiner goes, 'Now the patient is in V-fib.' I'm thinking, 'The hell that puts him in V-fib, what is this?' and I told him as much."

"Those sons-of-bitches are staring at me. Not so much as an 'OK' or 'All right' the whole exam; so by the end of the test, I'm copping an attitude with these guys; I couldn't help it."

"I know they're trying to trick me, so when they said the patient has no problems with his airway, I didn't believe them, and told them so by double checking the airway again and again. Of course, it was strange that we never got past that part in the preop section."

"I always do spinals for these cases. Then they say, 'How would you do a general for this case?' So I say, 'Look, a spinal's the way to go, that's all there is to it!'"

Lesson Learned: The examiners are there to *examine* you, not encourage you. The feedback that is a normal part of daily conversation is not part of the oral exam process. Furthermore, the examiners will take you to task. The exam is an *exam*, not a walk in the park with your pals. The examiners will push you, throw in complications, see if you can adapt to different circumstances. So adapt, explain, keep your cool. Fight with the examiners? Oh, that's a dandy way to impress them. If you win that fight, the grand prize is a trip back to the boards for another try next year.

Learn these hard lessons the easy way. Take practice exams, move on if you're stuck, don't cater to the examiner, and by all means don't get mad. Avoid these titanic mistakes and you'll sail right into your home port with board certification aboard, matey.

5

Hope Springs Eternal in the Human Breast

Yea, verily I say unto thee take heart; for I have known many who have passed through the valley of the shadow of the exam and lo, they have passed.

Some, there were, who passed the exam, who were people of great understanding. Knowledge flowed from their mouths like cool water from a bubbling brook. Their passing of the exam surprised no one in the land.

Some, there were, who passed the exam, who were people of lesser understanding. Knowledge flowed from their mouths, not so much like a bubbling brook, but more in fits and starts, like a leaky faucet. Their passing of the exam surprised some, but not all, in the land.

And finally some, there were, who passed the exam, who were people of little or no understanding. Knowledge did not flow from their mouths at all. The well ran dry. Their passing of the exam surprised all throughout the land. A multitude of voices joined as one to say, "Surely, if that person can pass the exam, then there is hope for such a creature as myself to pass the exam too."

6 | Ye Olde Format

Sun Tzu, a Chinese philosopher and author of *The Art of War*, wrote the following: "Know yourself and the enemy and you need not fear the result of a hundred battles." Well, the examiners aren't exactly your enemies, but it does pay to know what they will be asking and what they will be looking for.

You will have two exam sessions and, in each, there will be two examiners. Periodically, a third person may be in the room. That third person is auditing the other two examiners, not you. Before you go in the room, you will be given a stem question. You can scribble a few notes down, then you will be called into the room. Perfunctory introductions will occur (you'll be so zoned out you may not even remember the examiners' names), then you sit down at a table and have at it. It's not a malicious atmosphere, but it is all business. Most disconcerting is:

1. Lack of feedback like you have in normal conversation.
2. The examiners writing as you are answering. (Did the examiner just write down, "This guy is a moron"?)
3. The air of "we all know what we're here for" that hangs like musk in the room.

The two rooms have slightly different formats to their questions, though the bottom line is still the same—you need to know your stuff.

Session 1: A detailed question with all the preop workup done. You launch right into the intraoperative considerations for 15 minutes. Next, 10 minutes of postoperative care. The final 10 minutes will be a variety of grab bag questions on other topics.

Session 2: A less detailed question, without all the preop workup done. You will be quizzed on 10 minutes of preop questions, then 15 minutes of intraoperative care. The final 10 minutes are another round of grab bag questions on a variety of topics.

TO REVIEW

Session 1: Big, detailed stem question, 15 minutes intraop, 10 minutes postop, 10 minutes grab bag.

Session 2: Small stem question, 10 minutes preop, 15 minutes intraop, 10 minutes grab bag.

What are the examiners looking for? This comes straight from the ABA:

1. Sound judgement in decision making and management of surgical and anesthetic complications.
2. Appropriate application of scientific principles to clinical problems.
3. Adaptability to unexpected changes in the clinical situation.
4. Logical organization of an effective presentation of information.

Here's a look at those guidelines in action.

1. *Sound judgement.* Full stomach in a patient for appendectomy. Do a rapid sequence or an awake intubation. It is not *sound judgement* to ignore the risk of aspiration in the patient with a full stomach.
2. *Application of scientific principles.* The parturient doesn't empty her stomach, so consider her a full stomach. Tailor the anesthetic accordingly.
3. *Adaptability to unexpected changes.* A cholecystectomy patient looked easy to intubate and you induced. Surprise, surprise, she is difficult to intubate. You move on to plan B, in this case, you mask her with cricoid pressure until she is awake then perform an awake fiberoptic intubation. You adapted to an unexpected change, the failure to intubate.
4. *Logical organization.* A trauma patient has hypotension. Hypotension has a multitude of causes, but don't just flounder around for every possible cause. Note that blood pressure hinges on viscosity, preload, afterload, contractility, rate, and rhythm. Then go to the most logical causes in this trauma patient, hypovolemia either absolute (blood loss) or relative (pneumothorax impeding venous return). Boom, boom, you explain that you understand the *whole* picture, then you cut to the chase on this *specific* picture. You organize in a logical fashion.

Touching all four bases—sound judgement, scientific principles, adaptability, and logical organization—is not impossible nor fantastically tricky. Those four principles constitute your daily work day, after all. Each day, with each case, you use your sound judgement, you apply scientific principles, you adapt, and you logically organize your treatment. So none of the oral exam is foreign territory. We'll review these four grading criteria in more detail in Chapter 7.

All you have to do is explain what you do every day. All you have to do is say aloud what you do as an anesthetic consultant. The examiners, this we've emphasized again and again, are practitioners of anesthesia just like you are. Just lay it out for them the way you do every day at work. You don't need to quote 10,000 studies, don't need to do a chi-squared regression analysis. Just tell them how you anesthetize a diabetic for a BKA, an obese patient for a cholecystectomy, a child for a tonsillectomy. Tell them how you would handle a drop in saturation, a rise in blood pressure, wheezing in the PACU. The examiners have done it, and *so have you.* So tell them.

But what about all the sneaky, underhanded tricks and traps for the unwary? Don't the examiners throw you all kinds of curveballs, split-finger fastballs, wobbling knuckleballs? In a word, no.

For years and years, test takers have all said the same thing. "The test was fair." Whether they passed or whether they failed, all agreed that the questions were on the level. The examiners shoot straight. If you know your stuff and convey that, you will pass. If you don't know your stuff or if you can't convey that, you will fail.

Simple. Easy. Fair.

When you first submit your application to the board, you will get an exam packet. Read it from stem to stern. That packet has all the latest, so study it all the way through.

Also included in your exam packet is a practice exam. GREAT! TAKE IT; IT'LL BE YOUR FIRST PRACTICE EXAM. SEE HOW YOU DO. FORGET ALL THESE REVIEW BOOKS, YOU'VE GOT THE REAL MCCOY RIGHT THERE! No better time to take your first practice test than when you get your exam packet.

Does knowing the format really help? Yes. It takes some of the spookiness out of the test, some of the unknown.

Now you know yourself and the enemy, so you need not fear the result of a hundred board exams. With any luck you won't need a hundred tries.

CHAPTER

7 | The Wisdom of the Ages

By the end of this chapter, you'll know everything that you need to know to pass the oral boards. You may ask, "How is that possible? People study for hours and hours and hours. I can read this chapter in minutes." The study methods highlighted in this chapter are designed to help you study "smarter" not harder.

As mentioned in Chapter 6, there are four grading criteria during oral boards: judgement, adaptation, clarity, and application. Apply these four principles as you do the practice exams at the end of this book.

1. *Judgment.* Your *priorities* and your *timing* indicate your good judgment or lack of judgment.
2. *Priorities.* If you have to decide whether to do a cosmetic alteration of a toenail versus triple bypass surgery and both need to be done, the triple bypass surgery is more important. That shows your priority is protecting the heart, not the appearance of a toenail.
3. *Timing.* You have to decide not only if, but when you should do things. What should come first—placing the central line or putting in the airway? Someone in respiratory distress and near death will need the airway placed before anything else is done. (The first letter in ABC is A.)

   Timing also means when, or whether, you should do the case at all. Take the patient for lung surgery who had a recent MI, for example. Do you wait and reduce the risk of perioperative MI? Or does waiting increase the risk of the cancer metastasizing? If more information would help, you can "assume" it. For example, if knowing a dobutamine stress echo demonstrated little additional myocardium at risk, then proceeding with the case would make sense. Often there is no "right" answer, but the defense of your answer is what makes your approach score points.
4. *Adaptation.* There are basically only a few ways this part of the exam presents. There are a couple of constantly repeated scenarios: *a life-threatening scenario* (your patient develops tachycardia, what will you do?). Or *plan A doesn't work* (you

give your patient lidocaine and it doesn't work, what are you going to do next?). Or *a changing clinical scenario* (you decide to do an echo on someone with a history of three old MIs, and the examiners inform you that the patient walks 10 miles per day). Your answer should illustrate your ability to adapt. With a life-threatening event, use ABCs and algorithms. With failure of your initial plan, do something else (e.g., with the arrhythmia you redose or you shock if hemodynamically unstable). With a changing clinical scenario, readjust your assessment (if the patient has great exercise tolerance, you do not need the echo). That's all the examiners want to hear. They want to hear that you're moving step-by-step. When a bad thing happens, that does not mean you did a bad thing. When plan A does not work, it does not mean plan A was wrong. Making you adapt to changes is part of the exam.

A common life-threatening scenario is the lost airway. What are you going to do? There's an ASA algorithm for what you should do (Figure 7-1). You're going to ventilate, attempt to intubate three times, you'll call for help, you're going to use your LMA, then try a fiberoptic intubation if oxygen saturation permits, and eventually move to tracheal entry via a criocthroydoidotomy or surgical airway. Think through the lost airway before you enter the exam.

You will see a life-threatening scenario, and you will see a lost airway on the exam. Bank on it. The following are some common "plan A doesn't work" scenarios:

- You want to do a fiberoptic, but the patient's airway is full of blood.
- You administer an epidural, but the block is not effective.

You will need to work through these, you cannot simply say, "That never happens to me."

The following is an example of a changing scenario:

- You decide to transfuse the patient, but then the examiners inform you the patient is a Jehovah's Witness.

The board will do this to see how you adapt to a changing scenario. They will grade you on whether or not you get flustered, and what you come up with as an alternative response. (Colloid administration, increasing oxygen to 100%, and measuring the oxygen delivery/consumption relationship via mixed venous oxygen saturation monitoring might be appropriate steps.)

1. **Assess the likelihood and clinical impact of basic management problems:**
   A. Difficult Intubation
   B. Difficult Ventilation
   C. Difficulty with Patient Cooperation or Consent

2. **Consider the relative merits and feasibility of basic management choices:**
   A. Nonsurgical Technique for Initial Approach to Intubation   vs.
      Surgical Technique for Initial Approach to Intubation
   B. Awake Intubation   vs.
      Intubation Attempts After Induction of General Anesthesia
   C. Preservation of Spontaneous Ventilation   vs.
      Ablation of Spontaneous Ventilation

3. **Develop primary and alternative strategies:**

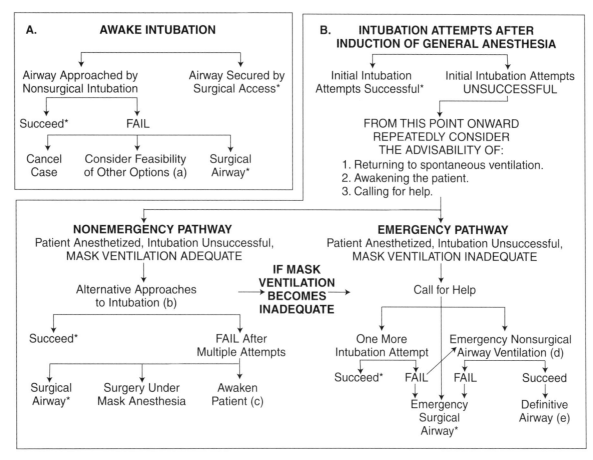

* Confirm intubation with exhaled CO_2

(a) Other options include (but are not limited to): surgery under mask anesthesia, surgery under local anesthesia infiltration or regional nerve blockade, or intubation attempts after induction of general anesthesia.

(b) Alternative approaches to difficult intubation include (but are not limited to): use of different laryngoscope blades, awake intubation, blind oral or nasal intubation, fiberoptic intubation, intubating stylet or tube changer, light wand, retrograde intubation, and surgical airway access.

(c) See awake intubation.

(d) Options for emergency non-surgical airway ventilation include (but are not limited to): transtracheal jet ventilation, laryngeal mask ventilation, or esophageal-tracheal combitube ventilation.

(e) Options for establishing a definitive airway include (but are not limited to): returning to awake state with spontaneous ventilation, tracheotomy, or endotracheal intubation.

Figure 7-1   ASA algorithm for a difficult airway. (Reprinted with permission from American Society of Anesthesiologists. Copyright © 1999 American Society of Anesthesiologists. All rights reserved. Reprinted with permission also from ASA Task Force. Practice guidelines for management of the difficult airway. Anesthesiology 1993;78:597–602.)

Clarity: Organize your thoughts before speaking. Do not launch into a list of possible problems a patient might have (people make this mistake all the time). The way you answer a board question is to:

1. Think about the case being done.
2. Think about what coexisting diseases the patient may have.
3. Organize your thoughts in a systematic fashion, with the most likely causes being mentioned first (more on that below). Reciting long lists proves you are a long-list memorizer, not a board certified specialist.

Application: Applying knowledge means knowing when to use what you know. Knowing that a low EF can cause shortness of breath is great, but applying that knowledge in a meaningful way to a clinical scenario is key to passing a question. For example, you get a previously healthy patient who is short of breath, and you've just put a CVP in. A low ejection fraction is on your exhaustive differential. But that's not it; shortness of breath due to a low EF in a patient with a high EF? That is not applying what you know. Hmm. He was *not* short of breath before I stuck him for the CVP. Now, after poking that needle near his *lung* he *is* short of breath.

Let us apply our knowledge base, specifically our "what can go wrong when a CVP needle goes near the lung" knowledge base. Aha! Chest X-ray looking for pneumothorax! Pneumothorax is the most likely problem, not a low ejection fraction. Remember, this is not rocket science.

Start out with the most likely thing, organize your thoughts, then, if your first impression is not the right fix, then go system by system in order not to miss some obscure cause. In this particular case, if they ask what you are going to do, "While providing supportive therapy such as supplemental oxygen, and after listening to breath sounds, I would order a chest x-ray to rule out a pneumothorax." That shows application of common sense and good medicine.

SCORING CRITERIA

Four examiners grade you between 70 and 80; a grade of greater than 75 is passing. The examiners are encouraged to give 70s or 80s. A definite fail is 70; a probable fail is 73; 77 is a probable pass; and 80 is a definite pass.

A passing grade is greater than 75 points, so you must convince more than two of the four examiners that you actually know something (two 70s and two 80s = 75 = fail). Avoid a 70 in any one room, at all costs. How? Keep plugging away.

KEY POINTS TO AVOIDING THE DREADED "70—THE MOTHER OF ALL BAD THINGS"

1. Organize your answers.
2. Make the patient healthy.
3. Do not question the examiners.

Organize Your Answers

How do the examiners want you to present information? For a model, look at Stoelting and Dierdorf's *Anesthesia and Co-Existing Disease*, especially the "Management of Anesthesia" sections. That's how to answer. That's how the examiners think.

Stoelting lays the answer out clean, system-by-system. If you want someone to mistake you for a smart person, imitate Stoelting's style.

Make the Patient Healthy

Some people make the exam more difficult than it has to be. Suppose the stem concerns a patient who has a history of an MI. Some examinees might say, "Oh, he could be in congestive heart failure, he could have valvular regurgitation. I mean, well, he could have unstable angina too, I guess." Yipes! The *examinee* has just made the patient rather unhealthy.

Try this instead. "If the patient did not demonstrate any signs of left ventricular dysfunction, and was otherwise stable, then I would check the EKG, make sure there were no interval changes, and proceed with surgery." This examinee made the patient as healthy as possible. If all manner of gruesome complications are not on the exam, then for God's sake leave them out.

Do Not Question the Examiners

You can be worried about a low EF, and there are two ways you can frame the question. If you ask a question on the Board exam, I can virtually guarantee you won't get a clear answer or you'll get an answer you won't like. Answer your own question when asking it.

For example, if you want to know if a patient has had their arterial blood gas checked, and you want the examiners to know you're thinking about that say, "I assume they've had arterial blood gases, and the values were normal." Boom, then move on. Remember, you have 35 minutes to impress these examiners.

Here's another example of avoiding a question. Say you wondered about the patient's EF. "I would make sure that the patient had a good EF before proceeding." There, you've got that cleared up, now move on to the next point. The examiners may interrupt you and say, "It turns out he has a cardiomyopathy and an EF of 25%." No problem, now you have that specific information, and you adapt to the new clinical scene. The main idea here is don't ask questions; make and state your assumptions and move on. If the examiners want to give you new information, they will.

This is difficult for some examinees, but worth the effort. To reiterate, don't ask a question.

Here are more examples to clarify:

WRONG: Does the patient have any wheezing?

RIGHT: Assuming the lungs were clear and the patient was doing as well as he ever does, I'd induce general anesthesia.

WRONG: Does he show signs of CHF? Are the cardiologists recommending ICU care?

RIGHT: From the information given, this man has poor ventricular function, so I'd monitor with an A-line and a PA catheter and would plan on post-op ICU care.

Let's take another look at organizing your answers. Three ways of organizing include:

1. Anatomy
2. Physiology
3. Time (sequence of events)

You might hear, "The patient is short of breath. Why do you think that is the case?" If you go into a "list everything on the planet that causes shortness of breath" mode, you may miss the one, most important cause. The cause the examiners want you to say.

So you have to make sure you don't miss something important. You have to be organized. If you just shotgun your answers (e.g., "It could be congestive heart failure; it could be pneumonia; it could be aspiration...") and you forget to say pneumothorax, then the answer the examiners want will be a pneumothorax. You will say everything but the right thing.

How do you avoid this? You have to answer in a simple, organized fashion, the same way each time. We recommend using the anatomic, physiologic, and time (time being least common) approaches.

PHYSIOLOGIC OR ANATOMIC ORGANIZATION

By organ systems:

CNS
Cardiac
Pulmonary
Hepatic
Renal
Hematologic
Endocrine
Other

or head to toe:

> Head
> Neck/airway
> Chest
> Abdomen
> Peripheral

Five organ systems stand out: CNS, cardiac, pulmonary, hepatic, and renal. Hematologic and endocrine are less common. Now look at the shortness of breath question. What could cause that shortness of breath? The CNS system? Not likely, but possible if following head trauma or in the post-op period. The cardiac system? Possible. Pulmonary? Highly probable. (Pneumothorax falls into the pulmonary system, so you would catch the problem there.) Hepatic? Yes, if ascites were huge. Renal? Yes, renal failure could lead to volume overload. This physiologic, system-by-system method makes sure you will at least hit the high points.

The anatomy approach goes: head, neck, chest, abdomen. Look at your examiner; that will be the model for your systematic review. Go back to the shortness of breath question. Look at the anatomy involved. The head as the cause of shortness of breath? Not unless it's been whacked. The heart? Yes, it could. The lung, with your misguided CVP needle stuck into it? That's it! That's the cause of your shortness of breath!

The time approach in this shortness of breath question? Before your CVP procedure, the patient had not pulmonary, hepatic, renal, or cardiac reasons for dyspnea. Then, in the *time* after you placed a CVP, the dyspnea occurred.

Review the pertinent anatomy head to toe, the pertinent physiology head to toe, and the sequence of events. That should help you organize your answers.

What about a more complicated question? What about diseases with multiple organ involvement? Same thing; go system by system. Organize your thoughts and you will sound like a professional. Now, on to analyzing the individual question.

ANALYZING THE QUESTION

The short-stem question (seen in the second half of your exam) is about three sentences long. The question describes the patient, the proposed surgery, the coexisting diseases, and some—not all—of the lab data, physical findings, and vital signs. This short-stem question will focus on the preoperative and intraoperative management of the patient.

The long-stem question (seen in the first half of your exam) will have a whole lot of information that relates to the preop evaluation. They skip any further evaluation of the preoperative period, and work on the intra- and post-op portions. The five-part analysis below should be adjusted to the type of question. While you don't have to worry about preop in the second room, at least noting if the patient is optimized, and saying you would attempt to do so before proceeding is appropriate.

Structuring Your Analysis

Five aspects go into the analysis of a stem question. Those five aspects are:

1. Reason—what is the gist of the question?
2. Timing—how much time do you have to optimize the patient?
3. Preop considerations
4. Intraop considerations
5. Postop considerations

Each question on the board exam is there for a particular reason. If you identify that reason, then you will know where the board exam is going (i.e., what they are going to ask you, and what are some of the crucial points you have to make in order not to fail). You probably will not fail the exam if you understand the *reason* for the exam.

One reason people fail is not understanding that reason. The examinee answers all sorts of answers correctly but misses the big point. People fail because they miss the thrust of the exam. Let's examine the reasons a stem question exists.

REASONS FOR A STEM QUESTION

There are three basic reasons for a board question to exist: multiple management problems/multiorgan system disease, conflicting diagnoses, and differentiation of common signs or symptoms.

1. *Multiple management/multi-organ system diseases.* Several considerations occur all at once—cardiac, pulmonary, renal, hepatic. So much is going on that the examiners can find lots to discuss.
2. *Conflicting diagnoses.* Raynaud's disease and hypotension (both vasodilation and vasoconstriction are indicated); coronary artery disease and asthma (beta blockade/beta-agonist); full stomach and asthma (deep intubation/rapid sequence intubation). Another classic example of conflicting therapies would be a patient with arrhythmias and asthma. Treating problem A aggravates problem B.
3. *Differentiation of common signs and symptoms.* What common symptoms can form a basis of an oral examination? Shortness of breath (cardiac versus pulmonary). Wheezing

(cardiac, pulmonary, incorrect intubation). Lethargy (drugs, metabolic, neurologic, i.e., leftover anesthetics, hypoglycemia, intracranial bleed).

It's amazing how the exam starts to make more sense once you put one of these three reasons down on paper. On to the timing aspects of a stem question.

TIMING

Timing affects how much you can do to optimize the patient. For any case you work in one of three time zones—emergency, urgent, or elective.

1. *Emergency.* Go to the OR without delay, even in suboptimal conditions. Vital signs are unstable; changing for the worse in the face of adequate resuscitation. Must have surgery to address the problem.
2. *Urgent.* Go to the OR after resuscitation; short-term optimizing. Life, limb, or sight is affected. Outcome is affected by a delay.
3. *Elective.* Go to the OR only after aggressive optimization. Really elective—a face-lift; kind of elective—a slow-growing cancer.

Emergency

There are a few definitions of emergency in a surgeon's mind. First is self-interest as in, "I've got to play golf later" (private practice surgeon). Second is self-importance as in, "I want to get this case done now, because when I want to operate, the rest of the world should do what I want" (academic surgeon). Neither of those really qualify as an emergency (unless that particular surgeon books half the hospital's cases and gets to pick his anesthesia team, in which case, go ahead, call it an emergency).

For the boards, however, you should understand what constitutes an emergency. First, vital signs are unstable. That means there are adverse changes in the face of adequate resuscitation, and the problem causing the vital sign aberration will be addressed by the proposed surgery. A lot of patients on the board exam have a blood pressure of 80. You don't know if they are just sitting there with a blood pressure of 80 and they're perfusing all their organs, or if their blood pressure was 120 ten minutes ago and they're bleeding to death. Unstable means a bad value changing for the worse. Resuscitation is ongoing but to no avail.

You can' t just say, "Oh my God, the patient's BP is low; let's get them to the OR quick!" Except in the case of open exsanguination, the usual approach is to do the ABCs, after you give them oxygen and give them adequate fluid resuscitation, and if the vital signs are still declining, then you do not wait any longer. You take them to the OR and you have the surgery—again assuming that the surgery addresses what the problem is.

For example, the patient is bleeding to death from previous tonsillar surgery and the IV has been pulled out—a classic scenario. What are you going to do? Well, you want to try to adequately resuscitate the patient first. But they're still bleeding to death and you can't get the IV. At some point after a short time trying to obtain venous access, it's time to do the surgery. No IV? It doesn't matter. You work on obtaining access and induction simultaneously. If the patient is bleeding to death, you do have to do something, right? You do anything that helps. You put a clamp on something. You temporize with endotracheal epinephrine. In this case you have all the makings of a true emergency—deteriorating vital signs, inability to adequately resuscitate, and a condition definitively treated with surgery. A ruptured AAA is a true emergency. You can name a dozen more.

Urgent

Urgent means life, limb, or sight is affected by delay. How urgent is urgent? That's a common way of evaluating your judgment. The answer is gray because "urgent" fits into a continuum.

A patient has an open fracture; you have six hours. You have a patient with a leaking AAA. Maybe you have a few minutes for optimization if the closed belly has tamponaded the bleeding; enough time to call for blood and place the arterial line. Maybe the leak is so slow you have hours. Maybe.

An urgent case should go to the OR after some period of resuscitation. If the patient is already five hours post open fracture and is grossly volume-depleted, and the surgeon says "we've got to put him to sleep before the sixth hour comes," that may not make a lot of sense.

There are no magic cutoffs. Almost everything in medicine is a continuum, and that goes back to priorities (i.e., deciding how urgent the surgery is versus how urgent and important optimizing the patient is—a key judgmental grading point in some exams).

If putting in a PA catheter pushes you over that six-hour mark (5 hours 55 minutes to 6 hours 5 minutes), that's not going to make the patient's risk of developing osteomyelitis change in any significant way. How long one can wait with an open fracture is not an absolute threshold, but a smooth continuum like all biologic processes.

Elective

What about elective cases? There are two types of elective cases. There's the face-lift that could wait until the cows come home. The second type of elective case (or very low urgency) is a slow-growing cancer. The patient has been diagnosed with lung cancer and has had a recent MI. How long do you wait? Sometimes it's not always possible to know how long you can wait. Sometimes you have to get consultants together to come up with the best guess. So, you get a cardiologist, an oncologist, and you all sit down together and you say, "So what are the risks here?" With their expert advice, together you make a judgment call. And that is an acceptable approach in both real life and on the boards.

Table 7-1   Preop Workup

Problem	Hx and PE	Labs	Tests	Consults	Further RX
CAD	Symptoms of ischemia, signs of LV dysfunction		EKG—new and old		
COPD	BS		Room air SaO$_2$		
Full stomach	What and when eaten				

Table 7-1 shows your preop workup. Everything you need to know—everything the examiners will ask—is predictable. It all fits into a formula. In preop, everything can be divided into history, physical, labs, tests, consults, and therapies. So…be prepared to answer questions on history, physical, labs, tests, consults, and additional therapies needed.

You'll also need to formulate a problem list. On an exam, your patient *will* have problems. For example, a patient had two MIs (problem)—you want to know his exercise tolerance and anginal history (history) and whether there are any changes between the new and old EKG (tests). Assuming his exercise tolerance is good (making the patient healthy), there would be no need for an echo.

For CAD patients, what are your concerns? You want to know if myocardium is at risk and you want to know of poor LV function. Most cardiac cases will focus on those two issues.

The following four concerns will make you call a cardiologist:

1. Ongoing angina that no one has evaluated
2. New angina
3. Unstable angina
4. Postinfarction angina

In an emergency, a consult does little good. If the case is urgent or elective, then timing enters into the equation. Will you gain by the cardiologist's wisdom?

COMMON PREOP PROBLEMS

When the board examiner asks, "Do you want any further information about the patient's cardiac disease?" examinees often make the question too difficult. There are only two parts to this question.

1. Is myocardium at risk?
2. What is the LV function?

Except in rare instances (like patients with arrhythmias or pacers), the two issues above are the only two things that affect outcome. Myocardium at risk and LV function matter. Myocardium at risk and LV function respond to therapies. Myocardium at risk and LV function require monitors.

With valvular problems you need to know if the valve is regurgitant or stenotic, and you need to know how regurgitant or stenotic. But for a heart without valvular problems, go back to the basics, myocardium at risk and LV function.

When the examiner asks, "What do you want to know about the cardiac system?" say, "I'd like to assess whether or not there's myocardium at risk and what is his LV function."

"How would you do that, doc?"

"I'd make sure that the patient doesn't have unstable anginal patterns, that the patient is well-treated for any existing angina, and I'd make sure that the patient has good exercise tolerance. If that were the case, I'd be satisfied. Other than that, I'd review a new and an old EKG to make sure that he didn't have any interval change."

Five seconds. Cardiac system fixed. It's the same answer every time. Practice saying this thing over and over and over again. The board examiners only hear it once, and if they hear it just like that, they will think that you're the genius you are.

INTRAOP

Monitors

During the intraoperative portion of the exam, they ask the same questions all the time. The formula reappears. If you understand the formula, you won't get upset when a bad thing happens intraoperatively. Bad things are planned. Like the bumper sticker says, "Bad things happen."

Your examiners don't make up the questions. They have a formula. They're given a script with the stem question at the top and all the questions they're supposed to ask. They will ask you about what monitors you're going to place. In this case, you do not need to say EKG and an NIBP. You can just say the ASA standard monitors (although you should know what those are). If you use something special, like 5-lead EKG monitoring or ST segments, that's not necessarily routine and must be noted if asked what special monitors will be placed. A Foley is also not routine, a capnograph is.

Induction

They're going to ask you, "Are you using general or regional anesthesia." Then, they're going to ask you, "What are you going to use?"

The examiners don't care if you're going to use 350 or 375 mg of pentothal. When they ask, "what will you give," they want to hear things like "pent-sux-tube," or "a reduced dose of pentothal followed by sux." You're supposedly way beyond knowing what dosages to give. If they ask, "How much are you going to give?" then that means they want a specific answer, which brings up another point. Make sure you answer the specific question the board examiners are asking. If they ask what, answer what. If they ask how much, give them an amount. If they ask for your differential, do not tell them what you are going to do next, give them a differential. Answer a directed question with a directed answer.

The Airway

If securing the airway might be difficult, it will be difficult. Expect difficulty.

You want to intubate? You can't intubate.

You want to do a fiberoptic? It's not going to work.

You ought to have plan B in mind before you walk in the room. Don't be flustered when plan A fails. You want to do a regional to avoid dealing with the airway? It's not going to work, or you'll precipitate a seizure. Does that mean that you should not do what you would normally do with a bad rheumatoid arthritic having a knee done? Does that mean that you shouldn't do a spinal? No. The best answer is the usual answer. Make sure you can explain your reasoning. When your suggested technique fails, the examiners are testing your adaptability.

If the airway is difficult, then have access to a difficult airway cart. Have access to a surgeon for placement of a surgical airway.

"But," you protest, "I don't do that because that annoys the surgeon."

Rubbish! This is the boards! Do whatever you have to for patient safety. This is a pretend patient. You can stick them and harass them and harass the surgeons as much as you want (for the sake of safety, of course).

Maintenance

What is there to ask? Propofol reduces nausea. Isoflurane is cheap. Sevo doesn't irritate the airway. That's about the only things they can ask. Occasionally there's something else like arrhythmogenic potential, but rarely.

Emergence

There are a lot of problems associated with emergence. Everybody has either a plan A that doesn't work or a life-threatening scenario. If you didn't get a bad problem yet, that bad problem will show up during emergence. Emergence will produce arrhythmias, hypotension, hypoxia.... And the ever present delayed awakening. That covers about 90% of the emergence problems.

Then there are some specific intraoperative considerations that you can expect with particular stems; e.g., with carotids you worry about the CO_2 and maintaining BP, with AAAs you will talk about aortic clamping physiology, and with cardiac surgery the heart-lung bypass machine is fair game. With renal cases and radical nephrectomy, you've got to worry about pneumothorax. With TURP, you've got to worry about hyponatremia. All of this is pretty straightforward, the stuff of weekly M and M conferences.

POSTOP

What can they ask you about postop? A few things include ischemia, weaning, oliguria, delayed awakening, high or low temperature, pain, and something specific to the case (low sodium post TURP, for example).

Postoperative problems are often related to the patient's pre-existing conditions or the surgery. If they had CAD preop, they might have ischemia postop. If they had a radical nephrectomy, they might have hypoxia secondary to a pneumothorax. If the patient recently had neurologic or carotid surgery, I'd bet dollars to donuts that you will have to differentiate surgical versus other causes of delayed awakening. Urologic surgery will present with some oliguria—determining volume status versus a surgical cause will be part of the exam. Common sense is all you need here. You've got to think, "Why are they asking me this?" If you cannot come up with an answer, rereading the stem question is often very helpful.

THE ANSWER TO EVERY VITAL SIGN PROBLEM

You are most likely going to have a life-threatening problem on one of your two tests. What that means is that your vital signs will deteriorate. You will have low blood pressure or high blood pressure. You will have really low oxygen or really high pCO_2. (There's more on this in the chapter, Vital Signs Are Vital, in the next section of the book. But this information bears repeating.)

The six-step answer below is the same for every single question:

1. Airway
2. Breathing
3. Circulation
4. Supportive therapy
5. Differential diagnosis
6. Definitive treatment

Fail the life-threatening scenario and you fail the exam. Try to avoid this disaster. Do the ABCs. Many examinees forget this simple lesson.

A—Airway
Place on O_2 (100%)
Make sure you have a patent airway

B—Breathing
ETCO$_2$
Pulse oximeter
Bilateral BS equal

C—Circulation
BP
HR
EKG—ischemia, rhythm

S—S*upportive therapy for aberrant vital sign problem.* If the blood pressure is 50, what to do? What would you do in the OR? Fluids, neo, ephedrine, epi. As you buy time with these measures, assure a patent airway, adequate air exchange, 100% oxygen delivery and check monitors—EKG, SaO$_2$, and recheck BP.

D—D*ifferential diagnosis.* Most likely diagnosis first. Don't list stuff; diagnose the problem. Give a list only if they press you.

"Well, what else doctor? What else? Can you think of anything else that this might be?" That question merits a list.

In that case, say, "Well, let me go back...." Repeat your most likely causes (in case they've missed your saying something, and THEN AND ONLY THEN, begin going through a list of possible, less likely causes in an organized fashion (e.g., organ system by organ system).

If the examiners are constantly asking what else is going on, they either:

1. want an exhaustive differential, or
2. you've missed it, or
3. are trying to rattle you even if there is nothing else (rare).

Go back and reread the stem. Remember it's *this* patient for *this* operation. It is not an athlete for a knee. It's not a 90-year-old for a bypass operation. It's a 60-year-old, history of MI for a cholecystectomy. It's *that* patient and *that* scenario for *that* operation. Make sure your diagnosis makes sense.

Even as you struggle, remember to continue supportive/resuscitative efforts.

D—D*efinitive treatment.* Treat the problem you've identified. Enough said.

Hypotension—The most common vital sign aberration. This occurs on almost every test. Again, there's a lot of different ways to think about it, but there's only five things that affect blood pressure.

This is it. Memorize it. One of the following five things is causing hypotension:

1. Preload (absolute—dehydration/bleeding; relative—obstructed filling of heart)
2. Contractility (ischemia, drugs)
3. Afterload (drugs, anaphylaxis, sepsis)
4. Rate (too low)
5. Rhythm (not sinus)

MORE TIPS—THE THREE TS: TREND, TITRATE, THRESHOLD

Trend

Focus on a trend; avoid fixating on one value, test, or number. "It's the trend, stupid." Nail down whether the trend is stable or unstable (stable pattern of unifocal PVCs versus new multifocal PVCs), chronic or acute (low potassium from diuretics versus a rapid loss of potassium from mannitol usage).

Titrate

Titrate everything to a specific endpoint. How are you going to make sure the anesthesia is deep enough? Drop blood pressure 30% below baseline while checking for ischemia. Avoid the vague phrase, "get 'em deep enough."

How much sedation will you give? Titrate to a BIS level above 80, or titrate to slurred speech, keeping the respiratory rate above 12/minute. Titrate to a clear endpoint.

Threshold

Have a threshold you can defend on the *high* and *low* side where appropriate. Mine are listed below. They may be different from yours, but I can say "below this is safe, above that is not," and give some reason to support that position. What is good support? "The patient's outcome is better/worse in this range," or "my anesthetic or monitoring technique will be different above (below) this value," or "my preop workup will change." The following is my cutoff for each one.

Thresholds

		Hi	Low
Na+		150–155	131
K+		5.5	3.0
Hgb		16–18	10–7
BP	sys	200	90
	MAP	(MAP 1510)	(MAP 50–60)
	dias	110	
HR		100 or EKG ischemia (lower is better)	40 or C.I. 2.2 L/min
Pulse Ox			Any change
ETCO$_2$ PaCO$_2$		40	25
INR		2.0–2.5 adequate for prophylaxis	
PT/PTT		1.2×	
PLT		100—major surgery 50—minor surgery 20—spont. hem. Expected	
Cr		1.5	
BUN/Cr		>20	
PIP		40	
RR		25	10

Dialysis within 24 hours.

The previous numbers reflect clinical impression based on reading. A lot is anecdotal. Few hard data exist, but you must pick something. So pick something and stick with it. "Stand by your plan." For example, why choose a potassium cutoff of 5.5 mEq/L? While private practitioners will proceed above 5.5 to avoid alienating surgical colleagues, (HEY, I SAW THAT LUBARSKY!) if you will bend your own rules and proceed with an operation at 5.6, why not proceed with an operation at 5.7, or 5.8, or 5.9?

If you fail to "stand by your plan," then the examiners will push you around. Pick a number and stick to it. Is 5.6 dangerous? No, but you may need to give blood, or you may need to give sux urgently. Both of those therapies raise your potassium into a range with potential cardiac problems (6.5–7); therefore, you don't want to start out higher than 5.5.

Now, consider the low threshold, a potassium of 3.0. Why 3.0? Because there is a study (Slogoff, et al. for those who care) that looks at patients both on and off digoxin who had potassium as low as 3.0, and these patients with low potassium had no increased incidence of perioperative arrhythmias.

What of the Hemoglobin Values?

Why is the upper threshold for hemoglobin 16–18? Vascular sludging occurs at that range. Why is the low threshold for hemoglobin 7–10 mg/dl? For a patient with no significant organ disease (a rarity on the boards), 7 mg/dl is fine. Why 7 mg/dl and not a lower number? Jehovah's Witnesses with a hemoglobin below 5 mg/dl for long periods of time die. And a Hgb of 7 is higher than 5, and otherwise healthy patients empirically seem to recover well with this value. Hence, you can defend this value of 7 mg/dl. It is also the consensus value of the NIH panel on transfusion medicine. By the way, the causes of anemia? Losing too much, making too little.

When and why do you pick a low threshold Hgb of 10? If a patient has compromised circulation to the head, to the heart, to the lungs, to the kidney, or to the liver, then the answer is 10 mg/dl. Why? Optimal oxygen delivery. The following is a common board exchange on this topic.

"Why transfuse at 10?"

"Because I don't want to add insult to injury."

"But aren't you worried about the transfusion risks?"

"Yes, but my main priority is this patient's critically compromised organ."

Emphasize that, while you are concerned about injuring patients with a therapy, the risk of a transfusion-related reaction is very low. Transfusion risks today are about 1 in 400,000 for AIDS, 1 in 200,000 for Hep B, 3 in 10,000 for Hep C, and almost 0 for any bacterial or parasitic infection. Immunocompromised patients who are CMV negative have real risk. So you recommend transfusion, balancing the risks (infectious) against the benefit (better oxygen delivery to a diseased organ).

Cutoffs for Blood Pressure Present a Thorny Dilemma

What blood pressure will cancel a case? A diastolic blood pressure of 110 mm Hg. Why is the diastolic blood pressure of 110 important? Because 30 years ago in England, seven patients anesthetized with that degree of hypertension had complications. Complications were serious, such as congestive heart failure, MI, and death.

But have things changed in 30 years? Esmolol was not available then, nor was labetalol. Hmm. That alone is enough to give you pause.

A diastolic of 110 is unlikely to cause congestive heart failure, MI, or death. We are just too good at treating hypertension now. However, for the purposes of the board exam, I would say that a diastolic blood pressure of 110 or greater indicates increased probability of a cardiopulmonary complication and delay for better control is appropriate. If the case is very urgent acute control using IV agents is a reasonable board answer.

What of the Thresholds for Heart Rate?

Heart rate of 100 or EKG ischemia. In the adult population, a lower heart rate is better. Beta blockade decreases both perioperative complications and increases long-term viability according to recent NEJM articles. A protective effect has been associated with a heart rate < 85 perioperatively in these articles.[1,2] There are two reasons why the heart rate is important. High heart rates cause ischemia; low heart rates affect cardiac output. (Forget for a while the rare athlete with a slow rate but superb cardiac conditioning.) How low is too low for cardiac output? A cardiac index of 2.2 L/min/m² is the cutoff for adequately perfusing critical organs. At a heart rate of 40, your output falls significantly and your heart may dilate, increasing wall tension and tending toward subendocardial ischemia. So too fast is no good, too slow is no good.

Now look at the threshold for pulse oximetry. There is no such thing as a drop in pulse oximetry on the board exam that is benign.

$PaCO_2$ low cutoff? Why 25? Because at 25 one gets such severe vasoconstriction of cerebral vessels, a lactic acidosis of the brain can develop.

Coags? INRs are useful for patients on coumadin. INR of 2–2.5 is adequate to prophylax against clot formation.

Another coag consideration is the PT ratio. A PT ratio of < 1.2 × normal is safe (and yet there's no data on this). Some physicians feel it's okay to slip a needle in a nonepidural space up to a PT ratio of 1.5 × normal. Not us. Bleeding complications lurk in the wings. Why risk the complications?

Can you defend the alternative approach? Yes. More important than your choice is your attention to potential problems.

The bleeding time is a test in search of an indication. Bleeding time does not correlate with anything. When they ask you, "What about the bleeding time, doctor?" just note the bleeding time doesn't correlate with any clinical status of coagulation.

On to More Thresholds

Creatinine. Creatinine > 1.5 suggests compromised renal function, and one should make sure the Cr is stable or decreasing so as not to increase the chance of ATN, which still carries a very high perioperative mortality rate. BUN/creatinine ratio greater than 20 suggests dehydration and possible therapy prior to induction of anesthesia (fluid replacement, CVP?).

That most vital of vital signs, respiration. Respiratory rate greater than 25 is my cutoff. Why? The patient can't maintain that type of respiratory effort against increased resistance of breathing for a long period of time. A respiratory rate less than 10. Why? Below that you will almost certainly retain CO_2 and possibly compromise oxygenation.

Thus endeth the discussion of the three Ts: trend, titrate, and threshold. Know your thresholds. More important, know the *why* of your threshold. Then "stand by your plan."

MONITORING

Monitoring indications—arterial catheters. There are only four indications for an arterial catheter. It's not "the patient is sick."

1. *Small blood pressure swings equal physiologic problems.* Recent MI, unstable angina, left main coronary artery disease, or critical carotid stenosis increased ICP. In these cases small blood pressure swings may lead to big problems, and one has to tightly control BP to avoid badness.

2. *Large blood pressure changes.* Trauma, massive blood loss, aortic cross-clamping, coronary artery bypass operations. Why not an automated BP machine like DinaMAP? It cycles 20 mm Hg above the last pressure, then cycles all the way down. If it can't find a blood pressure; then it cycles all the way up to 240; then it cycles all the way down. When you have no blood pressure it will take you 2 minutes to find out. Two minutes of zero blood pressure—not good.

   If you have an arterial line, you wait 0 minutes to see the blood pressure of zero. Better.

   If you have a sky-high blood pressure, it may still take you over a minute to find out. A minute of 350 blood pressure—not good.

   If you have an arterial line, you wait 0 minutes to see the blood pressure of 350. Better.

   So if you have really large blood pressure swings you can't follow that with an automated cuff, so you need an A-line.

3. *Can't get a reading from an automated cuff—arrhythmia/morbid obesity.* An automated BP machine cannot pick up irregular beat patterns and so often cannot perform its algorithm to yield a BP. Furthermore, also reason 2, large rapid blood pressure changes could happen suddenly with the onset of an arrhythmia. With obese patients, you can't get a good cuff fit.

4. *Frequent blood draws.* Intra- or post-op—if you need more than three samples for Hgb, glucose, electrolyte, or blood gases, then place an arterial line. An A-line poses extremely low risks of thrombotic complications, and even more rare are infectious complications.

There's not a single indication you can think of that doesn't fit into one of these four categories. So, when they say, "Why will you put an A-line in?" all you do is pick one of these four reasons.

CVPs

Three reasons. Fluid shifts will occur and

1. need to be followed on a timely basis (urine output lags actual fluid shifts, e.g., ruptured small bowel).
2. urine output is not available (urologic surgery).
3. urine output is an inaccurate reflection of intravascular volume (diuretics being administered).

These are the *monitoring* indications for a CVP. There are, of course, therapeutic reasons for a CVP.

1. No adequate peripheral access.
2. Need for central access for delivering inotropic agents or "caustic" goods (hyperal).

PA Cath
1. You need an invasive monitor of fluid status as previously mentioned *and* the patient's right and left heart pressures don't equal each other.
2. You need to optimize a variable (SVR, PVR, cardiac output, mixed venous oxygen saturation) you can only measure with a PA catheter.

Volumes are written about the PA versus CVP question. Be able to defend your choice. The mass of stuff written about this question proves only one thing—the experts lack a consensus on the issue. IF you are ever at a loss, always remember that mortality was *increased* in ICU patients with presence of a PA catheter for management, so you can always defend not putting one in on the grounds that you may actually be improving outcome (although, we don't buy that personally).

So much for the discussion of monitors.

FREQUENT POSTOPERATIVE PROBLEMS AND QUESTIONS

Extubation
When will you extubate? How you will evaluate for extubation?

If you anticipate problems extubating, get preoperative PFTs. How can you judge if a patient is ready if you don't know their baseline? So get PFTs to know their baseline status.

Back to the question, when do you extubate? Follow the *ACME Guide.*

ACME Guide to Extubation
1. Adequate level of consciousness. (This ties in closely with 2.)
2. Airway reflexes intact. (Extubating someone who promptly aspirates is bad form.)
3. The endotracheal tube is not acting as a stent. (Say a patient with post massive fluid resuscitation. Massive edema everywhere means massive edema in the airway too. You pull out the endotracheal tube, the stenting of the airway is removed, the airway collapses; all the king's horses and all the king's men can't reestablish an airway again.)
4. Stable hemodynamics. (Speaking of all the king's horses. Get it? STABLE hemodynamics? Man, I slay myself with this

humor! But seriously folks, if an intubated patient is hanging by a thread hemodynamically, the last thing you want to do is take away a nice, secure airway and add to their other stresses. If an intubated patient codes, at least you have the A and B of the ABCs already in place.)

5. Normal internal milieu. (Normal temperature, pH, electrolytes. Again, if you have a nice secure airway amidst a physiologic nightmare—DKA, wacked out electrolytes, hypothermia—don't add to the stress. Keep the airway until all the chemistries are back on track. Also, at your next cocktail party, try to fit the term "internal milieu" into the conversation. People will think you have panache and sophistication.)

6. Phrenic nerve control. (COPD patient who just underwent redo CABG with a difficult dissection? Make sure the surgical procedure didn't section the phrenic nerve. The loss of diaphragmatic function could prove the patient's undoing. It might even lead to an imperfect "internal milieu.")

7. Adequate pain control. (Splinting from severe pain, say after a thoracotomy, could lead to atelectasis, pneumonia, hypoxemia, the whole nine yards.)

8. Good weaning parameters. (Nothing beats the bedside evaluation, but keep the numbers in mind to guide your extubation. Look for tidal volume of 5 cc/kg, vital capacity of 10 cc/kg, respiratory rate less than 25/minute, negative inspiratory force of 30 cm H_2O, pO_2 greater than 60 on an FIO_2 of 40% and PEEP no greater than 5 {that is, the conditions you will be able to reproduce post extubation}, and a pCO_2 less than 50. No one of these numbers is etched in granite, the overall clinical picture plus an interpretation of the numbers is the key.)

You can find the physiologic numbers about extubation criteria anywhere. Remember that they often refer to ideal body weight with a slight increase for fat.

Take another look at 3, the endotracheal tube as a stent. For *any* surgery around the nose, the mouth, and the neck, decide whether the ETT is acting as a stent. Test this by putting a thumb over the tube opening, a stethoscope on the trachea, and putting the cuff down. You should hear air movement *around* the ETT. If you do not hear air movement around the ETT, then that tube is acting as a stent. Pull that stent and you lose the airway. Foolish move.

Delayed Awakening

Delayed awakening, lethargy, or combativeness are common preop and postop questions. Use the same differential diagnosis each time. Organize your thoughts.

First address the life-threatening causes:

- reduced oxygen delivery (primarily hypoxia)
- hypotension
- hypoglycemia

After that, consider the complete differential diagnosis:

- drug
- metabolic
- neurologic

Start with the most likely diagnosis. Consider their pre-existing diseases. Diabetic? Cirrhotic? Postpheochromocytoma removal? Check for hypoglycemia. Postintracranial surgery? Check for a rebleed.

Almost any drug you give and almost any aberrant lab value that you have can cause a problem in the brain. Supportive therapy is always indicated while you search for the cause.

BRINGING IT ALL TOGETHER

- Timing: emergent, urgent, elective.
- There's a reason: multiorgan system disease, conflicting therapies, and differentiating a common sign or symptom.
- Preop: organize a problem list, decide what further information you need.
- Intraop: monitors, induction, maintenance.
- Postop: know extubation and delayed awakening problems.

If you organize your board exam all the time by the format above, it will be like anesthetizing a healthy outpatient; everything is routine and expected. It's a formula; no surprises, no problems.

REFERENCES

1. Mangano DT, Layug EL, Wallace A, Tateo I. Effect of atenolol on mortality and cardiovascular morbidity after noncardiac surgery. Multicenter Study of Perioperative Ischemia Study Group. *N Engl J Med* 1996;335:1713–1720.
2. Poldermans D, Boersma E, Bax JJ, et al. The effect of bisoprolol on perioperative mortality and myocardial infarction in high-risk patients undergoing vascular surgery. *N Engl J Med* 1999;341: 1789–1794.

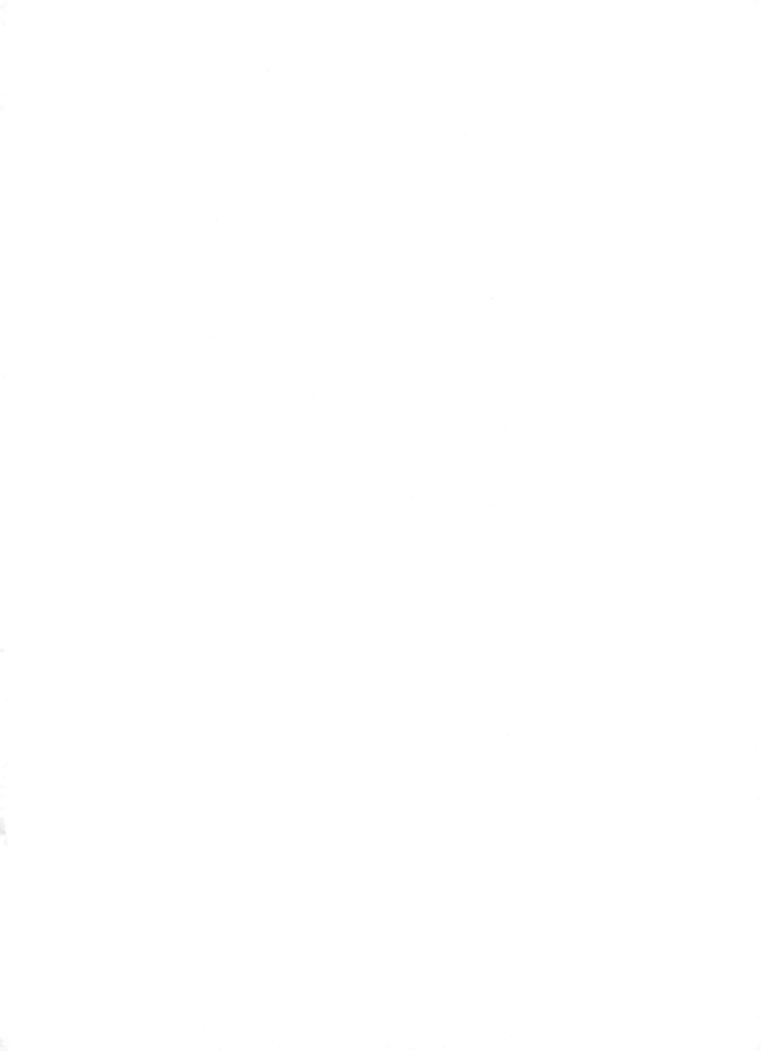

Mechanic's Manual

Part I: Driving School gave you insight into taking the test. A "how to" review. Now it's time to do a "what's inside" review. In Part 2: Mechanic's Manual, we will look at the major areas covered on the test—vital signs, peds, OB, neuro, the whole shebang. We seek out possible preop, intraop, and postop questions at each turn. All review relates to "How will this help me take the test?"

Keep in mind, what we cover in a few pages, others cover in entire books. So this section highlights only the tips of some icebergs, no more.

So roll up your sleeves, find the latch that pops the hood, and let's take a look.

Vital Signs Are Vital

"Hark, hoof beats!" the oral board examiner hints.

Bright eyed and ever alert, the examinee jumps all over that. "Must be a zebra! Or…or maybe a unicorn! Is not the great-toed sloth of prehistoric times a possible suspect in this hoof beat scenario?"

The two examiners look at each other, shake their heads knowingly, and then look back at the examinee.

"You flunk, professor, those hoof beats are from a horse!"

And so it goes with vital signs. Remember the basics. Common things are common.

EXAMPLE 1

A patient is tachycardic, hypertensive, well-oxygenated, and reaching up to grab the 11 blade out of the surgeon's hand. Tears are running down the patient's eyes and you notice the isoflurane vaporizer has run dry. Is the tachycardia from:

1. Light anesthesia
2. Epinephrine having been snuck into your IV bag, against your will
3. Light anesthesia
4. An occult pheochromocytoma
5. Light anesthesia

The answer is in the appendix under, "How do you spell the word 'duh'?"

Lesson learned: Go for the obvious stuff first. Light anesthesia is not the world's most exotic or rare phenomenon. Face it, light anesthesia accounts for a lot of hypertension, and too deep of an anesthetic accounts for a lot of hypotension.

EXAMPLE 2

The first examiner asks, "The patient develops tachycardia. What could it be?"

The clever examinee remembers safety first and says, "First and foremost remember the ABCs. Assure adequate oxygenation and ventilation. Would hate to go chasing other causes of tachycardia when it was hypoxemia causing the problem."

The second examiner says, "OK, the pulse oximeter says 99%."

The examinee says, "Well, I'd make damn sure the patient is well-ventilated."

First examiner, "He is, genius; now what's causing the tachycardia?"

"Remember the ABCs," the examinee harps.

Now both the examiners speak as one, "We said he's oxygenating and ventilating fine! What *else* could be causing this tachycardia, oh master of the galaxy?"

The examinee, now sheepish, says, "Well, you never can be too safe."

Lesson learned: Yes, yes, of course make sure the patient's respiratory status is optimized. Say it first, say it clearly, mention it, and then move on, please. Getting into a washing machine spin cycle saying "ABC, ABC, ABC" over and over again does you no good.

THE PROBLEM WITH STUDYING VITAL SIGNS IN ISOLATION

Studying a dissected heart from a formalin preparation is quite instructive. The valves wiggle, the thick left ventricle bespeaks a lot of pressure work, the thin right ventricle reveals less pressure work. Coronary vessels tell a story about the heart's blood supply.

Only problem—the heart does not function in a formalin jar! The heart works; it thunders when a tiger is chasing you, it slows down when you sleep. Input and feedback from the lungs, the brain, the peripheral circulation, the myocardium itself, all affect that slab of muscle sitting in that jar. So, studying the heart in isolation does not tell the whole story.

It's the same story with individual vital signs. Listing tachycardia alone, without considering all the other things going on, is like studying that heart in a jar. Vital sign aberrations occur within the flux of the OR—blood loss, fluid shifts, response to anesthesia, response to surgical stimulation. So keep that in mind as you study the lists of vital signs below. One vital sign alone cannot tell the entire story, so consider a vital sign just one facet of the entire picture.

WITH VITAL SIGNS AS WITH ALL THINGS, COMMON THINGS ARE COMMON

1. Gunshot wound; half the cardiac output is running all over your shoes. Tachycardia and hypotension. What is it? Hypovolemia, of course.

2. Patient moving, tachycardia, and hypertension. Light anesthesia? Of course. Common things are common.

COMBINATION PLATES

The other kicker with vital signs is, you can't always find a single cause for the problem. A cardiac patient, for example, may be getting ischemic. Ischemia can cause tachycardia or, for that matter, tachycardia can turn around and cause ischemia. Plus, the ischemic patient can have other, more pedestrian causes of tachycardia, such as light anesthesia, fluid loss, or anemia. So it can be tough to say, "Here is the one vital sign that has changed, here is the one cause for that one change. Thank you, hand me my board certification."

BEST APPROACH ON THE BOARDS

Take charge of any "vital sign" question by stating an assumption or two, then getting on with the answer. You are there to TELL THE EXAMINERS USEFUL STUFF, not to ask a lot of questions. (Recall in the previous chapter—"Don't ask the examiners questions.")

Compare the following two responses and decide who sounds like a consultant and who sounds like, Bud, the anesthetic mechanic.

Response Number One: "The patient's heart rate goes up, you say. Well, what's the blood pressure, oh, is the saturation OK? Um, how much fluid have I given? Has there been much blood loss?"

Response Number Two: "The patient's heart rate goes up, you say. After a check to assure adequate oxygenation and ventilation, and a tally of fluids in and out, I would check the EKG to make sure there weren't any changes indicative of ischemia, then I would deepen anesthesia. If this maneuver dropped the blood pressure, then I would assume hypovolemia and administer a 500-cc fluid bolus."

Response number one is going nowhere fast. Response number two is rocketing toward board certification.

THE SKINNY ON VITAL SIGNS

Groom yourself to handle every aberration in vital signs. In fact, that is the essence of an anesthesiologist's job. Work on a good, systematic approach to these vital sign aberrations.

- Tachypnea
- Apnea
- Tachycardia
- Bradycardia

- Hypertension
- Hypotension
- Hypoxemia
- Hypercapnia

TACHYPNEA

The most noticeable thing about respirations is you shouldn't notice them. Certainly under anesthesia it isn't noticeable; most of the time we just set the ventilator and that's that. So a tachypnea question is likely to come up in a preop question (less emphasized now than in years past) or in the postop area. Bottom line, if you notice, really notice the patient breathing, then that patient has a problem. Look for the following causes.

- Peripheral pain—What's the respiratory rate of a person writhing in agony? High. Treat the pain.
- Central nervous system—If your patient is so bad off neurologically that he has Cheyne-Stokes respirations, you'd better be at that bedside, or else intubating the patient, or else calling for the hospital clergy.
- Heart/lung—Overload, overload, overload, overload. What is the most common, the most common, the most common cause of labored breathing in the postoperative arena? Too much fluid that can be from a multiplicity of causes, depending on the patient's kidneys, heart, and lungs. During anesthesia, whether spinal or general, we tend to drop the pressure and tend to treat it with fluids. End of case, anesthetic gone, fluids not gone, boom. Patient is in fluid overload. What is the most sensitive sign of fluid overload, CVP, Swan, TEE? No! Respiratory rate! The damned respiratory rate!
- And if the patient has no kidney function? Is it easy to push them "over the edge" with your fluids? Yes.
- If the patient has emphysema, COPD, right heart failure, is it easy to push them "over the edge"? Yes.
- If the patient has had a boatload of MIs and is in and out of CHF all the time, is it easy to push them "over the edge"? Of course.
- And the respiratory rate will tell you! The respiratory rate will tell you. Hallelujah, let me hear it from the rooftops; let me hear you shout it all together, the respiratory rate will tell you. Amen, I say unto you.
- Compensation for a metabolic acidosis. (You wanted more explanation? Maybe. Well, we're not endocrinologists.)

APNEA

The most noticeable thing about respirations is that when there aren't any at all that can be a real bummer. There is one chief cause of apnea with several subcauses underneath it.

Iatrogenesis Imperfecta—yes, you are usually the culprit in this particular vital sign aberration, or should we say this lack of a vital sign. Drug and CNS causes highlight the list.

- Brain death. Stroke of the respiratory centers. You are encouraged to avoid causing this in your patient.
- Too much anesthesia stuff, be it narcotic, muscle relaxant, sedative/hypnotics, or just the vapors that haven't worn off yet.

TACHYCARDIA

The causes of tachycardia are so numerous that it pays to break them into two main categories; that way even if you miss one little cause you've hit the main points. Primary tachycardia means a fast heart rate from a pathology inherent in the heart itself. Secondary tachycardia means a fast heart rate from some stimulus to the heart.

Primary Tachycardia
- Supraventricular arrhythmia—A fib. WPW or some wiring problem with the heart's conduction system. These are unlikely to appear without earlier warning in the stem question.
- Ventricular arrhythmia—Again, some weird wiring problem could account for this as a "primary tachycardia," but such an arrhythmia is much more likely in the face of a secondary cause (electrolyte abnormality, blood gas aberration, ischemia).

Secondary Tachycardia (Sympathetic Stimulation from Somewhere)
- Hypoxemia—Always address this first. As mentioned before, don't belabor the point, but it is the one thing that needs fixing NOW before any other considerations.
- Hypercapnia—Less likely, and it's worth noting that people have survived astoundingly high pCO_2s (in the 100 or even 200 range!). Still, if something is awry, make sure that the CO_2 aspect of ventilation is addressed. The end-tidal gives you a clue, but a host of problems can make the end-tidal CO_2 inaccurate compared to the actual arterial pCO_2.
- Hypoglycemia—Diabetics are common on the boards.
- Decreased oxygen delivery (from anemia or decreased cardiac output)—If this is a concern, a Swan with mixed venous saturation is just the cat's pajamas. (Regarding anemia, I have never

in my life regretted drawing a hematocrit.) Remember all the places that blood can hide, the abdomen, chest, pelvis, in the thigh after a femoral fracture. Once oxygenation and adequate volume resuscitation are assured, tachycardia is due to hypovolemia until proven otherwise. Keep in mind one aspect of hypovolemia in the bleeding patient. A person can bleed to death and still have a normal hematocrit. As they bleed down, their entire blood volume is reduced to one cup of blood (with a normal hematocrit!) racing around in the circulation, trying to do the work of an entire blood volume.

- Hypovolemia—This can be absolute, meaning dehydration or hemorrhage, or relative, such as tamponade, pneumothorax, or PEEP.
- Pain—In addition to surgical pain, remember the sympathetic stimulation from a tourniquet or from a distended bladder.
- Another round of Iatrogenesis Imperfecta—Oops! Running that dopamine in too fast or not mixing the dopamine correctly in the first place.
- Left field possibilities—Pheochromocytoma, carcinoid syndrome, thyrotoxicosis. There's always a few rare things floating around. In all the exams we've heard about, no test taker has been tripped up by some "out of the blue" cause such as these.

BRADYCARDIA

After that exhausting trip through tachycardia, it is reassuring to know that bradycardia isn't so extensive. The old primary/secondary schtick works well for bradycardia too.

Primary Bradycardia

This is more commonly seen than its tachycardic counterpart.

- Sick sinus syndrome
- Complete heart block—Worth noting at this point is another Iatrogenesis Imperfecta maneuver—floating a Swan in a patient with a left bundle branch block. Hit that right bundle and voila! No heart beating. No blood pressure. Unhappiness all around.

Secondary Bradycardia

There are really only two reasons for secondary bradycardia—increased vagal tone or sympatholysis.

- Toxicity from digoxin
- Narcotics and neuromuscular blockers (vagotonic)
- Beta blockers (sympatholysis)
- Calcium channel blockers

- Vagal stimulation—from the oculocardiac reflex, traction on the peritoneum, laryngoscopy, or from a baroreceptor reflex (you give Neo, pressure goes up, heart rate goes down).

HYPERTENSION

Most of the causes here overlap with the tachycardia algorithm.

Primary Hypertension
Nothing we can't eliminate with our usual delicate induction.

Secondary Hypertension
Sympathetic stimulation from the usual causes, pain, hypoxemia, or an inotrope running in. The left-field causes of tachycardia also apply here—thyrotoxicosis, pheo, carcinoid.

HYPOTENSION

- Preload—absolute or relative. Not enough blood in the veins (e.g., hemorrhage, dehydration), or not enough of the blood in the veins is getting to the heart (e.g., tension pneumo, tamponade).
- Afterload—unclamping the aorta, sepsis, minimal hematocrit, and low viscosity, anesthetic or vasodilator overdose. Along with vasodilator overdose is the effect of regional anesthesia. Spinals and epidurals, with their accompanying sympathectomy, drop afterload.
- Contractility—CHF, ischemia, and once again, anesthetic overdose. Recall that inhaled agents are "cardiomyopathy in a bottle." Propofol is cardiomyopathy in a vial.
- Rate—too slow or too fast (inadequate filling time with a rapid heart rate, especially important if the patient has stenotic lesions).
- Rhythm—the best rhythms, in order, are sinus, then A-pace, then AV-pace, then V-pace, then asystole, which comes in dead last and with reason. Losing the atrial kick hurts output and blood pressure drops accordingly. Losing the ventricular kick hurts output to quite a noticeable degree also.

HYPOXEMIA

Whaddaya think the odds are of hypoxemia showing up on your exam? 100%. If you can't explain how you handle hypoxemia, don't bother going to the exam. Your grade will go

Boop
Boop
Boop

Boop
Boop
Boop
Just like the pulse oximeter does.

The geographic approach to hypoxemia covers all the bases. Go from the wall to the airway, from the airway into the lungs, then go back outside the patient and go from the outside of the chest all the way into the alveoli.

- Wall to airway. Wrong composition of gas. Oxygen turned off or some kind of crossover in the lines. An oxygen analyzer in the inspiratory limb of the circuit is a must here.
- Airway screwup. Disconnect. Obstruction. Misplaced tube. Ventilator disconnect (the alarms are *almost always* perfect, but just *almost*). The handle on the anesthetic machine is set on manual when you have the ventilator on (although newer machines have fixed that problem by linking the vent to the manual/vent switchover). Kinked, clogged, or misplaced endotracheal tube or LMA. Misplaced oral airway causing obstruction rather than relieving it. Endobronchial intubation. Thinking you're going to one lung ventilation during a thoracic case when you're actually going to NO LUNG ventilation.
- Thorax, outermost to innermost. **Diaphragm** and **chest wall** problems—hypoventilation on the patient's part due to weakness from neuromuscular blockade, flail chest, or kyphoscoliosis. In the **pleura**, pneumo-, hydro-, hemo-, or chylothorax can impede lung excursion. The lung parenchyma can malfunction due to **alveolar** malfunction—aspiration, pneumonia, atelectasis. The lung **parenchyma** can be congested from cardiac failure. The lung **airways** can be constricted or obstructed (aspiration, reactive airways disease, collapse of an anterior mediastinal mass). The **lung vasculature** can fail to deliver enough blood to the lungs to provide sufficient oxygenation—fat, amniotic, or regular pulmonary emboli, or right to left shunting in **cardiac** abnormalities. Note each **bold** topic is one layer in, and these eight areas can more easily be remembered than the 100 causes of hypoxemia that fall under those eight anatomic areas.
- CNS—Hypoventilation due to narcotics, residual anesthetic, or hypothermia. When the patient's CNS doesn't work, you'd better make sure *your CNS* is working. Start breathing for them!

HYPERCAPNIA

Again, be systematic rather than hit or miss. Break hypercapnia into big categories and subsets.

- Overproduction—Any metabolic supernova will generate more CO_2 than you can eliminate. Malignant hyperthermia, thyrotoxicosis, and sepsis fit this category.
- Decreased elimination—Hypoventilation, either due to the patient's own illness (weakness from a neuromuscular disorder, respiratory insufficiency secondary to CHF, asthma), or hypoventilation due to your crummy anesthetic (inappropriate ventilator settings, residual neuromuscular blockade or over-narcotization).
- Rebreathing CO_2—Not too common. A malfunctioning valve in your circuit will allow this rebreathing. This could also be thought of as a subset of decreased elimination.

There you have it. Vital signs in all their glory. For sure, for absolute sure, for superdeedooper sure, you will be asked to manage some changes in vital signs. Remember, vital signs are vital to both the patient and your certification.

From this point forward, the Part II: Mechanic's Manual will take on a new look. All review will be geared to thinking preop, intraop, postop.

9 | To Fly the Plane, You Must Know the Plane: Anesthesia Equipment

Scotty looks bent out of shape as usual. "But Captain, you can't mix the Dilithium crystals with Drano, it'll blow the Enterprise to kingdom come!"

"RED ALERT, RED ALERT!" The Enterprise's warning system is going bananas and people are running all over the place. Explosions rock the ship; smoke fills the air.

Captain Kirk rolls his eyes, "Oh Scotty, every week you tell me the same thing. 'But Captain, you can't mix the antimatter with the matter, it'll tear apart the ship!', or 'But Captain, if you continue to go warp speed 50 any longer, we'll disintegrate!'"

Scotty shrugs his shoulders. In his hand he holds Dorsch and Dorsch's *Understanding Warp Drive Equipment.*

Captain Kirk goes on, "And every week, I do what you tell me not to do, and the Enterprise never blows up. Isn't that right?"

Scuffing his feet, looking down at the ground, Scotty nods in agreement.

"Go back to your cabin and read Dorsch and Dorsch again, Scotty," Kirk admonishes, "I don't think you really understand the equipment in the Starship Enterprise."

Don't be like Scotty. Know your equipment. Here are some preop, intraop, and postop questions pertaining to anesthesia equipment.

PREOP EQUIPMENT QUESTIONS

What is the purpose of the line isolation monitor and what do you do preop if it sounds an alarm?

A regular electrical system is grounded. Touch a wire and you complete the circuit and ZAP! An operating room system is created by inductance and is not grounded, therefore if you touch a wire you will not complete a circuit and will not go ZAP! The line isolation monitor alarm goes off if there is a fault in the operating room electrical system somewhere. The short answer—you should not do a case in that room until the fault is found and fixed.

On the subject of electrical safety, what is the difference between macro- and microshock?

A decimal point tells a thousand words. Fifty *micro*amps applied directly to the heart can cause V-fib. Any patient with a central line is at risk (Spooky isn't it? Makes you think twice about that ungrounded boombox with a hangar antenna that's sitting right on your anesthesia machine).

Keep in mind the line isolation monitor can pick up electrical "leaks" of 2 to 3 *milli*amps. Catch that? We can tell when a machine has a problem in the *milli*amp range, microshock occurs below our radar, at the *micro*amp range—a thousand times lower. The lesson: Especially if a patient has any kind of central line, keep the room electrically clean. This is especially pertinent when placing multiorifice CVPs using an EKG machine for P wave monitoring to document correct placement. You are hooking that machine (and any current leaking from it) via a fluid filled column directly to the heart.

Before you start your case, you must pick a circuit. What are your circuit options?

Mapleson A, B, C, D, E, Jackson-Reese, Bain—who *are* these people? Why did they make such a menagerie of different circuits? Thank God for small favors, though. That stuff tends to be the misery of the written boards. Still, you should at least know the advantages of these various circuits.

1. Open system—such as open drop technique (you've done these a lot). Lightweight, portable, no complex equipment needed. You'll use this after World War III when we are plunged back into the dark ages, or when managed care dictates that we all have to use ether again.
2. Semi-open system—such as the Mapleson system, a Jackson-Reese (modified Mapleson E), or Bain (modified Mapleson D). These systems are lightweight, portable, and disposable. These systems lack valves, so resistance is low. Good for kids under 10 kg.
3. Semi-closed—which is the generic system you use every day in the operating room. Rebreathing is possible, so heat is conserved. Rebreathing is possible, so a CO_2 absorber is necessary.
4. Closed system—which is a semi-closed system with the pop-off valve closed. This conserves heat and anesthetic agent and is a useful system for teaching uptake and distribution. Truth to tell, there are closed system gurus out there who profess the greatness of this system, and they periodically go out and preach the word. Usually, a teaching program will do a few cases "that way" while the guru is around. Then, within days, things go back to the semi-closed, less demanding way.

INTRAOP EQUIPMENT QUESTIONS

Two clicks to the right on your vaporizer, then one click back. Just how does that vaporizer work? Should you care? I mean, you drive a car, and they don't make you draw the steering chassis before they give you a license. You use a computer, but cannot outline the motherboard (if you could, you'd be doing something lucrative now, like inventing a way to put anesthesia on the internet and make some *real* money.)

Luckily, you don't need an engineer's degree or a blueprint to draw the fundamental essence of the anesthesia vaporizer. Oxygen flows through the machine, some is diverted over the liquid anesthetic and some bypasses the liquid anesthetic. The more oxygen that flows over the liquid anesthetic, the higher the concentration of anesthetic delivered.

This knowledge helps you answer the question, "Why should a vaporizer not get tipped over?" Tipping a vaporizer would spill some anesthetic liquid into other parts of the machine and thus the concentration of anesthetic vapor would not be controlled. In all likelihood, the concentration leaving the vaporizer would be much higher.

Oxygen is good, or so you've heard. What helps us make sure we deliver oxygen?

1. Diameter indexed safety system (DISS). The coupling between oxygen and nitrous oxide is such that one cannot fit into the other, both at the wall connection and on the yokes by the side of the machine.
2. Colored tubing and cylinders.
3. Fluted handle on the oxygen control knob versus a sintered feel on the nitrous knob.
4. Oxygen on the far right of the manifold so that a crack anywhere in the manifold system should not produce a hypoxic mixture.
5. Fail-safe mechanism that alarms if the oxygen pressure falls below 25 lb./sq. in. (Note, this alarm assures oxygen pressure, but not oxygen flow.)
6. Oxygen ratio control monitor to link N_2O flow to O_2 flow.
7. Disconnect alarm on the ventilator. (Note, the ventilator may disconnect, fall against the drapes or the table, and the ventilator will merrily cycle away for a while.)
8. Apnea alarm on most monitors if the CO_2 fails to register.
9. Oxygen analyzer. This is a must, an absolute must. There is no way, just no way, of knowing that you are delivering oxygen unless you have an O_2 analyzer. The stories of crossovers and line screwups are legendary. Analyze what is going into your patient's lungs.

Your oxygen knob is on 2 L, your nitrous knob is on 2 L, but your oxygen analyzer reads 85%. What's up with that?

The bellows are powered by O_2. There is a hole in the bellows and O_2 is entering the bellows, yielding a higher FIO_2. Alternatively, the oxygen analyzer may be malfunctioning. Remember, if a monitor says something *odd*, then either *something odd is happening* or else *the monitor itself is odd*. Believe the worst thing is happening. This explains, by the way, *why* we use oxygen to power the descent of the bellows and not some other gas.

Back to our old friend, the line isolation monitor. It alarms in the middle of a case. What do you do?

If the line isolation monitor goes off, then the patient is at risk for macroshock. Find the machine at fault (the insulation is probably frayed) by unplugging the machines one at a time until the line isolation monitor clams up. If you ignore it and forge ahead, you could put the patient into V-tach or V-fib, cause burns, etc. Ouch!

Your reservoir bag keeps collapsing, what is happening?

The scavenging system is sucking too hard and pulling gases out of the circle system.

The reservoir bag keeps inflating despite low gas flows.

The scavenger system is clogged or else the pop off valve is closed.

Oxygen flowmeter reads 5 L, N_2O is 0 L, but the FIO_2 reads 21%.

Pipeline crossover or wrong cylinder forced into the oxygen yolk. Probably air is being used rather than O_2.

A cylinder is hanging crooked and hissing.

The cylinder is improperly connected.

The oxygen knob is turned off but the rotameter reads 5 L.

There is dust in the flowmeter and the bobbin is sticking.

The ventilator is cycling and no alarm is sounding, but the chest is not moving. What to do?

Something disconnected. The ventilator hose may be pressing against the drapes, so the low pressure alarm is not going off. *The answer is always*, when in doubt, hook them to an ambu bag and separate freestanding O_2 tank.

The ventilator does not fill. Your move?

A disconnect somewhere in the system. If you look all over the place and can't figure it, grab an ambu bag. The anesthesia machine holds a million little things, any of which can fail. If push comes to shove, you can't figure out the problem, and the patient is in trouble, don't waste time on diagnostics. Disconnect, get an ambu bag and an oxygen tank, and hand ventilate. You can always figure it out later, you can always anesthetize with IV agents, you can always suffer untold embarrassment as another anesthesiologist comes in and figures out the problem. Just save the patient, concentrate on the patient, and get that oxygen in there. Don't be like the pilot, trying to figure out why some little alarm is going off, in the meantime he forgets to fly the plane and BOOM!

With a hanging bellows (old machines) oxygen flow is 5 L, nitrous flow is 5 L, FIO_2 reads 25%, and the ventilator is cycling.

Hanging bellows is drawing in room air from a partial disconnect in any part in the circuit. No, we don't think that the archaic hanging bellows will be on the exam, but we just wanted you to know how old we are.

Capnogram shows inspired CO_2. What is your best maneuver, oh wise one?

One-way valve malfunctions and causes rebreathing or else the CO_2 absorber is exhausted. Channeling through the CO_2 absorber may have the same effect.

POSTOP EQUIPMENT QUESTIONS

The postop area doesn't lend itself as readily to board type questions. The only one we can conjure up relates to ventilator malfunctions in the intensive care unit.

After a CABG, a patient is connected to the ICU ventilator. With successive inspirations, the patient's chest rises and rises and his blood pressure nose-dives. What is happening and what do you do?

The exhalation valve in the ventilator is malfunctioning. Disconnect from the ventilator, watch for a big *WHOOSH*, and connect to an ambu bag while you send for a new ventilator. Barotrauma is a danger here, so examine for signs of pneumothorax, get a chest x-ray, and insert a chest tube if necessary. If a tension pneumothorax has occurred during this mishap and there is no time for chest tube placement, place a 14-g angiocath in the midclavicular line in the 2nd intercostal space.

In all likelihood, equipment questions will not constitute the lion's share of anyone's test. But to completely ignore equipment in your study may land you in a heap of trouble. Some examinees have faced equipment questions early in their test and were so rattled that they never recovered. The examiners weren't looking for electrical engineering Ph.D. answers, just some indication that the examinee had *some* understanding of the stuff we use every day.

OK Scotty, you can beam me back up now.

10 | Smoke 'em if You Got 'em

The year is 1621. Sir Walter Raleigh has just come back from the new colony in America. In his mouth is a device no one has ever seen before. And smoke is coming out of it! A smell fills the royal chamber as England's King James I looks on in amazement.

Tobacco has entered Europe.

King James I says, "A custom loathsome to the eye, hateful to the nose, harmful to the brain, dangerous to the lungs, and in the black stinking fume thereof, nearest resembling the horrible Stygian smoke of the pit that is bottomless."

PREOP PULMONARY QUESTIONS

A COPD patient presents for an elective procedure. How do you assess whether he is ready to go?

Evaluate the patient with the simplest yet best diagnostic tool—history. If the patient feels "as good as he ever gets" and there has been no recent worsening of symptoms, then the patient is about as optimized as he will get. If, in contrast, sputum color or production has changed, if the patient is more short of breath, if coughing has worsened recently, then the patient is not in optimal condition for an elective procedure.

If the patient has a regular pulmonary doc, then all the better. Have the patient see his/her regular pulmonary doc preop with two simple questions, "Is this patient as good as he/she can get? What else can we do to optimize the lungs preop?"

Which patient will get a pulmonary function test? Any patient undergoing a lung resection (lobectomy or pneumonectomy) needs a PFT, so you can have some prediction of residual pulmonary function. For other patients, PFTs may be an unnecessary expense and add little to the patient's treatment. Some recent data suggests PFTs might not be the final word on the ability to tolerate lung resection, however.

Which patient will get a pulmonary function test? Take two. Any COPD patient with severe COPD undergoing an operation involving large fluid shifts or postoperative ventilation should have PFTs with and without bronchodilators to see if there are further reversible components to their reactive airway disease. The information from the PFTs, which can now be done at bedside by a technician, will help guide postoperative ICU decision making. For example, if the PFTs are all borderline, the ICU doctor may be much less likely to discharge a "freshly extubated" patient to the floor.

Note that the PFT question had two opposite answers, each defended reasonably. That emphasizes an important point about the boards. Many questions are open-ended, with no absolute right or absolute wrong answer. The idea is to defend your answer with a reasonable explanation. Defending an answer with, "Well, that's the way we do it at East Bumblebee Memorial Surgicenter," or "An attending told me so," will not cut it.

Now another COPD patient presents for an emergency operation. What's your best move? Aminophylline in the acute setting will buy you only grief, rhythm disturbances, and little improvement, so avoid it. Inhaled beta agents and a steroid pulse may help. The beta agents work almost immediately. The steroids won't kick in for about 6 hours, but remember 6 hours from now you may be happy that something is working for you, not against you. Start treatment for any infection the patient may have. Again, in the acute setting, you're not going to get much immediate help from this, but the idea is to start optimizing whatever you can optimize.

A smoker is scheduled for a carpal tunnel release in 2 days. Do you advise quitting smoking? No. Smoking cessation takes months to make a real difference. To tell the patient, already nervous about an upcoming operation, to stop smoking will just make the patient more nervous. Stopping acutely will also cause increased pulmonary secretions at the time of induction.

A smoker is scheduled for a carpal tunnel release in 2 days. Do you advise quitting smoking? Yes. The only positive is a decrease in blood carbon monoxide concentrations. Although it is unlikely that this will make any practical difference to the carpal tunnel operation, it will optimize their oxygenation in the event of a pulmonary complication/exacerbation. Furthermore, you are a doctor with an obligation to advise patients on all their health, not just the anesthetic aspects of their care. So you should tell them to stop.

Get the idea? Once again, you've seen the same question answered two opposite ways, each answer defended in reasonable fashion. The boards are not looking for specific answers, they are looking for defense of reasonable answers.

INTRAOP PULMONARY QUESTIONS

You face a patient with reactive airways and must now do the anesthetic deed. What choice of anesthetic is best?

Regional if you can, with the usual caveats associated with any regional anesthetic.

1. No regional is guaranteed to work. Spinals fail, epidurals come out, and arm blocks wear off at the worst times.
2. Spinal or an epidural in a bad COPD patient can go high enough to take away some intercostals, robbing patients of important accessory muscles and throwing them into respiratory insufficiency.
3. Patients can refuse a regional technique.

General anesthetic but avoid instrumenting the trachea? Good, but again, not guaranteed.

1. LMA or mask is good and should avoid stirring up bronchospasm, but an LMA may not work. LMA or mask leaves the patient at aspiration risk. You want to see bronchospasm? Aspiration will give you bronchospasm like nobody's business.
2. Many cases require intubation—intra-abdominal procedure, insufflation, prone case, or a neurological case with the airway somewhere lost under drapes and headpins.

General anesthetic with intubation. Recall the old Latin maxim, "Primum non causum bronchospasm withum tooum earlyum intubationum."

1. Breathe the patient deep or get enough IV agent on board to prevent bronchospasm (an ounce of prevention is worth a pound of cure). How do you know what is "deep enough?" Well, there is the BIS, but that endpoint is not well-defined. A good rule of thumb is a decrease in BP (assuming adequate hydration) of 20% to 30% from baseline after induction. This implies some degree of adrenergic ablation and deep anesthesia. If you have a better answer, great. The point is, have an answer for the question, "How do you know when they are deep enough." No right answer here, just an explanation of how you assess the endpoints of titration.
2. Even with a rapid sequence, you can get the patient prepared with, for example, a few puffs of albuterol in the preop holding area, then IV lidocaine or some IV narcotics with induction. Imperfect? Yes, but the idea is still to "prepare" the trachea for the stimulation of an endotracheal tube.

Intraoperatively, an intubated patient starts wheezing. What is the diagnosis and treatment? Back to that old reliable chestnut—all that wheezes is not bronchospasm. Wheezing equals noise from nonlaminar flow through the airways. Anything that compromises the lumen of the airways or adds extra turbulence to airflow can cause wheezing. Kinks, secretions, pneumothorax, aspiration, foreign body, endobronchial intubation, can all cause wheezing. Diagnose and treat these causes first. If you have ruled out these causes, then proceed with treatment of bronchospasm.

1. Inhaled beta agents. Good stuff. Make sure your delivery system actually gets the stuff into the patient's lungs. If there is total lack of air movement, inhaled stuff does not work.
2. Steroids. Will take hours to kick in. Still worth giving, because heck, you might still be in trouble a few hours from now. And on the boards, you can expect to have trouble recur in the PACU.
3. Deeper inhaled anesthetic. Another good choice. All the vapors are good at bronchodilation…if you can move air.
4. Epi—the savior of anesthesiologists everywhere. Small doses are the key; 5 to 10 mcg to start, and quickly doubling until you see an effect or until you reach 100 mcg. If severe desaturation has already occurred, be bolder. Put a mg in a 250 bag and run it wide open until effect, and titrate down. If epi isn't improving bronchospasm, be thinking, why is my bronchospasm treatment not working? Is this not bronchospasm? But at the same time, continue to do something—escalate doses, change drugs, etc. Never give up. No IV? Both epi and atropine work down the ETT.

A word to the wise—just as there will be a question on "How do you treat hypoxemia?" (see "Vital Signs Are Vital"), so will there also be a question on "How do you treat intraoperative bronchospasm?" There are precious few guarantees in this world, but we can guarantee that you will see one or both of these questions.

Now, on to more pulmonary questions. How would you extubate someone "deep"? When no further muscle relaxation is necessary, allow the muscle relaxant to wear off, go to manual ventilation, allow the patient to resume breathing, maintaining anesthesia with a high percentage of inhaled agent (looking at eye signs to make sure the patient is not in stage 2, and at increased risk of laryngospasm). When ready to extubate, switch to 100% oxygen for a minute, then deflate the cuff and extubate. I would not extubate someone like this if I were concerned with my ability to reintubate them.

Not every question on the boards will be a gut-wrenching, super-impossible, "there are 10 right answers" kind of question. Some questions are like this; "How do you extubate deep?" The examiners just want to hear you explain how you do something.

POSTOP PULMONARY QUESTIONS

Bronchospasm occurs in the PACU. What now Captain?

If the patient is ICU bound and is still intubated, then look for the usual suspects—kink, clog, endobronchial intubation, pneumothorax. Complicating things in the postoperative period is the patient emerging from anesthesia and bucking on the endotracheal tube. If the patient's condition allows, then remove the stimulus from his trachea, that is, the endotracheal tube. If the patient requires continued intubation, then deepen his sedation with IV agents—narcotics, lidocaine, propofol—and institute care as noted above—inhaled beta agents, epi, if necessary.

In the intensive care unit, a patient with ARDS drops his pressure with increasing PEEP, but he needs the PEEP. What next?

The ventilator and the heart engage in a tug of war with oxygen delivery. The ventilator, pushing in the good air, increases the delivery of oxygen.

GOOD! Oxygen delivery is good.

But the ventilator, while pushing in the good air, decreases venous return, decreasing cardiac output, thus decreasing delivery of oxygen to the tissues.

BAD! Decreased oxygen delivery is bad.

What, then, to do? Do you go up, up, up on the PEEP? No. Taken to its extreme (say PEEP of 10,000 cm H_2O), the patient's oxygenation will be dandy, but their cardiac output will go to 0 and, furthermore, the patient will blow up all over the intensive care unit. Just imagine explaining that at your next M and M conference!

Titrate to "best PEEP" (optimal oxygen delivery). Counteract the hemodynamic effects of the PEEP by fluid loading (to increase venous return), inotropic support (to increase cardiac output, hence increasing oxygen delivery to the tissues).

Such a balancing act requires close hemodynamic monitoring. A Swan-Ganz catheter with continuous mixed venous oxygen monitoring and/or a transesophageal echo will help.

Also, you may need PEEP to counteract the toxicity of oxygen. Keeping the patient on greater than 50% oxygen can cause pulmonary damage, so you need that PEEP to be able to reduce the FIO_2. No mean feat this is.

> **Example:** You are on 75% oxygen and have a pO_2 of 60. You go from a PEEP of 5 to a PEEP of 10. That improves your pO_2 and allows you to drop the FIO_2 down to 50%, but now the cardiac index is down.
>
> Fluid loading helps, but now the PA pressures are high.
>
> Start dobutamine. That helps the PA pressures get lower and helps your cardiac index. As PA pressures fall and the cardiac index goes up, the mixed venous oxygen saturation

rises too, indicating better global oxygen delivery.

Congratulations, junior ranger, you have just done a demonstration (albeit oversimplified) of "best PEEP."

OK. That's enough work for now. Take a break. Smoke 'em if you got 'em.

11 | Hearts—Catch-22

In Joseph Heller's classic *Catch-22,* a pilot named Orr wanted to get out of World War II. Orr wanted a psychiatric release based on insanity. The danger of flying bombing missions was driving him insane and he couldn't take it anymore. But his psychiatric release was denied. Heller describes the denial in a stellar example of military/medical gobbledygook, which has given rise to the enduring expression "Catch-22."

> There was only one catch and that was Catch-22, which specified that a concern for one's own safety in the face of dangers that were real and immediate was the process of a rational mind. Orr would be crazy to fly more missions and sane if he didn't, but if he was sane he had to fly them. If he flew them he was crazy and didn't have to; but if he didn't want to he was sane and had to.

PROBLEM 1—CATCH-22 ANESTHESIA STYLE

Money spent and delays caused *before* a case raise eyebrows and anger surgeons.

"What do you mean he needs this cardiology consult, he didn't tell *me* he had chest pain! God damn it, I'm calling Dr. Smith, he'll sleep ANYBODY. You can go to hell!"

If you fail to insist on the workup and something goes wrong *after* the fact, the surgeon will become a paragon of humility and deference to any concerns anesthetic.

"Well, if you had been so worried, you should have *told* me. I would *never* proceed in the face of a genuine concern for the patient's welfare. And now, here we are, *your* patient had a big MI and is sitting on a balloon pump in the ICU. I hope you have a good lawyer. Remember, *you* said it was OK to proceed. I'm just the surgeon, after all." Catch-22 anesthesia style.

CATCH-22 NUMBER TWO

Ischemia runs silent and deep. Diabetics, with their neuropathies, can have all kinds of ischemia and show nothing until they go into CHF or something shows on EKG. On the other hand, you can't do a mega workup on all diabetics.

EKGs themselves cause headaches aplenty.

- Normal in the face of major coronary pathology.
- A bundle branch block can hide ST abnormalities.
- Nonspecific ST-T wave changes mean...exactly what?
- Old EKG for comparison? Great if you find it. And, on the boards, you should certainly try to find an old EKG before proceeding. But, in today's outpatient how-do-you-do-5-minutes-before-the-operation world, that old EKG can be hard to find.
- Cancel on the basis of a mild abnormality in the EKG? Not very realistic, unless supported by some sort of clinical sign.

However, on the board exam, there is no right answer, it's how you defend your answer. You could say, with silent ischemia so prevalent, any abnormality necessitates a dobutamine stress echo to determine the amount of myocardium at risk. Why? So that you can suggest angioplasty prior to surgery if indicated, and thereby reduce ultimate patient morbidity. Or you can say...the risk of a perioperative MI with minor surgery is very low, and if an EKG sign is unsubstantiated by any clinical signs, there is little likelihood that an abnormality will be diagnosed with more advanced testing. Furthermore the probable treatment of choice, an angioplasty, has not been studied to show that it reduces the perioperative risk (although we believe it does).

CATCH-22 NUMBER THREE

Old studies, new technology.

Everyone and their brother can cite the Rao and EI-Etr study. MI 0 to 3 months ago, risk of MI 30%; MI 3 to 6 months ago, risk of MI 15%; MI greater than 6 months ago, risk of MI 6%. And all these periop MIs had a mortality of about 50%.

All fine.

But nowadays, say you had an MI 2 months ago, were found to have single vessel disease, and that was successfully angioplastied. Now your risk is...well, they weren't angioplastying people in Rao's time, so, uh, the risk is...what is it?

Should you delay now?

Once again, make your case, and stick with it. Basically, you do what you do to minimize patient morbidity. That's always the answer. The best approach is to analyze the potential amount of "myocardium at risk" and, if minimal due to treatment like angioplasty, I would personally feel confident proceeding.

On the other hand, if this is a totally elective procedure, you can get the surgeon, the cardiologist, you, and the patient to all sit down and have a big powwow about the best course of action. (Right, as if that could ever happen in this day and age.)

CATCH-22 NUMBER FOUR

Hypertension and reality. (Review the "Threshold" section of Chapter 7 to get another take on the blood pressure question.)

Go ahead during the boards, get on your high horse and say you would cancel a case if the patient came in with uncontrolled hypertension. Hope the examiners cannot look into your eyes and see the hundred times you hooked a patient up, took the first blood pressure, saw it was 190/110, and you said, "Oh, heck with it, a slug of propofol and that pressure won't be so high."

You proceeded, handled a few wobbles in the blood pressure, the patient survived and lived to fight another day. The old study (another throwback to the 1960s before nitroprusside and esmolol) says cardiopulmonary morbidity increases if the diastolic is greater than 110.

That's why, on the boards the blood pressure is always exactly 110 mm Hg diastolic. Right at that old cut-off.

If the case is elective, cancel and medically optimize the patient. This will decrease lability and subsequent bouts of myocardial ischemia if the patient is at risk for that.

If the case is urgent, proceed. Defend yourself saying, "The studies that demonstrate increased morbidity are old and perhaps not applicable to today's practice with quick acting IV antihypertensive agents."

Obviously, don't lower the blood pressure when the pressure is the driving force behind just enough blood flow to the brain. That comes up a lot too, as a carotid patient or CNS tumor patient will present with a very high BP on the boards.

FYI—on the carotid case, if the patient has a stenosis, high BP is good. If the patient has 70% blockage and an endothelium that looks like its throwing emboli, then the high BP is not necessary and can be lowered. Gross postoperative lability is bad due to an increased risk of postoperative intracranial hemorrhage with a sustained BP > 200 mm Hg systolic following carotid endarterectomies.

CATCH-22—CHF

Tuning up and reality. "Patient's not optimized, he's in CHF." The surgeon sighs, agrees to a postponement, the patient goes back to the HMO maze and comes back in—guess what—CHF, no better off than when you sent him to be "optimized."

Now you're really ticked. Some internist is dragooned into helping, gives the patient a slug of Lasix or two, and now the patient comes back to you "optimized." The Lasix has dried him out so badly that you can't get a central line for love nor money. You induce and the pressure plummets. The whole case you're trying to breathe life into pruned out kidneys. Fluids are the only way to save the day and the patient ends up in, you got it, CHF.

If you'd have just done the case in the first place, given a little Lasix at the end of the case yourself, this whole charade could have been avoided.

Can you just sweep these real-life "Catch-22s" under the rug during your exam? Well, uh, that's a tough one. The examiners *aren't* ninnies and they *are* great detectors of nonsense. The best you can do is break the cardiac question down into digestible parts, do the best you can do with the information provided, enumerate your concerns and explain your decision.

Keep in mind, the examiners across from you face those same questions every day in their practice. There are no perfect answers in this arena. The examiners aren't looking for perfect answers. They are looking for reasonable answers that a consultant in anesthesia would give. They know you can't say, "Cath everybody on the planet and do CABGs on all those with positive findings!"

The current format for the oral boards emphasizes the intraop course, but it's worth taking some time to review the preop concerns.

Cardiac Preop Question

A cardiac patient is scheduled for a procedure. How do you steer the preoperative evaluation?

In these cost-conscious days, the history still yields the most information. If angina is present (recalling the caveat about silent ischemia in the diabetic), then assess whether the angina is stable or unstable. Unless contradicted by the stem, assume it is stable by saying so.

Stable angina is a chest pain pattern that is not changing. Stable angina does not occur at rest. Unstable angina occurs at rest or is a chest pain pattern that is worsening. A patient with unstable angina is not a candidate for elective surgery. A patient with stable angina is a candidate for elective surgery.

(Catch-22 consideration floating in the back of your mind—the term "stable angina" is an oxymoron. No matter how unchanging the chest pain pattern, that chest pain means myocardium at peril!)

Next look for congestive heart failure. A patient with congestive heart failure is not a candidate for elective surgery until the CHF is as fixed as it can get. A patient without congestive heart failure is a candidate for elective surgery.

A note about congestive heart failure—consider the scope of the operation.

The key in all this consideration of angina and congestive heart failure is your desire to preserve myocardium. Myocardial preservation is *minimizing* stress; minimizing the imbalance of myocardial oxygen supply and demand. So if a peripheral, low volume shift procedure is planned (a haircut, for example), then pursuing the million dollar workup is not worth it if you have a low index of suspicion for "hidden" coronary disease.

If, in contrast, you suspect that coronary disease is lurking beneath the surface and an intra-abdominal extravaganza is planned (major volume shifts, possible anemic periods, near the diaphragm so lots of respiratory embarrassment, long immobilization with possibilities of pulmonary emboli), then it makes more sense to do a more thorough workup or have the patient see a cardiologist before the operation.

View these preop concerns as being on a continuum with no clear cutoff, just areas where it makes more or less sense to pursue the big workup.

No need for further workup.	Clear cut need for further workup.
No angina.	Unstable angina. Recent MI.
No risk factors.	Lots of risks.
Minor procedure.	Major procedure.
Haircut.	Intra-abdominal whackola.
History alone suffices.	Angiography, echo, the whole 9 yards.

You get the idea. Anything the examiners will ask you will be somewhere in the middle. If you explain your reasoning, you will sound like a consultant. Even if the examiner him/herself would do it differently, you will pass if you make your point in sound, intelligent fashion. On a technique note, remember that you are *always concerned*, especially about potential cardiac complications, but must consider the need for the surgery.

Cardiac Intraop Questions

A cardiac patient is scheduled for a procedure. What invasive monitors do you see in the patient's future?

The continuum idea helps again.

Minor procedures in patients with good cardiac function need no special invasive monitors. (Think again of the haircut. Joe at the corner barbershop doesn't need an A-line and Swan-Ganz catheter every time he clips someone's hair, no matter how bad their hearts.)

Major procedures in sick patients need the works. No liver transplant is done with a finger on the pulse and an EKG alone.

CVP versus Swan? This debate will go on until we have to pay for Swans out of our own pockets, then we'll all get comfortable with CVPs real quick. Traditional wisdom says you need the Swan when right sided pressures do not reflect left sided function. So, if the patient has bad lungs and/or a bad LV, then you need a Swan. The advent and more common use of TEE may be causing some rethinking, because the TEE will tell us how the ventricle is functioning and just how full the heart really is. (As opposed to the Swan telling us a number and we draw the conclusion, "Oh, we must be overfilled.") Furthermore, certain places, such as the Texas Heart Institute for example, do about a zillion hearts each year and rarely use a Swan. Can you argue with such numbers or their outcome?

So what is the right answer? That's up to you. A few outs remain. Placing a CVP doesn't mean no way, no way, no way can you use a Swan. If you're floundering with a CVP, you can always put a Swan in later. Bottom line here, the Swan versus CVP question is yours to defend as you see fit. Just make sure you have a physiologic reason for your explanation.

A-line? Easier to defend—If you need to watch beat-to-beat blood pressure or will be drawing gases, you need an A-line. This issue was discussed in detail in Chapter 7.

Describe an induction tailored to the needs of a cardiac patient.

It's all in the physiology. Cardiac ischemia happens when oxygen supply—coronary blood flow and oxygen carrying capacity of the blood—is insufficient for the myocardial oxygen demand. There are only a few things you can do on the supply side of the equation:

1. Insist on and get an angioplasty or CABG preop.
2. Make sure the blood going through those coronaries is well oxygenated.
3. Nitrates to dilate the coronaries (arguable whether this really happens, the beneficial result is more likely from unloading and releasing wall tension in the heart itself).
4. Make sure the blood going through those coronaries has the optimal "internal milieu" for cellular function. Adequate hemoglobin, sugar, and acid base status are a must. A hematocrit of 4, a white out on the D-stick, and a pH of 7.03 aren't doing your myocardial cells any favors.

Of more utility on a board question is the myocardial oxygen demand. You, the inducer of anesthesia, control the myocardial oxygen demand.

1. Tachycardia? Bad business, that tachycardia. Avoid it. Tachycardia increases the work of the heart and decreases the resting/nutrition time of the heart (diastole). Even the shortest case, say, bronchoscopy, can elicit damaging tachycardia. Short acting beta blockers such as esmolol, or short acting narcotics, such as remifentanil, provide just the ticket for short acting control of tachycardia in a brief but stimulating case such as bronchoscopy. There is data that suggests that esmolol will not induce bronchospasm in patients with reactive airways disease (if you need to beta block on the boards, it is likely that the patient will have reactive airways disease).

2. Hypertension or overfilling the heart? Again, bad business. Avoid it. (Don't we sound like a cardiology consult?) With any induction, judicious use of the goodies we have should avoid a rocky induction. How, specifically? Pick your poison. Intravenous induction with propofol, then breathe the patient down. Narcotics up front with esmolol at the ready. Close watching of the A-line and regrouping at the first sign of trouble. (For example, you place the laryngoscope, the pressure starts climbing. Stop, pull the laryngoscope out, give more agent, then try again in a minute or two.) The idea is to present a plan that focuses on controlling what you can control with the heart's physiology in mind.

3. Hypotension? The coronaries are pressure dependent distal to their occlusive disease. Avoid hypotension, too. (If we say that enough, we'll be board certified in cardiology before the chapter is over.)

The biggest bugaboo of the above mentioned is tachycardia. Avoid that or, more realistically, treat tachycardia as soon as it appears. What anesthetic you use is much less important than how you monitor and treat the potential ill effects of your anesthetic.

A cardiac patient has a difficult airway. How do you reconcile the horror and pathos of an awake intubation with myocardial protection?

How about an awake intubation as the perfect "cardiac induction"?

WHAT? Stop the presses! Blasphemy! Burn them for witches!

If you spend 5 minutes in a catch-as-catch-can topicalization and proceed to battering ram your way down a struggling patient, then awake intubation is anything but a perfect "cardiac induction."

But, if you explain the procedure to the patient, administer an anti-sialagogue with sufficient time to dry the patient's airway, adequately topicalize, and sedate, then an awake intubation can have the smoothest vital signs you've ever seen.

If, halfway through, the heart rate or blood pressure is going up, do you panic and force the intubation through? No. Stop. Give some esmolol or labetalol. Start nitro. Topicalize some more. As the wicked witch of the west reminds us, "These things must be done delicately, delicately, my pretty."

In the middle of a case, the EKG shows the tombstone sign of ischemia. You are too far along to bail out of the case. What next?

Fix what you can fix, concentrating on the old oxygen supply versus myocardial oxygen demand.

Supply

Keep the blood flowing through the coronaries well oxygenated.

Although this will come later, keep the possibility of postop cath, all the way to emergent coronary angioplasty or bypass, in mind.

Nitrates to, perhaps, dilate the coronaries.

If, by chance, an internal mammary has been placed recently, start diltiazem in case the internal mammary graft is in spasm.

As mentioned earlier, fix the chemistry of the blood. It would be a shame to place someone on an LVAD when they just needed an amp of glucose or a few amps of bicarb.

Demand

Fix those vital signs you can fix.

Tachycardia, the monster for causing ischemia. Of course, treat any *cause* of tachycardia first (pain from light anesthesia, anemia, hypoxemia, hypovolemia, an inotrope running in too fast). Once you've fixed that, get a handle on the volume status. If you're overfilled, you're placing a strain on the patient's heart. If you're underfilled, you won't be able to adequately perfuse. The best initial volume monitor is a Foley. If a Foley's not in already, place one now.

Institute invasive monitoring as needed (falling blood pressure in the face of ischemia mandates vasoactive agents, which means you'd better have at least a CVP. If that doesn't work, then it's Swan time). Then shift into cardiac gear. If they need an epi drip, they need an epi drip.

Of course, the whole time you are informing the surgeon of what is happening and what you are doing. Enlist his/her help if necessary (cut down for a femoral A-line, for example, or placement of a volume line in the field).

A specific for this worst case scenario? Chris's favorite—a bolus of milrinone with institution of a norepinephrine drip to maintain blood pressure is a lifesaver.

At induction, before the case has started, you see signs of unsuspected ischemia. Do you bag the case?

That depends. If your induction was patently moronic and you dropped the pressure to 50 and the ischemia promptly disappeared when blood pressure returned to normal, then you can forge ahead. The ischemia was from anesthetica imperfectans, not from the patient's anatomy.

But if you suspect the patient may have coronary disease (say, a long-standing diabetic who could easily have silent ischemia) and nothing at induction was *so* out of whack, then you have just done the equivalent of a strongly positive stress test. Some might say that this case should wait for another day and this patient needs a cardiac workup pronto. Others would say that as long as the surgery is not particularly stressful in itself, the major stressors are induction and emergence, therefore, they would treat aggressively, monitor the EKG constantly, and proceed. For an elective or slightly urgent case, no one would proceed if the ischemia did not resolve easily.

What special considerations are there for valve problems?

Aortic stenosis—Really, really avoid tachycardia. There is not enough time to squeeze blood through that little orifice. Also, maintain

SVR. A spinal or epidural may plummet the pressure and then you're stuck doing CPR on someone whose cardiac outlet is the size of a pinhole. That's why CPR resuscitation rarely works on the severe aortic stenosis patient.

Mitral stenosis—Same consideration for tachycardia as in aortic stenosis. The heart needs time to fill through a narrow opening. Tachycardia does not allow that time.

Aortic regurg or mitral regurg—If the coronaries are clean, then you want to avoid bradycardia, as this prolongs the time of regurgitation and minimizes forward flow. Odd as it sounds in the cardiac discussion, tachycardia, or at least high-normal heart rate (how's that for a dodge?) is preferable. The patient's baseline is always a good goal to shoot for.

The smartest anesthesiologist is not as smart as the body's compensatory mechanisms.

Intraoperatively, what is the best detector of ischemia?

The EKG as detector of intraop ischemia is imperfect by any measure. The best detector is the TEE. If you see a reversible wall-motion abnormality, you've picked up ischemia. But there are a couple of problems with the all-knowing, all-seeing TEE. Most cases won't have a TEE. If one is in, you need to be trained in its use and need to be looking at nonstop feedback films to pick up that wall motion abnormality. Tough to do in most settings. Studies suggest that on-line (i.e., diagnosis as it occurs) pick-up of ischemia is poor. Another problem is the fact that marked alteration of load conditions (pre and after) can produce wall motion changes that mimic ischemia.

A Swan will pick up early ischemia by increasing PA pressures suggestive of a stiffening ventricle. A pathologic V-wave may also develop on the PCWP trace due to papillary muscle dysfunction with acute mitral regurg. However, these are not necessarily early signs of ischemia. They also assume a PA catheter is in place, and that you are constantly performing wedge measurements. A regional ischemic event may not be picked up by your PA catheter. Multiple studies show that it is extremely difficult to distinguish ischemia from other causes of PA pressure changes (like fluid loading). Construction of a starling curve with a given preload, and with no changes during the surgical course may yield an answer, but again, it is difficult to perform as surgery does not stop for you to obtain various steady-state measurements. Most of the time you will have to *settle* for the EKG. Multiple ST lead analysis (including V5) is most sensitive. The PA catheter may aid you in heightening/lowering your index of suspicion for ischemia, but is not a foolproof measure of early ischemia by itself.

You settle in for a long winter's anesthetic, and what to your wondering eyes should appear? An arrhythmia! On lido! On procaino! On bretylio and cardizo! What the hecko do you do?

THIS IS A FOR SURE QUESTION. FEW GET THROUGH AN ORAL BOARD EXAMINATION WITHOUT SOME RHYTHM DISTURBANCE IN THE INTRAOP PHASE OF THE TEST.

Rhythm disturbance means *find a cause.* Yes, give lidocaine by instinct if it's V-tach, go through the electrical zappage as demanded by the patient's vital signs (synchronous if V-tach has a pressure, asynchronous if it's pulseless V-tach or V-fib. Know your ACLS!). But *find that cause.*

- Artifact? Feel a pulse, look at the other vital signs.
- Interference with the pacemaker by the bovie?
- Hypoxemia? Always, always.
- Hypoglycemia? A diabetic under anesthesia on, say, beta blockers may not reveal signs of hypoglycemia until major wipeout. Do a D-stick.
- Hypokalemia, or, its less thought-about companion, hypomagnesemia?
- Surgical compression? Lung cases, especially, can have iatrogenic rhythm problems from pushing down too hard on the mediastinum.
- Anestheticus imperfecticus? Did you succumb to the devil and give aminophylline for wheezing? Is your Swan pulled back into the right ventricle? (Think of this in real life, especially at the time of transport, when lines get yanked and you're distracted by other things; on the boards, I just don't see them asking this question.) Is your CVP too far *in* and tickling the right ventricle?
- Too many catechols running around—light anesthesia, pheo, your drips, etc.

Think, think, think, like Winnie the Pooh says. Think of a reason for that arrhythmia, be it multifocal PVCs, a run of V-tach, or V-fib. Find that reason and treat that reason. Do the supportive, antiarrhythmic stuff too (lido, procainamide, bretylium, ACLS, whatever it takes), and then go for the underlying reason. Often, something in the stem gives away the expected cause (like the patient was on Lasix or had an NG tube in—think hypokalemia). The board folk do not try to fool you, and they often give you hints. If you are stuck, look at the stem.

A cardiac transplant patient arrives for a nonrelated operation. What special considerations for this case?

- Stress steroid coverage.
- Remember the new heart is denervated, so atropine won't speed up the heart, nor will ephedrine. For BP support you'll need phenylephrine. For heart rate support you'll need either an isoproterenol drip or else you'll need pacing.
- There is some evidence that selective reinnervation can occur, and arrests following reversal with neostigmine have been reported. A mivacurium drip is a great idea in those cases. Don't know the dose? Even on the boards you can say you would look the dose up.

- Not that you usually spit on your needles or anything, but note that you would observe strict aseptic technique during line placement.
- Because of the lack of normal compensatory mechanisms for HR changes in response to BP, some suggest mandatory arterial lines. Some say there is no reason unless other pathology dictates its necessity. Anecdotal experience is that minor cases do not routinely require an art line for safe management.

A patient arrives to your operating room, smiling and jovial—and paced. What precautions do you take intraop?

The primary faux pas in pacerdom is ignorance. You either fail to ask the patient if they have a pacer, or else you fail to notice that lump in their upper chest that says, "PACER!" (This failure to notice a pacer is not an idle concern in a busy OR with fast turnover, where cases get switched around all the time.)

Keep the grounding pad away from the pacer, as the electrical current could screw up the pacer. Pay special attention the first time the bovie fires. In as calm a voice as possible, inform the surgeon that his bovie is causing asystole in the patient and tachycardia in the anesthesiologist.

Pacers are better now than in days of yore and less likely to go awry intraop, but still, anything can happen when electricity starts floating in and around the patient.

Have a magnet in the room. A magnet *should* make the pacer go to VOO at a fixed rate of about 70, though that's not an absolute guarantee. In the best of all possible worlds, you'll even have a pacer doc (electrophysiology jockey) around. No such luck? In the cath lab, there's always someone there who can help you out.

If headaches persist with the bovie, tell the surgeon to just tie everything off, like they used to in the good ol' days (right!). More realistically, suggest a bipolar bovie. The common bipolar bovie has the current go from one part of the bovie to another, rather than from the bovie and out through the patient's grounding pad (unipolar). For this reason, less current in a bipolar runs around the body, and less often causes pacer problems.

Try moving the grounding pad again if you must. If all else fails, just use short bursts. This constant movement of one solution to another is the type of adaptation the board examiners are looking for. And yes, finally, you can insist that the surgeon go back to the dark ages of sutures for hemostasis.

If the patient has an AICD (Automatic Implantable Cardiac Defibrillator), then you really do need a special EP guy (electrophysiology) around to turn the darn thing off. You don't want the AICD firing every time electrical cautery current flows. Keep in mind that turning off an AICD doesn't remove the patient's propensity to life-threatening arrhythmias. Have a Zohl defibrillator hooked to the patient so you can cardiovert or defibrillate the patient intraop. Immediately postop, turn the AICD on again.

A reading note here—Pacer considerations change as newer, more complicated gizmos get placed in people. Read all about it in the ASA Refresher course. That always has the latest.

You must have offended someone in another life, for your stem question concerns a pedie heart. (And yes, the grapevine reports that rare pedie hearts have appeared on the boards.) May the force be with you as you discuss this question. What are your concerns in a pedie heart?

Just so you won't draw a 100% blank, here's some info to help you tread water until (you hope) the examiners move to another topic.

1. Pedie hearts, first and foremost, demand a real, live, honest-to-God pediatric specialist. Not some schmuck who, yeah, every now and then breaths down a 2-year-old for ear tubes.
2. Monitoring is, with the exception of pedie TEE, some of the old-fashioned stuff, like color of the nail beds, palpation for peripheral perfusion. The old reliables like urine output, blood gases, and blood pressure are crucial, because there is no Swan to guide you.
3. An understanding of the anatomy is more important in pedie hearts than in a run-of-the-mill adult heart. Most adult cases are bypasses or valves. Pedie hearts are a dizzying array of flip-flops, transpositions, truncations, inundations, confusionations, and God knows what else. The road map has to be clear and a plan outlined before the case begins.
4. Although considerable discussion goes into "preserving pulmonary resistance with this kind of lesion" and "maintaining systemic perfusion with that kind of lesion," the fact is, most little bitty kiddie hearts are induced by mask so they'll hold still for the (heroically difficult) invasive line placements.
5. Volume and vasoactive infusion rates must be under tight and air bubble–free control. Volume overloads can be catastrophic, as can air in the lines. The air can lead to paradoxical emboli as the bubbles flow through the complex web of the pediatric heart and end up on the left side of the circulation.
6. Hypothermia is highly likely as the child's surface to volume ratio is high. As well, any premie with heart problems has poor fat reserves, and, therefore, has little brown adipose to mobilize for warmth.
7. Retrolental fibroplasia is always a concern. So FIO_2 is reduced. Countering that, though, is the fact that the child's SaO_2 may already be low, due to compromised pulmonary circulation. Some procedures "stage" the reintroduction of said pulmonary flow, so the goal is *not* to get real high SaO_2

out of the case. And all the time, the mantra must be going, "the brain goes soft before the eyes get hard." Sound tough to figure the right course? It is.

The authors re-emphasize that this *review* book is no *textbook*. Never truer than the above, a woefully inadequate, barely introductory glimpse at the distant glimmerings of pediatric cardiac anesthesia. Perhaps the most useful thing you can take away from the discussion is this:

> You may see a pedie heart, so be ready for it. It is, though, thankfully, *very* rare as a stem question. Much more likely, if it were to happen, would be a kid who had tetralogy of Fallot (corrected or uncorrected) appearing for a minor operation like hernia repair.

Take care of the minor things, and that will take care of the big things.

1. Do a good preop, including a consult with the cardiologist. Ask the cardiologist, "Is the lesion fixed? Is there a communication between the right and left sides? Is the child medically optimized for this operation?" All the usual stuff of the preop arena.
2. Warm the room, and warm up to the patient and parent. Keeping the child calm, avoiding crying, screaming, and high oxygen demand, are all to the good.
3. Have phenylephrine drawn up, to treat a Tet spell. (Usually you do not draw up phenylephrine for a pediatric case.)
4. Get all air bubbles out of the IV tubing. A paradoxical air embolus could cause end organ damage anywhere in the arterial tree. An air embolus to the end arteries of the brain could mean catastrophe.
5. Induce in the usual way. Not meaning to sound glib here; the idea is to induce the patient with the tools you use best. If that means preop with midazolam syrup or rectal methohexital or if that means a straight inhalation induction, just do what you do the most. Freaking out and doing something "special" or "different" because this is a "heart patient" will lead you to badness. You'll lose the airway, get hypoxemia, and that is a *for sure no no with any patient let alone a "heart patient."*
6. Get help with the IV. These patients may have had a million cutdowns in their earlier days and may be a tough go in the intravenous access department.
7. Then round up the usual suspects, keeping an eye out for a Tet spell. Treat that with phenylephrine, the increase in systemic

vascular resistance will (you hope) push more blood into the pulmonary circulation and increase oxygenation.

8. Check with the cardiologist whether the patient needs SBE prophylaxis.

Cardiac Postop Question

After an ischemic event in the operating room, with the patient doing fine in the PACU, what do you do?

No one will hassle you now if you ask for the cardiologist. At least you have that going for you. After that, it's the typical stuff for an ischemic event—EKG workup, initial troponins, and go from there. If all is OK, further workup can be referred to a cardiologist.

Recommendations for treatment of ongoing ischemia/MI change all the time. Heparin? Thrombolytic therapy? Go right to cath/PTCA? Wait until an MI plays out and let the patient cool off? Go right to bypass surgery?

Complicating all this is the patient's just-completed surgery. Say your patient just had cerebral aneurysm clipping. Is he a good candidate for thrombolytic therapy? Will you take him to the OR and give him 30,000 units of heparin? Not likely. This is one time when you really punt to the cardiologist.

Cardiac considerations in anesthesia can box you in, can make you as insane as the pilot named Orr in *Catch-22*. There may seem to be no escape for you as you wrestle with the "what ifs" of ischemia, congestive heart failure, and arrhythmias.

By the way, in Joseph Keller's book, did Orr make it?

Yes. He crash-landed his plane in the water off Sweden and paddled to safety.

Orr made it. So can you.

12 | Well, First of All, I'd Trach Him

Board exams from all different specialties have spawned their own legends. This first legend comes to us from radiology.

Radiology conducts their oral board much like we do. Two examiners in a hotel room. A viewing box is in the room for looking at x-rays. The examiners hand over the x-rays, the examinee looks at them, questions are bandied about, and the exam concludes.

One examinee in just such an exam asked to go to the bathroom. Minutes passed, then more minutes. The concerned examiners finally went to the bathroom and knocked on the door.

"Are you OK in there? Time's a-wasting."

"Yeah, I'm just so nervous, I can't come out," comes the plaintive cry from the bathroom.

The examiners looked at each other, then came up with a solution. They slipped the x-rays under the door.

"Hold them up to the light in there and tell us what the diagnosis is."

The nervous examinee took the x-rays, held them up, nailed the diagnoses, and passed the exam.

Anesthesia legends? Here's one that, if it's not true, it should be true.

Everyone sits down at the table, the examinee has the question in front of him. Then, before the examiners can say word one, the examinee says, "Well, before we start, let me say this. I'd trach the guy right away. I figure we're going to get there anyway, might as well go right to it."

No one knows whether that examinee passed or not.

The airway is, of course, our stock-in-trade. Once you have secured the airway, you can hack your way through most circulatory and anesthetic problems. What is the scariest part of any case? What accounts for the lion's share of anesthetic disasters, both medical and medico-legal?

The airway. All else pales in comparison.

So what's the best oral board preparation for this, most germane of questions? And yes, in this world of no guarantees, we can guarantee you that a difficult airway question will appear on your exam.

First, get the ASA algorithm for a difficult airway in your head (see Figure 7-1). Second, listen to the single best *Audio Digest* ever—May 1, 1998, Vol. 40, No. 09 "The Difficult Airway" Part II. In this, Dr. Benumof from UC San Diego goes over the toughest aspect of a bad airway, namely, the options when you're in the "cannot intubate, cannot ventilate" arm of the algorithm. Think about it, what oral board exam is not going to eventually get you to that point?

AIRWAY PREOP QUESTIONS

What in the preop evaluation will tip you off to an impending airway difficulty?

History

1. "Doc, they couldn't intubate me last time." That is a good clue.
2. (Here's another one that happened to Chris) "What's that scar from in your neck?" "Oh, last time I went to sleep they couldn't put that thing in, so they had to cut a hole in here real fast they said." That is also a good clue.
3. A more subtle variant is, "Last time I had a really sore throat for a long time." That may be the generic sore throat that accompanies intubation. But if the patient makes special note of the sore throat, then that may indicate multiple attempts at intubation with a variety of blades, tubes, and practitioners.
4. "You see those chipped teeth, Doc? They weren't chipped before my last operation!" That is called the "dental hint" of difficult intubation.
5. Old anesthetic records—worth their weight in gold. There is nothing so reassuring as seeing an old intubation note. Caveats here:
   - Change in status from previous surgery. The patient may have worsened his airway since the last intubation. Arthritis, for example, can worsen the airway over the years. Obesity can also alter the picture as time passes.

Physical

1. Large incisors, receding chin, short neck, large tongue.
2. Mallampati with his class 1 to class 4 system gives us a good way of communicating from anesthesiologist to anesthesiologist just what you saw. As always, nothing is guaranteed, but a class 4 airway will pose, on average, more difficulty than a class 1.
3. Airway pathology—trauma, Ludwig's angina, radiation, surgical scars, tumors. Of great use in such a case is a talk with the patient's ENT. The ENT may say, "I did indirect laryngoscopy in the office and the nodule is no big deal." Or, the ENT might say, "There is a fungating, friable tumor the size of Kansas right at the base of the patient's tongue."

4. Limited jaw opening or neck extension as with the arthritic patient.

5. Tightly packed fat in the submental area. (This is an observation of Chris's and we haven't seen it written anywhere else.) If, in an obese patient, the submental area is easily wiggleable, then you will be able to lift that area. Intubation shouldn't be difficult. If, in contrast, the submental area is tight—doesn't move around when you try to wiggle it—then it will be hard to lift with the laryngoscope. Hence, intubation will be difficult. Although not really part of the board exam, we thought we would throw in something useful. We apologize for being relevant.

6. Certain specific genetic conditions—Pierre Robin syndrome, any of the mucopolysaccharidoses, Trisomy 21. All of these present airway obstacles due to upper airway anatomy.

Examine the patient from the following point of view—How easy will this patient be to mask ventilate if I can't intubate? Morbidly obese? Hmmm. After a failed intubation the morbidly obese patient will desaturate in no time flat.

Unstable neck? Will you be able to crank the neck back if the mask starts going PPPPPPPFFFFFFFFFFFFTTTTTTTTTTTT! No? Hmm. Remember, the airway exam has to have an element of the crystal ball in it. Look into all the future possibilities, especially your ability to mask the patient if intubation fails.

A final note on the airway exam—you're planning a regional. So the airway is no big deal, right? Oops! The regional didn't work.

Oops! The spinal went too high or the epidural went intravascular.

Oops! The regional didn't last as long as the operation.

Oops! Tourniquet pain has made the procedure unbearable. Now you *must* handle the airway.

So, even if planning a regional, make sure you have done all the necessary fact-finding and planning to handle the airway as an emergency. There are probably more hypothetical high spinal apneas during board exam week than in this country for the last 10 years.

How do you explain an awake intubation to a patient in the holding area?

"For this operation I'll need to put a plastic breathing tube into your windpipe so I can help you breathe while you're asleep. There are a few things about the way your mouth and neck are shaped that make it a little hard to place this tube after you are asleep. So before you go all the way asleep, while you're comfortable and sleepy, I'm going to spray you with some stuff like the dentist uses to make your mouth nice and numb. Then I'm going to use a plastic, bendable special flashlight to look in your mouth and place this tube. It'll be a little unpleasant for a bit, but not too bad, then you'll go all the way asleep."

As with some earlier questions, this one is not complex, controversial, or convoluted. You merely explain in concise fashion a routine procedure in anesthesia. You may choose a less Pollyanna-like explanation to use on the examiners.

AIRWAY INTRAOP QUESTIONS

So, have you trached the patient yet, or what?

Just kidding. No matter the airway case, no matter the airway question, just don't burn bridges. That means an awake intubation if the airway exam looks scary. Another option (let's say it's a child incapable of cooperating with an awake intubation or a mentally impaired adult also incapable of such cooperation) is to keep the patient breathing spontaneously. Sevoflurane, with its nonpungent smell and quick uptake, is great for this approach.

If you get in trouble, at least the patient is still breathing.

Succinylcholine? Sux does burn a bridge, but at least it wears off quickly. (Heaven forbid you should get a rare combination of a difficult airway and a pseudocholinesterase deficiency.) Many argue that you shouldn't use Sux, but in a gray zone, it does get you a good, relaxed view of the airway. Provided you can mask ventilate for just a few minutes, you can get out of trouble quickly.

Long-acting relaxants? If you're thinking difficult airway, not one of the brighter ideas.

You induce a patient, try to intubate, and can't. What is your sequence at this point?

The best answer here is to go through the difficult airway algorithm all the way (see Figure 7-1).

1. Can't intubate, can ventilate.
   - Wake the patient up? This is safe, gets you back to ground 0. Now you can use your fiberoptic expertise.
   - Do the surgery under mask anesthesia or its surrogates (LMA or Combi-tube)? Eeeeeeek! Pretty scary. What if the patient vomits, or if the airway worsens and you get into the "can't intubate, can't ventilate" situation? One possible exception (I said possible) is the stat C-section. No less an authority than Benumof himself says you could proceed with mask ventilation with cricoid pressure. In 3 minutes the baby is out, and masking gets easier. We agree that, in this awful scenario, you could do the case under mask anesthesia. We dropped Benumof's name in case you didn't believe us. This particular airway problem (stat C-section, can't intubate, can ventilate) will always be controversial.

2. Can't intubate, can't ventilate.
   - If you haven't gotten help yet, get on it.
   - Often the very person hard to intubate can take an LMA quite easily. Through this LMA (and its new cousin, the intubating LMA) you can pass a fiberoptic then pass an ETT. Doesn't always work, but a good bailout plan.
   - Cricothyrotomy. The best take home lesson from Benumof's *Audio Digest* lecture is, (paraphrasing here) "Consider the option. The patient will die. So, sticking a 14-g catheter in the trachea, however messy it may seem, is preferable to the patient dying. Don't fret too much where you enter the trachea, though the cricothyroid membrane is the easiest, most accessible spot. Just make sure you're in (e.g., sucking air up through a small amount of liquid in a 3-cc syringe, similar to the PTX maneuver). Insufflating under high pressure with the catheter subq will make bad things worse, wasting precious time, possible anatomic alteration of the neck from subq oxygen, and no oxygen in the blood.
   - Trach. Back to Benumof's words, "Consider the option. The patient will die." Cut, open, shove in a small endotracheal tube. So what it bleeds, so what you nicked this or that? Cut. Cricothyroid too high? Bull. It's easiest there. Some clever ENT surgeon can clean up the mess later. Your job is to get that airway and get that oxygen in. Better yet, anticipate a difficult airway, ask to have an ENT doctor available before you start (or at least a surgeon trained to do a trach on premises).

Not to sound like the pitch man for *Audio Digest*, but I just can't sing the praises of that all-important, all-encompassing difficult airway tape. Want to order it? Call 1-800-423-2308 or order by fax 1-800-845-4375 (No, they're not paying us).

A SLIGHT DEVIATION FROM THE PREOP, INTRAOP, AND POSTOP QUESTIONS.

We have already discussed the gist of the airway questions you're likely to see on the boards—the preop evaluation, the intraop management of failed intubation, plus the "can't intubate, can't ventilate" scenario. Since the airway is so critical, the authors step out of "board preparation" mode and into "real world" mode. The following is advice for your real life airway stuff. Call it the culled wisdom from 10 plus years of airway fretting.

1. Do all you can to make the mask ventilation and preoxygenation easy. Specifically, a little reverse Trendelenburg takes the weight off the diaphragm and makes ventilation easier. That ease of mask ventilation keeps the patient oxygenated just a little bit longer. And that good oxygenation makes the difference between a cool, calm move to plan B and a rushed, panic-stricken move to plan B.

2. Airway looks a little iffy, but you don't want to go gonzo with an awake intubation? Look in your crystal ball. If your first attempt at intubation should fail and you have to wake the patient up, what will obstruct your view through the fiberoptic? Saliva and blood. So do what you can to eliminate saliva and blood. Give a little glycopyrrolate IM and give some neosynephrine nose drops (neo in case you have to go through the nose).

3. It's easier to call *across the room* than *across town* for help. If you are spooked, think you might need help, might need an extra pair of trained hands (for example, one pair of hands holding the mask on, one pair of hands squeezing the bag), then get your help close by before you get into trouble. Have one of your anesthesia partners stick around until you have the airway secured.

4. Think you may really and truly need a trach? Same advice applies. It's easier to call *across the room* for an ENT than *across town* for an ENT. Have an ENT in the room, have the trach set ready, and make sure the trach set has everything in it. (Chris's misadventures again—in one such case, they opened the trach kit and had no blade!)

5. Once badness happens, badness happens fast. If you need special equipment, (fiberoptic, intubating stylet, any of the specialized blades, a Combi-tube, an LMA), make sure it is right there and working. In the middle of a disaster, you don't want to be explaining to the nurse, "Go to the third room down on the left, open the second, no, I mean the third drawer, somewhere in back there is a Bullard scope, do you know what it looks like?" On the boards, luckily, you can assume everything you will ever need is right nearby.

6. No, there is no such thing as a difficult extubation, but there sure as hell is such a thing as an *inappropriate* extubation, with subsequent and catastrophic attempts at reintubation. The difficult intubation is sure to be difficult to reintubate, so assess the timing of extubation carefully. Midnight? No one around? I don't theenk so, Bubba Looie. No specialized equipment on hand? Again, not a good idea. The extubation has to be done with all the care and preparation as the intubation. That may mean passing a tube changer or fiberoptic scope

down the endotracheal tube before pulling it out, so that you have a bridge to reintubation already there. Also, in the case of a traumatic airway, remember to suction, deflate the cuff, and make sure the patient can breathe around the tube (finger over the hole, steth on the trachea to assess).

7. There are a thousand excuses during residency for not getting facile with the fiberoptic. "My attendings didn't use it much." "I did it a few times, usually the pulmonary guys would do it." WAKE UP AND SMELL THE SEVOFLURANE! Get good at fiberoptic intubation! If there is anything you need to be able to do, it's handle a difficult airway, and in this day and age, that means getting good at the fiberoptic. Make it your business to perform a lot of fiberoptic intubations. Use it on easy patients, once they're induced. Get used to the normal look of things so when you *have* to use it, when the airway's bloody, or distorted, or clogged with tumor, you will be able to navigate that airway.

8. Awake trach? An option not lightly undertaken. But if the upper airway pathology is bad (a fungating tumor on the epiglottis) then you are best served by securing the airway by awake trach right from the start.

COMBINATION PLATES

Shakespeare wrote, "When troubles come, they come not as single spies but in battalions." So it is with the difficult airway. Bad enough the airway is hard to secure, but what of other diseases that impact on your ability to secure the airway?

1. Asthma and difficult airway.

The last thing you want to do with an asthmatic is place an endotracheal tube in them awake.

The best thing for a difficult airway is to place an endotracheal tube in them awake. So, in an asthmatic with a difficult airway you should…uh…you should…uh um uh…. Herein lies the dilemma. Best approach here is to optimize the asthmatic patient medically, which may mean some blasts of aerosol beta agent right there in the holding area. Steroids, ideally a few hours before the operation so they will have "kicked in." Airway trumps reactive airway, so the best thing is to proceed with the awake intubation, but *take your time*. This is no time to rush the topicalization. Sooner or later, the patient will cough as they get lidocaine into the trachea (transtracheal, nebulized, through the fiberoptic, however) and that may stir up a reaction but, with luck, that same coughing will spread the lidocaine around and prepare them for the real aggravating stimulus, the endotracheal tube. Nebulized lidocaine, delivered just as a breathing treatment, lays down a fine mist of topical in their airway, and is the least "reactivating" way to topicalize an asthmatics airway.

Alternative plan? Breathe the patient down with non-aggravating sevoflurane. Place the fiberoptic in the still-breathing patient and secure the airway that way. That, of course, runs the risk of airway loss through obstruction as the patient loses consciousness. One nice advantage of sevoflurane in this instance is that its level falls quickly once it stops being inhaled, so the patient should wake up quickly if the airway obstructs, regain consciousness, and regain airway patency. But no plan is free of risk when you have two conflicting needs such as asthma plus a difficult airway. And things don't always work the way you expect them to on the boards.

2. Heart disease and difficult airway.

As detailed in the earlier chapter, the hyperdynamic response to an awake intubation is avoidable. Topicalize, topicalize. Sedate, sedate. Leave an out in case you oversedate (romazicon, narcan). You can't reverse propofol and you can't reverse droperidol, so don't use those in your sedation regimen.

The main point is, don't rush it. Treat hypertension or tachycardia right away, don't just buffalo past it during the intubation. Have vasoactive drugs ready to go (esmolol, 20-mcg boluses of nipride or nitro).

3. Open eye or increased intracranial pressure and difficult airway.

Coughing and struggling worsen intracranial pressure. Coughing and straining can also harm the open eye. So a savage awake intubation could hurt patients with either of these conditions.

Then again, if you induce anesthesia, lose the airway, and cause a hypoxemic insult, you have exacerbated the problem in the patient with increased intracranial or intra-ocular pressure.

For the open eye, topicalize, take a quick awake look, and if it looks bad, proceed with the awake intubation. Or do the long, time consuming topicalization noted under heart problems.

For the increased ICP dilemma, consider a recommendation that comes from the Maryland shock/trauma people. Big time bucking and coughing really could cause herniation and kill these neuro patients, so the shock/trauma people do the following. Prepare for a trach (they do so many of these that they have surgeons right there who can open the neck in a hurry—you may not). They do a modified rapid sequence with (gulp!) a nondepolarizing muscle relaxant, then if they can't intubate right away, they go right to trach.

This is definitely a toughie. Talk it over and come up with your own best management. Just don't think of it for the first time *during your oral board exam*. You want to go in there having *already thought it through*. When these issues present on the boards, the key is to show your knowledge of the potential problems, your ability to prioritize, and your ability to develop a plan. It is *not* to come up with a perfect plan. It does not exist.

There you have it. The difficult airway, in all its glottic glory.

Now, go forth into the exam and create your own legend.

Hatchets in the Head and Other Mishaps

The following is a little heartwarming anecdote to emphasize an important point about trauma.

"Holy s—! She's got a hatchet in her head!" goes the cry in the emergency room. Gawkers that we are, a dozen doctors, nurses, and technicians rush into the big trauma room of the ER to see the latest mayhem from the streets. The handle of the offending hatchet sticks way out and presents some practical problems.

How to secure the airway with a hatchet handle pointing right at you? Will the CT scanner admit such a large, bulky object? CT scanners were not designed with hatchets in mind. Do we "wiggle" the hatchet out first? Risk hemorrhage in an uncontrolled setting? Saw the hatchet handle off first? Hmmmm. Many heads were scratched as we pondered the problem of "Our Lady of the Hatchet."

The issue takes a turn for the worse when the patient codes, dies, and is transferred to the refrigerated surgical suite downstairs.

Diagnosis from our friends the pathologists? Cardiac tamponade from the knife wound hidden under the patient's left breast.

Everyone was so mesmerized by the (admittedly impressive) hatchet in the head that we forgot the prime directive with trauma.

Trauma means *associated injuries*.

Anyone who would plant a hatchet in someone's head might visit some other less striking, but more deadly, injuries on their victim.

Remember that if your exam question involves a trauma victim. Remember *associated injuries*. Yes, of course, ABC first. But if the question involves an injury, remember to look for other injuries too. This *Hunt for Other Injuries* occurs in the preop arena.

TRAUMA PREOP QUESTIONS

Into the ER comes a trauma victim and you are called to evaluate. In systematic fashion, how do you help your ER colleagues?

In any trauma, once ABC has been addressed and with due respect to the C-spine, get a look all over the patient. Gunshots in the head can (and have) been missed under a tangle of hair.

"I thought the blood was coming from his bleeding shoulder!"

We're not talking the world's most thorough physical exam; we're talking *lay eyes on all aspects of the patient.* Bullet wounds, stab wounds, electrical injury exit sites, can all hide under crumpled clothes, in pools of blood, and in the general chaos of trauma.

But you are just the anesthesiologist, not the ER Doc? No excuse—real life or boards. If that patient goes to the OR, you're going to pay if there is some hidden trauma that suddenly gets "uncovered" intraop.

What special considerations accompany head trauma?

Head trauma means neck trauma until proven otherwise. Falls from trees, deceleration injuries, missiles to the head—all can snap the neck. Clear that C-spine before you manipulate the airway. On a converse note, knee to the dash, head to the windshield is a common MVA scenario on the boards. But they only tell you initially about the femoral fracture.

Clearing the C-spine has been described as a "pain in the neck." What are the issues with potential C-spine injuries?

Clearing the C-spine is easier said than done. In real life and on the board exam, you rarely get a good view of all seven vertebrae. And 20% of C-spine problems are down low, in the hard-to-see C6-C7 area. Topping that off is another problem—neck injuries that don't appear on C-spine films. Ligamentous torsion can occur. The spinal cord itself is injured or its blood supply is jerked loose, and there is neural injury in spite of a "normal" x-ray. Diagnosis of such a "normal C-spine but injured spinal cord" can only be made on clinical grounds. Surprise, surprise, such a patient is often unconscious or else cannot cooperate due to injuries, drugs, or alcohol. This explains the maddening stance of your friendly surgical colleague. You say, "Is the C-spine cleared?" He replies, "Yes." "Can I take the collar off?" "No. Well OK, for intubation, I guess you can if we hold in-line traction." "But that's what we would do if it wasn't cleared!" Right. The x-ray really just gives you some indication of whether you can actually do some neck extension if you cannot intubate or ventilate.

The C-collared, uncooperative, C-spine patient is just the one who is desaturating in the ER. Blood, emesis, broken teeth, and the frenetic atmosphere of the ER all add to the joys of this clinical scene. Then, add associated injury physiology.

"He may have blood in his skull, too. Increased intracranial pressure. Just the person who cannot tolerate hypoxemia and hypercarbia."

That C-spine gets you up to your ass in alligators, and they're all snappin'.

Best approach? Keep the neck aligned, avoid extension (again, easier said than done) and have plan B ready to go. Yes, that means have that trach kit ready, a surgeon ready to open that neck.

Worried that you might be *overreacting* by saying, "Cut that neck. I don't want to extend this person's neck and risk a C-spine injury"?

Consider the alternative, you crank back on the neck and make the person quadriplegic. Quadriplegia is better than a possibly unnecessary tracheostomy? I don't think so.

On the boards, they expect you to act, and to understand the consequences of your action. Yes trachs have all sorts of problems—bleeding, infection, subsequent scarring with stenosis—but in a "back to the wall" trauma, with intracranial, spinal cord, and patient survival at stake, a trach may be the only alternative. Showing consummate skill as an examinee, you could say, "while concerned about the potential complications of trach such as bleeding and infection and possible future stenosis, my priority here is securing an airway without causing iatrogenic injury to the spine."

Damn, you sound good!

Prior to the tumultuous cavalcade to the OR for abdominal exploration, a trauma victim displays a disquieting tendency towards the hypotensive. Enlighten us as to possible causes.

Trauma means associated injuries. Trauma means associated injuries. Trauma means associated injuries.

Hypotension in the trauma victim. Think fast, there's a lot of reasons for it, and they can all kill the patient before you get through the differential diagnosis. The primer under vital signs says it all.

1. Preload (absolute loss of preload from hemorrhage, the most common cause of hypotension; relative loss of preload due to pneuomothorax, tamponade, or fat embolus). It's worth remembering that any sick trauma patient will be on positive pressure ventilation. That positive pressure will convert a pneumothorax into a tension pneumothorax right quick (that equals relative loss of preload from obstruction of return).
2. Contractility (hypoxemia, myocardial contusion, myocardial ischemia from coincident myocardial infarct).
3. Afterload (sepsis from opened bowel in the abdomen, this is less likely to develop, of course, in the acute setting).
4. Rate (brady or tachy in the face of stenotic heart lesions).
5. Rhythm (non-sinus).

Blood loss as cause of hypotension is most likely and should be stated as such. Yes, oh, yes. Remember the *associated injuries* mantra. Splenic rupture, bleeding from the long bones or the pelvis, tear of the aorta. An injury in one place can mean an injury in another place.

Congratulations, you've survived the trip upstairs in the elevator and have plunked into the operating room.

TRAUMA INTRAOP QUESTIONS

As the surgeons start slashing from stem to sternum, you notice the

Boop
Boop

Boop

Boop

of the pulse oximeter. In this trauma setting, how do you diagnose and treat this spooky trend?

Obviously, it can be from any of many causes, and the differential is listed in Chapter 7, hypoxemia. What's most likely? If it is not positive pressure induced tension pneumothorax, then second on the list would be…

Trauma often means loss of consciousness and that means aspiration risk. In an oral board setting, you could see this sequence—in comes the trauma victim, uneventful intubation, intraop or postop hypoxemia.

What's the gig? Think aspiration. You don't have to see aspiration happen at intubation; aspiration may have happened before, out in the field, at the site of the accident, and is just being manifested now.

Treatment? What you always do. Make sure the ETT is positioned correctly, not in a mainstem bronchus.

1. Suction—suction with the fiberoptic, if necessary, irrigating with saline if you really need to clean them out
2. High inspired FIO_2
3. PEEP

Supportive therapy in short. Major, major aspiration? May need rigid bronchoscopy to clear particulate matter. Endotracheal tube completely occluded by aspirate and unable to ventilate? Replace the endotracheal tube, you have no choice. Even if that means pulling out and masking for a while. This of course would be rare.

You are treating an isolated head injury patient and hypotension develops. What do you do, Sherlock?

Trauma means associated injuries. Trauma means associated injuries. Trauma means associated injuries.

Before you start the hunt for associated injuries, make sure you're not doing obvious dumb anesthesia things. Agent up too high. You just gave too much propofol. You had a rough time putting in the CVP (and caused a pneumo). Do the routine "fix hypotension" things first; then start looking for other causes using preload, contractility, afterload, rate, and rhythm.

A head injury by itself is unlikely to cause enough blood loss to account for hypotension. That "isolated" injury might not be as isolated as you think. Go over the entire patient again. Pneumothorax, bleeding in the chest, the abdomen, the pelvis, the thigh. Still nothing? Go over it again. You just might be missing something.

TRAUMA POSTOP QUESTION

In the PACU, a patient with long bone fractures galore develops respiratory distress. What specific to this case may be going on?

Fat emboli. Treatment is supportive—intubation, PEEP, and circulatory support.

Days after a thrash of a trauma case, a nurse calls from the ICU. "The patient says he remembers the whole operation." What do you explain to the patient?

Intraop recall is a possibility in any anesthetic. Risk of recall is higher in a trauma case with an unstable patient. Precious little anesthetic can you give in such a case. As the patient hangs onto their last shred of sympathetic tone, any anesthetic—inhaled, intravenous—can put them over the edge.

So, what are your approaches to preventing recall in such cases? And if recall occurs, how will you explain it to your patient?

"Faking it" with a little scopolamine is no guarantee of an erased memory. For that reason, one of the best things you can do in such an operation is talk to the patient, reassuring them that everything is being done to help them. If they have recall, they will also recall that reassuring voice of yours. And of course, make sure that all conversation in the OR is professional. In this as in every case, assume the patient will hear everything said during the operation.

Psychologically, patients with recall seem to have the most trouble when their concerns are dismissed. "That's crazy, you didn't hear them talking!"

The best approach is a straightforward discussion of what happened and why. And validate their concerns. "Yes, you were so sick that we had to concentrate all our energies on saving your life, and we couldn't give any sleeping medicines for fear it would drop your blood pressure lower. You did hear the doctors, nurses, and technicians who were working to save your life."

Remember that trauma means associated injuries and the board examiners won't do a hatchet job on you.

I'm a Brain Surgeon

Imagine this scene, which actually played out in an Atlanta bar in the early 1980s.

The Time

Atlanta is booming. Money from looted S&Ls is flowing like water in the financial community. (That bill won't come due until the 1990s.) Everywhere, young, newly rich MBA guys are making the fern bar scene, hitting up on secretaries, paralegals, anything that moves. In the power/sex/cool guy world, the big thing is impress the women with your dizzying credentials. They'll love you.

The Setting

One of Emory's neurosurgeons, a young woman recently divorced and thrown into the singles quagmire, goes to one of Atlanta's night spots. She is "spotted" by one of the MBA macho men. He approaches her, puts on his smarmiest lounge lizard grin, and says, "Say, I'm a lonely fella with a BMW parked outside and an MBA from Harvard hanging on my wall at home. What do you do, honey?"

The Greatest Line Ever Said in All of History

Without batting an eye, she said, "I'm a brain surgeon."

Any specialty that could spawn such understated genius merits a few anesthetic considerations.

NEUROANESTHESIA PREOP QUESTIONS

You are in the holding area, about to start a cerebral aneurysm clipping. As you are starting your right IJ Swan, a colleague comes by, gestures you aside, and hisses, "You'll cut off drainage from the brain by putting that big old sheath in there." How do you respond?

Venous drainage is one aspect of keeping the brain from swelling during an intracranial case. But one sheath in one IJ will not cause the supratentorial equivalent of superior vena cava syndrome. There is still plenty of drainage on the other side of the neck.

Of more importance is the need for adequate line access before the case starts. Once the patient is in pins and is in some weird position, draped all over the place, you will not have easy access to placing additional lines if you need them. Ask yourself, "If the aneurysm bursts, will I have adequate access to save this patient?"

Peripheral access has the distinct disadvantage that the IV may infiltrate without your noticing. You'll also need a guide for intravascular volume assessment since you'll be giving diuretics and mannitol and you cannot count on the urine output to give you information on filling pressure.

Long arm CVP? The long, narrow path makes for slow flow and it is not appropriate for a volume line. Because of the long distance, it is not that great for vasoactive infusions (long dead space and long time to realize changes in infusion rates). However, combined with large bore peripheral access, a long arm CVP is a reasonable suggestion.

A diabetic patient about to undergo a long spinal cord instrumentation asks if he'll need blood. He would prefer not to receive any. He will be in the prone position for 8 hours, at least.

A real concern in a long prone case is optic nerve ischemia. In the diabetic, already prone to ischemia in many organ systems, optic nerve injury is a real possibility. Even with adequate padding and no pressure on the eyeballs, the patient may still emerge from anesthesia blind. The best management, though by no means guaranteed, is to keep the pressure up and the hematocrit above 30 for the entire case. This is not the case to use controlled hypotension to control bleeding.

This patient will need blood.

The surgeon may squawk a little, as he will want that hypotension if he is laying open a lot of bone. But the needs of the eye, in this case, outweigh the desire to minimize blood loss.

NEUROANESTHESIA INTRAOP QUESTIONS

Halfway into a neuro case the surgeon says, "The brain is tight." Discuss the options for improving the surgical field.

Multiple factors affect brain size and anesthetic technique can affect all of them.

Hypoxemia. Before any erudite discussion of CO_2 response curves, inhaled versus intravenous agents, barbiturate comas, and the relative merits of mannitol, let us not forget the basics. Keep that patient oxygenated! Hypoxemia increases cerebral blood flow (until the patient expires, then the cerebral blood flow drops precipitously and the entire issue becomes moot). Plus, hypoxemia will worsen any injury to brain or spinal cord cells. This is not good! We have it on highest authority. Before you go to any more exotic methods of brain shrinkage, make sure you're getting good air into that neuro patient. Check the pulse ox.

Hypercarbia. Here is where knowledge from the written boards has most overlap with the oral boards. You don't have to know the exact numbers, but you must know the detrimental effects of hypercarbia (increased cerebral blood flow) and beneficial effects of hypocarbia (decreased cerebral blood flow). Hence, once the airway is secured, hyperventilation is the thing to do in the brain-injured patient.

One warning. Don't initiate hyperventilation until the dura is opened in another kind of neurosurgical patient—the aneurysm clipping. Hyperventilation in such a patient may alter the shear forces on the aneurysm. A marked decrease in interstitial brain pressure may actually increase the transmural pressure across that thin walled aneurysm causing it to burst. This, also, is not good.

Mannitol and/or diuretics. Get the fluid off, "dry out" the brain. Does it really and truly work? For the boards, assume so. But...do you often (we're talking in the real world here) dry out the patient, watch the pressure drop, then end up tanking them up again, all the time wondering to yourself, "Am I just fooling myself?" Mannitol requires an intact blood-brain barrier to "draw off" fluid from the brain. But most injured brains *lack an intact blood-brain barrier.* Hmm. OK, there are some holes in neuroanesthesia thinking, but recite the litany at board time.

Head position. No doubt on this one. Elevate the head, and make sure the neck is not cranked around such that the venous outflow is impeded.

Potent inhaled agents. Cerebral vasodilators. Keep them below ½ MAC and use IV agents. Recall the brain itself has no pain receptors, so once through the scalp, periosteum, and dura, it's not that painful of a case.

Bucking and straining mid-case will swell the brain, anger the surgeon, and embarrass you. Keep the patient anesthetized, of course, but this is one case where keeping them paralyzed is critical too. So keep them relaxed. Watch that twitch monitor!

Wake-up at the end. Although impossible sometimes (e.g., severe cranial injury requiring long-term ventilatory support), a quick wake-up and exam is a real plus at the end of a neuro case. For example, the patient may awaken and be unable to move an entire side, indicating that the wrong vessel was clipped during an aneurysm operation. Get the vapors off early, then run on a propofol drip for the last half hour or so. That is one of many methods to getting a quick wake-up at the end. Remifentanil, sevoflurane, BIS monitoring, can all be employed in pursuit of this worthwhile goal. Think to yourself now—what do I do to ensure a timely wake-up after a long surgery and why do I do it that way. Any reasonable answer is a good answer.

During a sitting craniotomy, the vital signs take a turn for the nonvital. What specific to this case is happening and what do you do about it, oh sagacious one?

Anytime the operative field is above the heart, air can entrain into the circulation and cause an "airlock" with sudden, catastrophic hemodynamic collapse. Neuro cases, especially, say a craniotomy with the head up or a sitting cervical laminectomy, are setups for venous air embolisms.

Diagnosis. Best made by precordial Doppler. You hear a rushing sound, like being a spectator as Ichabod Crane rides by. Major league spooky. End tidal nitrogen appears (air bubbles communicate with alveoli, pushing some nitrogen into the alveoli, which are then breathed out) and end-tidal CO_2 drops (blood to the lungs is blocked off by the air bubble, reduced blood flow to lungs, reduced CO_2 getting out of the lungs).

Treatment. Tell the surgeon to flood the field, aspirate air from your central line, if you weren't on 100% O_2, get on it pronto (nitrous would expand the air bubble) then hope you can provide sufficient supportive therapy so that the patient makes it. Get them into "CPR position" (no mean feat when they're in pins and in a weird position) *OR* put the patient in the left lateral position to get the airlock out of the way of the pulmonary outflow track? Well, yes, in theory, but if things are that bad, you probably want them on their backs for CPR anyway. Mechanical compression of CPR may have an additional benefit. The physical force of the compression may break up the airlock and save the day.

A surgeon requests that his carotid endarterectomy be done under local. What do you see as the advantages and disadvantages of such an anesthetic?

A carotid under local or regional block—when it is good, it is very, very good.

1. No blood pressure plummet with induction.
2. No blood pressure skyrocket with intubation.
3. You have the best cerebral perfusion monitor—patient cooperation with talking or squeezing a squeak toy. (I love that squeak toy. In this day and age of gazillion gigabyte computers, we still make a toy go "squeak" to know what's going on in the brain.)
4. At the end of the case, there is no dilemma of "I want to make sure the patient is awake before I extubate, but I don't want the patient bucking on the tube or getting hypertensive as they emerge and causing a big hematoma at the surgical site."

Only problem with a carotid under local or a regional block, when it is bad, it is very, very bad.

1. Hard to get at the airway, with the head turned, drapes up, and neck open.
2. If the carotid cross clamp goes on and ischemia occurs, the patient may suddenly become uncooperative or confused. You now have to induce general anesthesia under difficult conditions.

Which method of anesthesia do you choose? Dealer's choice. As with so many other "there is no absolute right method" situations, you will have to defend your choice rationally.

NEUROANESTHESIA POSTOP QUESTION

After a big kahuna intracranial case, the patient is slow to emerge. How do you evaluate this?

The neurosurgeon's request for a "quick wake-up" is appropriate. The neuro exam tells legions, and a failure to emerge quickly may mean a rebleed, increased intracranial pressure, and the need to reoperate.

Surrendering the secured airway in a critically ill patient represents any anesthesiologist's worst nightmare.

So the surgeon's need clashes with the anesthesiologist's tendency to cling to the endotracheal tube. The best approach is logical, stepwise, and deliberate. Tailor the anesthetic to a quick wake-up, using, for example, a propofol drip (or a little remifentanil) toward the end of the case. Get the patient back breathing on his/her own, and consider lidocaine IV right towards extubation time or maintain very low dose remifentanil to keep the patient from waking up thrashing.

If the vapors are off, the CO_2 has returned to normal, the narcotics and muscle relaxants have worn off, the temperature is normal, and metabolic things are in order (make sure the glucose is OK; it's easy to fix but disastrous if allowed to go too low), then there should be no "anesthesia reason" for slow emergence. At that point, keep the airway secure, go on the assumption of rebleed, and hyperventilate, assuming increased intracranial pressure. CT to look for a bleed. This is the most conservative approach, but the most logical and safe approach.

CHAPTER

15 | The Wheel of Diuresis

Yes, the following actually happened at a prestigious institution that shall remain nameless. The Red Sox play there, and there was a famous Tea Party there, and baked beans are a popular food item there, but that famous institution will forever remain anonymous.

Phone calls from the ICU were deluging a certain resident of the anesthetic persuasion. Most of the calls were the old standby, "Mr. Smith's urine output has dropped off."

What innovative response does the resident come up with? Rather than analyze each individual case of low urine output, the resident invented the "Wheel of Diuresis." When someone's urine output fell, the resident would tell the ICU staff to "spin the wheel." Whatever the arrow landed on, the staff would do. They kept this up until the patient's urine output picked up. Amazingly, the "Wheel of Diuresis" usually worked! Here's what the "Wheel of Diuresis" looked like.

Lasix

Mannitol   Dopamine

Fluid Challenge

In the center of these was an arrow set on a spinner.

The genius of it.

Are we suggesting you pull the "Wheel of Diuresis" out when the board examiners ask you the (guaranteed) low urine output question?

YES! Do it! Come on, you only live once, this is the stuff of myths! You will be an immortal in the board's eyes forever! Granted, you will flunk, but hey, you get a couple more tries. Be a sport!

Unconvinced? All right. Here's the straight answer. (But I still think it would be so cool if someone spun that damned wheel.)

We'll skip the preop, intraop, postop format for the oliguria question. The question is always framed the same, is usually asked as a postop question, and always boils down to, "After her hysterectomy, Mrs. Jones' urine output falls below 10 cc/hr. What do you do?"

Decreased urine output classically falls into one of three categories, pre-renal (hypovolemia or decreased cardiac output), renal (acute tubular necrosis or anything else that has damaged the kidneys themselves), and post-renal (any block in the flow of formed urine, from the ureters to the bladder to the bladder outlet to the Foley to the OR tech standing on the Foley).

Post-renal is the easiest to peg. From a practical standpoint, unless the ureter has been operated on, this means trouble shooting the Foley. Is it kinked? Is there a clot? Was it placed correctly in the first place? Does it need to be irrigated? God forbid, has bladder rupture happened? In a freshly operated on urinary system (a renal transplant, for example) could the ureter be kinked inside the abdomen? It's important to make sure the flow of urine goes uninterrupted before you go to measures designed to increase urine production. A kinked or misplaced Foley, followed by a tremendous urine production from your well-meaning Lasix and dopamine, can spell catastrophe.

Next easiest to assess is pre-renal oliguria. Assess fluids in and fluids out. If need be, place invasive lines. Dry is easy to fix—give fluids. A few special cases merit attention. Burn patients can have astounding fluid requirements. Patients with liver failure may require higher than "normal" cardiac outputs to perfuse their kidneys. For example, a cirrhotic patient may normally have a cardiac output of 10. When his output falls to 5 (still "normal") that may be insufficient cardiac output for him. So inotropic support is necessary to perfuse his kidneys even though it doesn't seem necessary.

Another point to remember in fluid replacement is a consideration of the hematocrit. If you have a borderline hematocrit and the urine output is tailing off, that is a valid reason for transfusing. Further crystalloid or colloid will just drive the hematocrit lower. A low oxygen delivery may cause adrenergic output leading to renal vasoconstriction.

A final note on pre-renal oliguria. If you're worried about overdoing it, putting the patient into pulmonary edema, remember the old adage, "Pulmonary edema you treat with an endotracheal tube and Lasix, renal failure you treat with dialysis." (This glib, yet snappy approach might not fly with board examiners.) In the exam, you might say something like, "While understanding the consequences of overaggressive fluid replacement, the danger of ATN due to kidney underperfusion is my primary concern here."

THEN SPIN THE WHEEL OF OLIGURIA!

Sorry, we just couldn't help ourselves.

Renal oliguria. This is a diagnosis of exclusion, after you've done what you can to assure post-and pre-renal causes have been fixed. Certain special cases:

- Crush injuries. Myoglobin can gum up the works, keep up a brisk diuresis to flush out the evil humors.
- Nephrotoxic drugs. Especially in an ICU where patients can be on a million drugs, don't overlook potentially nephrotoxic medications, such as gentamicin. Most hospitals have clever

pharmacology Ph.D.s to keep track of the peaks and troughs and dosing regimens of those nasty drugs.

The oliguria algorithm follows a standard if-then line of reasoning. (Looking eerily not unlike that Wheel of Diuresis.)

MANAGING OLIGURIA, ONCE YOU'VE MADE SURE THE FOLEY IS OK

- Oliguria? Try a fluid challenge. Make sure fixable stuff is fixed (hematocrit, for example).
- No luck? If further fluids are possibly hazardous (overload, CHF), get invasive.
- Filled to the gills and still no luck? Try dopamine or try to increase cardiac output.
- Still no luck? Try Lasix to convert oliguric to nonoliguric renal failure. Why? It's easier to manage.
- Yipes! Still hurting? If all your efforts can't make it happen, you may have to dialyze for a while and hope against hope that the kidneys come back to life.

True renal experts will pop a gasket at that microexplanation of oliguria management, but that is a practical approach to handling low urine output in the perioperative arena. If you really want to see a graphic illustration of this algorithm, you'll have to find the first edition of *Board Stiff*.

MYTHS YOU MAY OR MAY NOT WANT TO MENTION

The boards are not the time to mention the great clinical debates of our era, but for completeness, we have to mention some aspects of oliguria.

Has giving mannitol, even in the "pre-clamp" time before an aneurysm resection, ever been shown to do anything? No.

Has giving Lasix ever been shown to make a difference in renal outcome? No.

Has the sacred cow of all sacred cows, renal dose dopamine, ever been shown to make doodly difference? No.

Is appropriate volume resuscitation the only thing with any semblance of a track record? Yes.

In conclusion, there is more myth than meat in our complicated oliguria algorithms. Do we ourselves follow the algorithms, knowing they're mostly anecdotal? Yes. That is our current best standard of care, no matter what the thin threads of reasoning are that bind them together. And on the boards, you explain the current standard of care.

So there.

PATIENT ON DIALYSIS?

Make sure that they are dialyzed within 24 hours of an elective operation. Keep in mind that dialysis and renal failure imply poor platelet function. What is the K post-dialysis? If it is higher than 5.5, you could make an argument for postponing the case. Also, if the K is that high, you may want to avoid the use of Sux, with its attendant slight rise in potassium (0.5 to 1 mEq/L). That's the conservative approach. However, the acuity of the rise in K levels determines the relative membrane irritability, and attendant risks of problems (like widened QRS, peaked Ts, etc.). So that slight rise in K level may not make a difference.

In case of doubt, use the EKG. If there are no peaked Ts and there is no widened QRS complex, then (of course with careful attention to the EKG) with some concern, consider proceeding if there is any urgency at all.

RENAL TRANSPLANT CONSIDERATIONS

Central monitoring is important, because you don't want to underhydrate the new kidney. Establishing a brisk diuresis early is important to preserving the donated kidney.

Know the kidney. Like the difficult airway question, the oliguria question is a for sure question you will face. And if you're bold, do the thing with the "Wheel of Diuresis." We'll buy you dinner if you do it! We won't, however, pay for your inevitable return trip to the boards.

16 | I Don't Know Nuthin' 'Bout Birthin' No Babies Miz Scarlett!

"Yea, I have heard the voice of woman in travail." —*The Bible*

Examiners expect, rightfully so, for you to know the physiological changes of pregnancy. There are a million. Concentrate on the changes that impact on our anesthetic. Know the time course for these changes as well—like when it is normal for a patient to get her dilutional anemia. Shnider and Levinson's book on obstetric anesthesia is our favorite. At risk of sounding repetitive, remember that our review of this and all other topics is *brief* and does not constitute a *comprehensive* look at the subject.

The physiologic changes of pregnancy fall into the preop area of questioning.

OBSTETRIC PREOP QUESTIONS

A 25-year-old multipara is admitted to your hospital for delivery of her third child. What are the physiologic changes of pregnancy that will affect your anesthetic?

Cardiovascular:
1. Increased intravascular volume.
2. Increased cardiac output.
3. 1 and 2 combine to throw pregnant patients with valvular disease into failure. (Mitral stenosis is the classic example.)
4. Dilutional "anemia" (fluid volume expands more than red cell mass).
5. Supine hypotension from the gravid uterus compressing the vena cava and decreasing venous return. (A classic trap would be to get you talking about something else, not mention that the patient is lying flat on her back, then fetal heart

rate drops. Unless you have the supine hypotension idea floating in your head, you may go through all sorts of crazy machinations, including a C-section, without doing the obvious—left uterine displacement to relieve the venous obstruction. If you have an OB question, be sure to write LUD in big capital letters across the top of your exam.

Pulmonary:
1. Increased minute ventilation and oxygen consumption.
2. Decreased FRC and residual volume.
3. Swollen upper airway (dilated capillaries/veins) with a tendency to bleed if massacred in an intubation attempt.
4. 1, 2, and 3 combine to make the airway the number 1 headache for the anesthesiologist, in which case a general anesthetic is needed. Failed or refused regional technique, toxic reaction to local anesthetic, stat C-section. (Some controversy here—is there time for a regional when the fetal heart rate is "nonreassuring" in the worst way? Most suggest not.)

Gastrointestinal:
1. Decreased gastric emptying.
2. Increased gastric volume and pressure.
3. Gastroesophageal junction is looser, more prone to reflux (progesterone effect).
4. All the above combine to make a pregnant patient a "full stomach" after the first trimester.
5. All of the above make you as nervous as a long-tailed cat in a room full of rocking chairs if you have to mask, or Combitube, or LMA a stat C-section you can't intubate.

Neurologic:
1. Engorgement of the epidural vessels.
2. Decreased local anesthetic needed for spinal or epidural as compared to nonpregnant patients (about 1 cc per dermatomal level versus normal 1.5 cc).
3. Local anesthetic mishap, such as a high spinal or intravascular injection, tosses you into the teeth of all the above problems—full stomach, rapid desaturation, possible difficult airway, supine hypotension syndrome if you have to quickly get the patient on her back to be intubated. And all this can be happening in the worst place, the patient's room with the shocked and amazed family looking on! Or, on the board exam.

Understand the physiology, know all the changes and how they impact what we do. The examiner will be able to come up with some question, some twist that all the review books in the world will miss. But if you understand the physiology, you will be able to apply that knowledge to figure out the examiner's question and answer like the consultant you are.

An 18-year-old is admitted with a 31-week pregnancy and a diagnosis of preeclampsia. What are the implications of preeclampsia?

Study the preeclamptic inside and out. A complete knowledge of all the changes of preeclampsia assures that you know the toughest of the tough questions pertaining to pregnancy.

First, the pathology, then, an approach to the tough aspects of their management. Here again, let us make a plug for Audio Digest. About every fourth or fifth one is on "Current Controversies in Obstetric Anesthesia." No matter which lecturer, they cover the field with attention to all the "oral boardable" questions. A few hours' listening in your driver's seat on the way to work could put you in the driver's seat during the test. (Chris is in private practice and spends a lot of time driving from his mansion to the workplace. Steve and Dave still have to live in the ghettos surrounding their tertiary care center with no time to be swaddled in Lexus leather luxury with *Audio Digest* screaming from eight surround sound speakers. Just in case you were wondering which of the authors most liked *Audio Digest*.)

Preeclamptic Pathology
Panvasculopathy, the normal transudation barriers are broken down. If you look at the circulatory system as a whole, then fill in the organs served, you can get a grip on the widespread nature of preeclamptic problems.

1. Cerebral—visual disturbances, headache, all the way to seizures (eclampsia) and intracranial bleeding. If intubation occurs for a stat C-section, the preeclamptic can shoot their blood pressure to the moon and cause an intracranial bleed— the most feared morbidity in the preeclamptic patient. So, if you need to go with a general, the usual Pent/Sux/tube gig might end in badness. Careful preparation to treat/prophylax hypertension.
2. Pulmonary—easy to overload.
3. Cardiac—can have LV dysfunction. Can get hard to separate pulmonary from cardiac, bottom line is volume management is problematic, may be difficult to differentiate the pulmonary and cardiac causes of desaturation in the preeclamptic.
4. Liver—Glisson's capsule can get tense and rupture (rare though). Serious bleed. If Glisson's capsule ruptures, you will measure the blood loss in decibels as the blood splashes on the floor. If Glisson's capsule ruptures, you will remember that day. Hepatic enzymes can be markedly elevated, consistent

with active hepatic inflammation. "Would you administer an inhaled anesthetic agent to a patient with active hepatitis? Does regional anesthesia result in less hepatic injury than general anesthesia?" (See Chapter 19 for answers to these questions.)

5. Renal—oliguria, proteinuria, can progress to renal failure. What happens to volume management when the kidneys function poorly, plus the pulmonary circulation is impaired? It's easy to give too little fluid, making things worse, and it's just as easy to give too much fluid, making things worse. Oy vay! Such a disease! PA catheter management is a consideration when you encounter evidence of CHF or urine output nonresponsive to your best guess as to appropriate fluid management.

Coagulopathy or "How Low Can You Go on the Platelet Count?" Major league vexation in this area.

The platelets can drop, drop, drop. And platelets tend to drop more the worse the preeclampsia gets, so you get painted farther and farther in a corner.

If you take the high and mighty road and say, "No way will I place an epidural if the platelet count drops below 100,000!", then you're stuck managing some preeclamptic's pain with…what? Fentanyl? Demerol? Now the pain relief is inadequate and their pressure goes up further. Now they're getting decels (the placenta, too, is affected by the panvasculopathy) and you're thinking, "This may go to C-section."

Going to do a spinal now? Hmm, platelets are low. A general? With the swollen upper airway of pregnancy, made even more swollen by preeclampsia? And don't forget the possibility of an intracranial bleed if the response to intubation is hyperdynamic, which it probably will be. If intubation is difficult, do you think the upper airway will bleed, get more swollen, get harder to intubate? Now are we talking about doing an emergency tracheostomy on a swollen neck with bad bleeding from the low platelet count? And who will do this trach—the obstetrician? When was the last time the OB-GYN did a trach?

Golly. OK, so we have no answers. However, some obstetric anesthesiologists will consider an epidural with platetlet counts as low as 50K with close neurologic monitoring during and after the pregnancy for signs of an epidural hematoma. It depends on the patient, how well they are doing with an alternative form of pain relief, and an informed discussion of the risks and benefits of proceeding with an epidural in these circumstances.

Uteroplacental insufficiency—as noted above, the placenta is not spared the vascular damage of preeclampsia. (Again, think of preeclampsia as a *panvasculopathy*.) So, for example, if you place an epidural and the blood pressure drops, say 20 points systolic, a healthy placenta could handle such a reduction in blood pressure.

Not so with the preeclamptic placenta. Such a small drop in blood pressure may cause fetal distress—oops, a nonreassuring fetal heart rate pattern.

The possibility of a C-section, which attends all pregnancies, is increased in the preeclamptic. And with the placental problems inherent in the disease, the possibility of a stat C-section hangs over your head like the Sword of Damocles.

What labs would you order on a preeclamptic?

As with all other labs, the best "lab" is the history. Have they had easy bruising and bleeding? And as with so many labs, the net gain from the lab results is fuzzy. Say you get a coag profile along with platelet count. Say the tests show abnormalities. You still have to face the ogre of a stat C-section with a swollen, friable upper airway. So is it worth getting a coag profile?

YOU ARE ENTERING A GRAY ZONE. CAUTION, YOU ARE ENTERING A GRAY ZONE.

Get a coag profile with special attention to the platelet count. Will a bleeding time help if the platelet count is low? Well…the bleeding time has been shown not to correlate with bleeding, so almost everyone now doesn't bother getting a bleeding time.

The bottom line—get a coag profile, just so you can know where you start. There will be no perfect cutoff, no epiphany of revelation when one lab comes in, but you can add that information into the whole risk/benefit picture. Scientific data on specific cutoffs in this population does not exist, with the exception of knowing that the lower the platelet count, the more likely the chance of an epidural hematoma.

OBSTETRIC INTRAOP QUESTIONS

What monitors would you place in a preeclamptic?

If preeclampsia is severe, with a blood pressure greater than 160 systolic, you need an A-line. Recall, if you have to go to a general, the *big bugaboo* is hypertension with an intracranial bleed. You will be needing an A-line for such an anesthetic.

CVP? Yes, if oliguria is present.

Swan? If oliguria persists or there is evidence of LV dysfunction, such as rales or impaired oxygenation.

Would you place an epidural in this preeclamptic patient?

This is controversial. We would place an epidural even if the platelet count goes below 100,000 with no clinical signs of easy bleeding (hint: examine the IV site), but *not* below 50,000. Why? A well-placed epidural that works and can get you through a C-section is worth its weight in gold. Below 50,000 it's pretty clear the risk of a bleed goes even farther up, and the relative benefits are outweighed by the potential neurologic disaster of an epidural bleed.

Or you can simply be prepared for general with a nipride drip and a syringe of esmolol, and not put in the epidural with a platelet count of less than 100,000 because of the possibility of neurologic sequelae. Hey, you're the consultant, so decide what *you* want to do in a controversial situation and defend it by putting yourself on the side of minimizing patient morbidity. The point is to know that the consequence of not having the epidural in is to have to deal with HTN, and to have the epidural in means having to deal with the possibility of an epidural bleed. It's your attention to *those* details that make your answer right or wrong.

Dosing the epidural in the preeclamptic must be slow, with close attention to signs of uteroplacental insufficiency with any blood pressure drop.

Spinal—in the preeclamptic? The rapidity of the blood pressure drop may be too much. So traditional physiologic wisdom went like this: since the preeclamptic's volume status can be so iffy, so tight between too little volume and too much volume, the lightning sympathectomy of a spinal is too dangerous. A more incremental sympathectomy as with a slowly dosed epidural makes more sense.

As always, there is a flip side.

Spinals use smaller needles, lowering the risk of hematomas with regional anesthesia, particularly as the preeclamptic's platelet count drifts lower and lower. The alternative to regional, a general anesthetic with the risks of lost airway and intracranial bleed is ever present.

There may not be time to place and dose an epidural, particularly if the fetal heart rate tends toward the nonreassuring. So does the theoretic risk of a spinal (too fast sympathectomy) outweigh the risks of epidural (big needle, time consuming) or the risk of general anesthetic (lost airway, intracranial bleed)?

This is tough stuff.

Although on the boards, you hesitate to say, "A recent study showed…," the fact is, this year's *Anesthesiology* looked at this very question. Is it safe to place a spinal in the preeclamptic?

The answer is yes; it is safe.

Even without that study, though, you can still defend the logical choice of a spinal. By citing the risks associated with not doing a spinal, and by explaining how you would treat the sympathectomy that would result from a spinal, you can reasonably and rationally defend this choice of anesthetic. And that marks you as a consultant, a board diplomat.

Be prepared on the orals for this question—preeclamptic, general anesthetic, C-section for fetal distress, difficulty intubating. This is, face it, about the hardest problem you could face as an anesthesiologist, and about the hardest question you can imagine on the boards. Let's call this particular question *the question*.

THE QUESTION

But before we tumble right into *the question*, let's hem and haw a little.

Choice of anesthetic: for all the reasons mentioned, we would do all possible to avoid a general anesthetic. That swollen airway, the rapid desaturation, all lay the groundwork for the ultimate disaster.

Couldn't get the spinal in with a little 25 gauge? I'd use the 22 gauge; the headache I can treat later, that's not life and death. A lost airway *is* life and death.

No time for a regional in a stat C-section? Some say yes, some say no.

- Yes, there is time for a regional in a stat C-section. If you are quick, get the patient on her side, go right with a bigger 22-gauge needle, and go like thunder, you can do a regional in such a case.
- No, there is no time for a regional in a stat C-section. No obstetrician will countenance the perceived delay. Stat means stat and that means go to sleep *NOW*.

As you see, you can defend either of these choices. Keep in mind, you are the consultant, and on the boards, you must make the tough choice and defend it. The examiners have the luxury of taking you to task on your choice.

- So you did a regional and the Apgars are low; the obstetrician blames you. Your response?
- So you "saved time" with a general and lost the airway, what will you do now?

Again, weigh the pros and cons, if you "save time" going to a general then lose the airway and kill the mother, just how much time have you really saved? In a jam, you can get the patient on her side, skip the local, and go with a big needle and move like Jackie Chan in a kung fu movie. Getting just 50 mg of lido in can get you operating level anesthesia pretty darned fast.

Or you can say, the baby is at risk, there is too much time lost trying to get a level, so we must proceed with a general. Our opinion is irrelevant, defending your approach is the key thing.

All right, so you *have* to do the case with a general anesthetic, no more hemming and hawing. No more skating around *the question*.

Have the *all important* antihypertensives right there. Mix up some Nipride ahead of time and have a syringe at 20 mcg/cc right on your cart. Have labetalol or esmolol drawn up. Remember *left uterine displacement*. With induction, watch that blood pressure like a hawk and give a dab of Nipride and esmolol to take the tops off those blood pressure peaks. Preoxygenate, induce with cricoid, cheat a little by giving a few puffs of oxygen through the cricoid (that's what you're going to do if you can't intubate, aren't you?) and give it your best shot. Have all specialized equipment on hand (Eschmann intubating stylet, fiberoptic, Bullard scope, whatever helps you). Make sure the head is in optimal position by building up a neck with pillows, blankets, or anything else that will align the axes for you. At this point, be prepared to go through the difficult airway algorithm (see Figure 7-1).

Can't intubate, can ventilate well, still in fetal distress?

- Keep cricoid, mask ventilate, and tell the surgeon, "No joke, this is not a teaching case, get the kid out fast." In three minutes the ventilation will be easier.
- Wake the patient up and do an awake intubation. The mother is your patient and the baby comes second. Killing the mother with a lost airway helps no one. We've heard it said, not meaning to be glib (for a change), "The mother can have another baby, the baby cannot have another mother."

Note the two different responses. You choose. You defend the one you believe. You have to make your choice in this situation and live with it.

Can't intubate, ventilate only so-so?

- Place a Combi-tube or LMA, do the case that way, again telling the surgeon to make believe it's already past his tee time.
- Wake the patient up. Do an awake intubation. The mother is your patient.

Tough choices and different avenues of response. You will make that call.

Can't intubate, can't ventilate?

- Cricothyrotomy to buy time, then go to trach.
- LMA—if that works, do the case under LMA.
- Wake the patient up as you infiltrate with local and remove the baby in that way.
- Cricothyrotomy, do the case under jet ventilation.

As things get worse, the decisions get harder. And always there is more than one alternative. We present all of them, but you will have to pick one. Any thinking creature knows this is rugged business. Your best bet is to *think these killer questions through ahead of time.* Then, in the luxury of the "before boards," you can straighten out just how you'd explain yourself. Don't figure these monsters out "intra boards," or else you'll stumble and end with the "see-you-again" boards.

Consider the ethical dilemma of saying, "Forget the baby, the mother is my primary concern."

That sounds good in a lecture hall or during some erudite discussion, but in a practical sense, no one is going to do that with the OB screaming, "We gotta get this kid out *now*!" Unless the mom is dying, you would probably go ahead. However, your prime concern *is* the mother. You can always ask for the baby who needs resuscitation to be brought to the head of the operating room table.

What about stopping and going fiberoptic? The swollen upper airway and easy bleeding make the fiberoptic option less appealing than in the nonpregnant patient. Now, in the same breath, if I saw a patient with a difficult airway before the stat C-section went down, I would think about doing the intubation awake from the start. An oral fiberoptic approach should be contemplated as the initial approach given the swollen nasal membranes, the possibility of inducing bleeding, and consequently making futile all further fiberoptic attempts secondary to blood in the airway.

Sedation? Sedating the mother is not fatal to the baby. Unsupported respiratory depression *after birth* is fatal to the baby, so if you had to give the mother sedation to conduct an awake intubation, tell the pediatrician that the baby will need ventilatory support until the absorbed sedation wears off. Again understanding the consequences of each action and clearly communicating that to the board examiner is key when taking a controversial approach to anything.

MORE BOARDABLE QUESTIONS

Having tackled *the ultimate question* in all of anesthesia, it may seem like a letdown to take on more mundane questions. But, face it, every question on the boards is not going to be a killer, oh-my-God-every-option-is-fatal question. You must reason with the examiners on more prosaic questions too. Each of these, in its own way, is a dilemma with its own set of pros and cons, its own "don't forget the important stuff" aspects. Don't overlook these.

A 20-year-old is admitted with placenta previa. What special concerns attend this condition?

1. Access, access, access.

Big blood loss is the danger here. Puny IVs will sink you. Patient's morbidly obese? Take the time to put in a central line if nothing's available peripherally. Better to place a central line electively than later on when the bleeding starts and the CVP is minus 3.

2. Regional? *Before* they do the exam.

The sympathectomy from a spinal will accentuate blood loss, therefore you should not place a regional. Ever, ever, ever, ever, right?

Well, er, not so fast.

Ruling out a regional means your C-section will have to be general. Have we already forgotten about the airway problems? Also, ruling out a regional means you will allow the patient a long, painful labor. Hmm. That might not go over too well. Ruling out a regional has some consequences.

Go ahead. Place a regional, but be prepared for the blood loss. Furthermore, the sympathectomy can be treated. Can we not use (gasp!) phenylephrine to replace the lost sympathetic tone? (Yes, ephedrine is the agent of choice, but if the blood pressure loss is linked to the sympathectomy of a spinal or epidural, then phenylephrine to restore blood pressure is OK.)

Note, once again you have two reasonable, physiologically based answers that are opposite. This is the essence of the boards.

A 36-year-old is scheduled for VBAC, what specific problems can occur with a vaginal birth after C-section?

Watch for uterine rupture. The abdominal pain may be severe and unremitting, versus the episodic pain of contractures. The kicker is, if your epidural is working really well, that pain might be masked, or you might "top it off" without realizing you're hiding a catastrophe. Fetal distress—there I go again!—nonreassuring fetal heart rate, may be the first tip off to this potentially fatal complication.

As you are rolling into the OR, the patient asks you for a candid discussion of the advantages of spinal and epidural.

For a C-section, a spinal gives a denser block, patients tend to moan less when the uterus is extroverted. But you can't redose a spinal. Say it's a repeat C-section and the surgeon finds a loop of bowel around an old uterine scar. If it takes a long time to take the bowel down, you've just bought a general anesthetic. The spinal will wear off too soon and there is no way to "top it up."

A spinal has the advantage of using a small dose of local anesthetic and, hence, no risk of a toxic intravascular injection.

Epidurals require huge doses of local anesthetics. Intravascular injection of that dose can result in prolonged vascular collapse as well as CNS complications.

If the patient is an anesthesiologist, you can tell her about ropivicaine. Ropivicaine, a new local anesthetic trying to knock bupivacaine off its pedestal, promises less adverse cardiovascular effects in the case of an intravascular injection. Ropivicaine hasn't yet set the world on fire, as many think that in equipotent doses, it actually has a very similar profile to bupivacaine. Nonetheless, it's a reasonable choice if you are familiar with it, and easy to defend as potentially less toxic (though 10 times more expensive than its generic cousin).

A spinal has the disadvantage of possibly causing a headache. The epidural is less likely to cause a headache, but if you get a wet tap, you've got a whopper of a headache.

OBSTETRIC POSTOP QUESTIONS

A patient complains of a headache after a spinal for a C-section. How do you evaluate and treat?

First, evaluate the headache to make sure something more sinister is not going on. Hard neurologic findings could point to an intracranial bleed, sagittal vein thrombosis, a burst AV malformation, or some other misfortune.

If the headache looks truly spinal in origin (worse sitting up), your response is:

- Blood patch right away. Who are we kidding with this conservative stuff? The blood patch is unlikely to cause a complication and is the closest thing to a miracle cure we have.
- Conservative. Fluids, generic analgesics, and caffeinated drinks. Why do an additional procedure when the conservative approach will eventually work?
- Conservative, then a blood patch later if necessary.

Same question, different answers. Be prepared to defend the one you think is best.

After an epidural, a patient complains of leg weakness.

Examine the patient for signs of an epidural hematoma—pain at the site, motor and sensory loss. If any of these signs even remotely indicate the outside chance of an epidural hematoma, get neurosurgical consult and studies ASAP. To prevent permanent neuro loss, you must evacuate the hematoma *now*. Don't tell the nurse to tell the unit clerk to call the office to get Dr. Whatshisname the neuro guy, then page you when he calls back; you'll be at lunch.

You make it happen, all else falls by the wayside while you make sure the CT gets done and the surgeon is all over this like a duck on a June bug. Time is of the essence.

A more likely cause of weakness is stretching of nerves over the pelvic brim. The baby's head pushing down plus the patient's legs pulling back can result in temporary weakness of hip flexion.

So, in your studying of obstetric anesthesia, prepare for the gut-wrenchers, preeclampsia with its multiple complications, the failed intubation in a stat C-section. But don't neglect other questions pertinent to the area. Be the complete consultant, not just the crisis consultant.

Yea, you have heard the voice of woman in travail.

Prepare, lest ye hear your own voice travail at the boards.

17 | A Burned-Out Wreck

A darkened lecture hall, a slide projector, a podium, a speaker. Pens, notepads, and water glasses on the tables. Coffee and danish available for the break. Ho hum. Another lecture at another meeting. Will this lecture be any different from a thousand others? Will this lecturer say anything that will stand out, will fire the imagination, will solder itself into by memory banks?

The lecturer stands up and speaks.

"Many of you think pediatric anesthesia is just anesthetizing little adults. Many of you view a child as a little adult. Wrong. For a child is not a little adult. An adult is a burned-out wreck of a child."

Oh, brave new world that has such lecturers in it.

PEDIATRIC PREOP QUESTIONS

How does the physiology of a child affect your anesthetic?

Airway
- You don't have to think about endotracheal tube sizes with adults too much. Not so with kiddies. Simple rule for size 3, 4, and 5. A newborn takes a 3, a 1-year-old takes a 4, a 2-year-old takes a 5. Simple rule for depth 10, 11, and 12. A newborn should be about 10 cm at the gums, a 1-year-old at 11, a 2-year-old at 12. Each of these is a starting guideline and modified to circumstances. You can also use those three lines at the end of the tube. Placing the double line at the cords is a good way to be in the right place all the time (although you still have to listen). As the child gets older you start getting into the formulas of age/4 + square root of 12 raised to the third power of the potassium level minus weight in slugs {actually (16 + age)/4}. Try the old standby of measuring the child's pinkie. That pinkie width is about the width of their trachea. Then have a size above and a size below handy.
- The narrowest part of the child's trachea is subglottic, hence the uncuffed tubes.

- The epiglottis is small and at times hard to lift (angled across the line of view). And knowing the differences between a child and an adult airway is a common question on the exam.
- The difficult airway in the child is most often linked to a specific genetic or metabolic abnormality (Pierre-Robin, Treacher-Collins, the mucopolysaccharidoses among others) versus the more prosaic and widespread causes of difficult airway in the adult (obesity, arthritis). Going "right to a trach," the ultimate option in the adult difficult airway, is much more problematic in the child. The trachea is smaller, and a trach at an early age could lead to terrible problems with stenosis as the child grows up.
- Cooperation in the case of an awake intubation is much more of a problem in a child. All the reasoning in the world cannot make a 2-year-old hold still for an awake fiberoptic intubation.
- So that's why they all get breathed down—with caution of course.

IV Access

- 99.9% of adults have an IV placed before induction of anesthesia. Most children (with an approximate cutoff of 10 years old), full stomachs excepted, are induced without an IV.
- Lack of cooperation and small size of veins can make IV placement difficult. This has a real impact on such conditions as the bleeding tonsil (volume can be low, you need that access to safely induce, and the more the child struggles and cries, the worse the bleeding and airway compromise), epiglottitis (starting an IV could set off a crying episode that loses the airway), and obesity (it's hard to see any veins, you hesitate to "breathe down" a 9-year-old who weighs 200 pounds). Whatever you do, make your decision and go with it. EMLA (local anesthetic cream) may help, but EMLA takes 45 minutes to work, and then, only imperfectly. Plus, you "EMLA" one place, miss, then you have to go to an "EMLA free" zone. Groan. Smart money always EMLAs two potential vein placements.
- Central lines—as noted with peripheral IVs, lack of cooperation makes this procedure a challenge. Back to the obese child. If you can't get a peripheral IV and multiple attempts have reduced the child to tears and thrashing, getting a central line now is impossible.

Desaturato instantanicus (Latin terms make us look so "doctor-like.")

- Kids have an alarming ability to desaturate in the blink of an eye and scare the living bejeepers out of the most hardened anesthesiologist. Ratios of FRC to cardiac output/oxygen metabolic requirements are lower in kids than adults. *So* they use up their smaller reserve more quickly.

Cardiac

- Unlike the burned out hulk of an adult, kids have clean coronaries, so tachycardia isn't such a bugaboo.
- Speaking of heart rate, a kid's cardiac output is linked to its heart rate. The stroke volume is more fixed in a child's less elastic heart.
- Premies have a maladaptive response of going bradycardic when stressed (the spooky apneic-bradycardic spells so common in the neonatal ICU). Whereas an adult under some stress, such as hypoxia, would get tachycardic, the premie will go brady. Decompensation can happen in a...well...a heartbeat.

Neurologic

- The mature adult neurologic system requires no special considerations regarding FIO_2. Not so, the premature infant with the ever-present (and poorly understood) threat of retrolental fibroplasia. Often in the sickest child, where you want the largest margin of safety regarding inspired oxygen, your hands are tied for fear a high FIO_2 (and attendant high SaO_2) will cause damage to the retina.

PEDIATRIC INTRAOP QUESTIONS

You are called to the delivery area to participate in a neonatal resuscitation. What are your primary concerns?

- An arrest in a newborn is respiratory, respiratory, respiratory in origin. The next three causes in order are respiratory, respiratory, and respiratory, respectively. Forget, in a resuscitation, the retrolental fibroplasia concerns—you have to save the baby's life. Getting drugs IV can be tough, and in a newborn code, there might not be the luxury of placing umbilical lines. Epinephrine, lidocaine, and atropine can be delivered and taken up by the endotracheal route. These resuscitative agents, though, take second place to the all-important need to ventilate the child.
- Choanal atresia. Easy to fix *if you think of it*. The nasal route to breathing is obstructed, so an oral airway and some support is the magic bullet here, as the neonate is an obligate nasal breather.
- Meconium aspiration. There is always a bit of a tug-of-war here. Yes, better to intubate and suction before the baby takes the first breath, but, man, it is hard not to slam that mask on

and puff a *little* oxygen in them while the peds resident is fumbling with the intubation. On the boards, intubate, suction, breathe. If no can intubate, breathe, understanding the danger of pushing meconium further into the airways, possibly leading to atelectasis, hypoxemia, and infection later.

A child is scheduled for repair of a congenital diaphragmatic hernia. How do you assure adequate oxygenation during such a case?

- Decompress the GI tract with passage of a gastric tube. Positive pressure with a mask may further inflate the loops of bowel in the chest and worsen respiratory distress.
- The shriveled up lung on the side of the diaphragmatic hernia is *not* going to magically inflate with a big puff. All you're going to do is pop the good lung.
- Have the art line and oximeter on the right side. The left side will possibly get "contaminated" with persistent fetal circulation blood and inaccurately reflect the brain's and the eyes' oxygen supply. Keep the PaO_2 at 50 to 80 mm Hg to try to avoid (there is no guarantee) retrolental fibroplasia.
- Hypoxemia, hypercapnia, crying, acidosis, and light anesthesia can all increase pulmonary artery vascular resistance and shunt blood flow away from the lungs through a patent ductus arteriosus. That worsens hypoxemia and you can get into a vicious spiral. Advice? Avoid all badness. (If it were only that easy.) Keep the patient warm, quickly treat suspected pneumothorax, and check gases for acidosis.

A young man is scheduled for repair of pyloric stenosis. You rock right into the case, ignoring all other considerations.

Just kidding. Wanted to see if you were paying attention.

- Pyloric stenosis is a medical, not a surgical emergency. Correction of the hypokalemic, hypochloremic, hypovolemic metabolic alkalosis must precede surgical correction.
- Full stomach precautions. Awake intubation, though it sounds good on paper, is usually too much of a struggle, especially once the kid's volume status is restored and they're able to put up a hell of a fight.

How do vital sign considerations differ in the younger crowd?

A board examiner could toss a "scary" vital sign at you. "The blood pressure is 50/30 in this newborn. Will you give albumin, blood, LR, or Hespan to volume resuscitate this newborn on the verge of cardiovascular collapse?"

Your response? "I wouldn't do a damn thing, buster, that's a normal blood pressure in a newborn. Try again, you weasel!"

Good answer in its content, you might want to work on style, though.

You need not memorize the entire vital sign table, but it's worth knowing at least the range for some ages so you won't get thrown on a vital sign question.

Age	Heart Rate	Blood Pressure
Newborn	120	50/30
4 years old	100	100/60

Any attempt to memorize more than that will short circuit your brain.

What are the approximate doses you use in a pediatric code?

The boards aren't real big on doses, but the following rule of thumb at least puts you in the ballpark for kiddie code doses. (To tell the truth, we include this more for your "real world" knowledge than your board stuff.)

- A newborn gets about one-tenth of an adult dose.
- A 7-year-old gets about one-half of an adult dose.

That will at least give you a starting point so you won't be utterly clueless in such unfamiliar territory.

A child is admitted with suspected epiglottitis. How do you induce the anesthetic?

- Keep the kid calm. Starting an IV or scaring the child may close off what little you have left of an airway.
- Don't send the kid off to x-ray, CT scan, MRI, gamma photodetection, dilithium posiquark cyclotron megasupraimaging, or any other radiology place. The diagnosis is clinical and you must act *now* to secure the airway.
- Inhalation induction (yes, even with a full stomach), then the gentlest laryngoscopy. Use a Mac and hike up the epiglottis indirectly, do not lift the epiglottis itself or there will be a bloody inflamed mess.

Trach set ready, surgeon gloved and ready. (On a clinical note, trach kits sit around and may not be used for long periods. When the moment of truth arrives, that is not the time to find out that someone in some distant past time forgot to stock it completely. Sorry—that was relevant again, and irrelevant for the boards.)

Six hours ago, a 4-year-old had a tonsillectomy and was sent home. Now that patient is back for reexploration of the bleeding tonsillar bed. How do you manage this anesthetic?

- Get another pair of hands if you can.
- Get access. The blood loss is, what? The kid could have been swallowing blood all day. Femoral stick? Do it if there is nothing peripheral. In a bad jam, it's often easier to hold the legs down and get a femoral line than the arms, and you can do it "blind." Cross for blood. Kids can bleed to death from a bleeding tonsil.
- Full stomach. Rapid sequence. If volume loss is tremendous, may need to induce with ketamine. Ketamine induction can be done IM, and IV access obtained immediately following intubation with a cut down if necessary. Again, understand what is important. Get to the OR, and do whatever is necessary to get the bleeding stopped and that IV in.
- Airway. Can be bad news with tons of blood in the way. Show the examiners you are prepared. Have an additional sucker ready, in case one suction apparatus is not enough. This airway can go to a trach. Make sure, as with the epiglottitis patient, that there is a trach kit ready. Fortunately, your surgeon is an ENT so a trach is not so foreign a procedure.
- IM ketamine if the kid is really wild and there is just no way, *no way* to get a line anywhere? Yes, we'd do it. Not an optimal thing to do, but if vital signs were deteriorating, we'd go with the ketamine dart.

Note, the bleeding tonsil is to pediatrics what the stat C-section is to obstetrics. Tough question with tough, controversial explanations required. Work on your response; practice it aloud. Run your explanation of the bleeding tonsil past the peds experts in your department. You may see this tough question at board time.

Do you avoid Sux in your pediatric practice?

The manufacturer's recommendation to avoid Sux in kids "unless necessary" brings to mind an important point. Do you ever need Sux in a kid? Well, do you? If their airway looks in any way bad, you should perhaps breathe them down and maintain spontaneous ventilation without any relaxants at all. If their airway looks good, then a medium duration muscle relaxant should be safe. The reason for the warning? Sux, in addition to triggering MH, can also trigger massive potassium release if a child has a yet-undiagnosed neuromuscular disorder, such as Duchenne's muscular dystrophy.

If you do use Sux, and the QRS suddenly widens and progresses to cardiovascular collapse, know that the presumptive diagnosis is hyperkalemia and institute treatment with calcium, insulin, glucose, and CPR.

You can say you use Sux, just be able to defend its need and be able to discuss the implications of using it.

In the middle of an orthopedic procedure, the end-tidal CO_2 rises out of proportion to any ventilatory changes. What is your presumed diagnosis and what do you do?

Malignant Hyperthermia

- Triggers are potent vapors and Sux.
- Think of MH as a metabolic supernova, with O_2 consumption going way up, CO_2 production going way up. Everything is on full throttle. Temperature rise may be a late manifestation. Look for the earliest signs, an unexplained tachycardia or a rise in end-tidal CO_2.
- Treatment is stopping the operation (if possible, you can't exactly stop an appendectomy), cooling the patient, monitoring and maintaining urine output (think of this as a kind of modified "rhabdomyolysis" and you don't want myoglobin gumming up the kidneys), hyperventilating with 100% O_2, getting a clean machine, or just a clean ambu-bag, and starting dantrolene. Dantrolene is the key. Mortality from MH plummeted after dantrolene use started. But even with dantrolene, people still die from MH. Better to sound the alarm and treat unnecessarily (the only side effect of dantrolene is weakness and the skin turning orange) than to hold off treatment until it is too late.
- Mixing dantrolene is a pain in the butt and time-consuming. If you've never done it (and most have not), grab a bottle and waste a few bucks. You'll see. Get extra hands to help you with this. You'll need extra hands anyway, to place invasive lines (you'll need to follow blood gases so get an A-line). It won't be hard to get help because MH is such a "novelty"—people will come running from near and far anyway.
- The patient and family will need Medic-alert bracelets postop.
- Trigger free anesthetics are no big deal. No vapors, clean machine, no sux. Especially with propofol, it's not that hard to do a trigger free anesthetic.
- Who needs a muscle biopsy? It's cavalier and impractical to say, "Anyone you suspect should wing off to places far away and get a muscle biopsy test." Who will pay for this? Get a biopsy for social reasons (can't get a pilot's license, an armed services appointment, or life insurance). The test itself is a procedure with risk, expense, discomfort, and, worst of all, false-positive and false-negative results. And if the results are equivocal? You'll just do a trigger-free anesthetic anyway.
- Masseter spasm, what does it mean? Have you just not waited long enough for the relaxant to work, or is it a "precursor" to

MH? The conservative approach is to consider real masseter spasm (jaw clenched, no way can you open the mouth) a precursor to MH, cancel the case if practical, or proceed with a nontriggering anesthetic if the procedure must continue. This question is batted around each year in, for example, the ASA refresher courses.

PEDIATRIC POSTOP QUESTIONS

After a successfully treated case of MH, how long do you keep the patient in the hospital?

The creepy thing about MH is, it can recur, hours later, and flare up just as badly as the first time. So if a patient has done OK through a bout of MH, then they must still be observed for at least 24 hours, looking for any signs of recurrence—tachycardia, rigidity, desaturation. As with the initial occurrence, waiting for a rise in temperature means waiting too long.

In the PACU, a child displays signs of upper airway obstruction. Your management?

Go to the bedside, this is no over-the-phone gig. Administer supplemental oxygen and examine for objects in the upper airway (a sponge from a tonsillectomy, a loose tooth) before administering positive pressure ventilation. You'd hate to push an object farther down. If the child has aspirated a foreign object, such as a tooth, then the child will need rigid bronchoscopy to remove it.

If the child is displaying "croupy" signs from upper airway edema, then administer humidified air and a racemic epinephrine nebulized treatment to try to reduce the swelling. Does the epi actually help? It may. If none of these treatments work, then reintubate, realizing that you may need a smaller tube than the one placed at the original operation.

So concludes another hour of "The Kiddie Hour," with an all too brief look at some of the highlights of the physiology of kids versus adults, and a brief listing of "boardable" questions pertaining to children.

Now, take to heart the lesson of the lecturer at the start of this chapter. Look in the mirror, and what do you see? Face the truth.

You see a "burned-out wreck of a child."

18 | What a Pain

Never had a toxic reaction to local anesthetics? Guess what? On the day of your oral boards, you will! Congratulations.

REGIONAL PREOP QUESTIONS

A patient presents for an ORIF of the finger. He prefers "not to be asleep." Discuss his options.

A finger operation can be done with a finger block. Tourniquet pain, though, could be problematic, so an axillary block is a good option. If the patient is a difficult airway, then a regional anesthetic presents a problem. If the block should fail or if the block should wear off, you face establishing an airway in a patient under non-ideal circumstances.

Patient severed his ulnar nerve in an accident and presents months later for additional repair work. Do you perform an axillary block?

In a patient with pre-existing neurologic loss, placing a needle in the axilla could be viewed as folly. If the ulnar nerve remains injured, some unscrupulous lawyer could blame the axillary block needle. In such a case of pre-existing nerve damage, you can argue to avoid a block. (Absolute contraindication? No.)

REGIONAL INTRAOP QUESTIONS

You inject local anesthetic for a regional block and the patient stops talking and seizes. Your treatment?

First things first, give oxygen, support the airway. Don't panic and jump right into intubation gear, you may be able to get by with mask ventilation *if the patient does not have a full stomach*. Support the good old ABCs.

Give pentathol to stop seizures, succinylcholine to stop the muscle movements if they are so severe you can't ventilate. (A point of neurophysiology, even if you "mask" the seizures with muscle relaxants, the seizure activity is still going on in the brain, with high cerebral metabolic oxygen requirements, so you still need to treat with antiseizure medication.)

To support pressure, you may need volume and pressor support. Bupivacaine-related cardiovascular collapse has gone all the way to cardiopulmonary bypass until the local anesthetic wears off. If you must, you must!

Discuss the relative merits of the interscalene versus axillary versus Bier block.

Interscalene is best for procedures at or above the elbow, axillary blocks for procedures below the elbow.

The interscalene approach most often concentrates the local anesthetic on the superior and middle trunks of the brachial plexus, assuring a good block of the musculocutaneous, axillary, radial, and median nerves. And the high approach covers the cervical plexus too, assuring good anesthesia for shoulder operations. The "lowest rung" at the trunk level of the brachial plexus, the inferior trunk, is sometimes missed in the interscalene approach. Thus, the ulnar nerve is not blocked.

(Can you draw that spaghetti junction of the brachial plexus?)

The axillary approach is more likely to nail the ulnar, median, and radial nerves, though you may miss the musculocutaneous (its takeoff may he higher than your local anesthetic reaches). Unless you put 3 gallons of local anesthetic in, you're not going to get the cervical plexus by this approach, so the axillary approach doesn't work for shoulder operations. A Bier block is limited by how long the patient can tolerate tourniquet pain. Interscalenes can result in a dropped lung, carotid puncture, or intrathecal tracking. A transarterial block in the axillary approach can result in continued bleeding and hematoma formation after the block.

Is regional "safer" than general anesthesia?

Orthopedic experience seems to be showing that, for hip procedures and total knees, a regional technique may indeed be safer. Pulmonary emboli are less in total hip patients with epidurals versus general anesthetics.

Is the jury in as regards other areas, for example, cardiac risk in fem-pop patients? No.

One thing may make a difference—pain relief with intrathecal or epidural narcotics is much better than traditional IM routes or even PCA (although in most studies patient satisfaction does not differ between PCA and epidural pain relief due to the higher control factor with PCA; PCEA may be the ultimate answer). What clear-cut answer can you give the examiners? The answer of a consultant is to say what the state of the art is, and to apply that knowledge to the particular case being examined. As the state of the art is in flux, there is no absolute way of telling whether one technique is safer than any other. Personally, we would recommend to a regional supplementation and postoperative neuraxial pain relief for a thoracotomy, an abdominal procedure such as a radical prostatectomy or AAA repair, and major orthopedic procedures. We would feel comfortable telling the patient that such pain relief procedures will aid in respiration (better PFTs, not lower complication rates), may prevent blood clots (only shown following hip surgery as decreased PEs and fem-pops with decreased graft occlusion), and ease of recovery. You can choose otherwise, noting a lack of hard outcome studies in general.

Board examinees are telling us that chronic pain questions are appearing more and more. Though no pain experts, we share these ideas about chronic pain management.

General considerations on the chronic pain patient:

1. Chronic pain does not mean popping in a block and "see you later." The difficult, protracted, and often poorly understood area of chronic pain requires a real pain clinic, a thorough evaluation and follow-up, not just a block jock sticking needles someplace.

2. Just like any other disease, a pain evaluation starts with a history and physical, followed by appropriate lab tests. Don't assume the neck pain is just some trigger point. Could it not be a tumor, pressing on nerves?

3. Provocative tests to "prove the patient is faking it" are of limited or no utility.

4. Multimodality treatment is the way to go. Blocks, physical therapy, psychiatric counseling if necessary, medication for sleep loss and depression all go together to help the chronic pain patient.

5. Goals are to return the patient to work or at least to improve function in daily life. At the outset the goals should be laid out, without unrealistic expectations such as "We will get rid of all your pain." That is often impossible.

Specifics of pain management:

1. Reflex sympathetic dystrophy can stem from relatively minor trauma, but result in debilitating loss in function of upper or lower extremity. RSD progresses from hyperesthesia all the way to muscle loss. Interruption of sympathetic flow to the affected extremity via lumbar sympathetic block for the leg and stellate ganglion block for the arm, is the current best treatment. A series of blocks is usually necessary. Even if you do not perform these blocks, you should know about them, and might be asked to describe them.

2. Lower back pain is the most common of the chronic pain complaints. Assuming etiologies requiring surgical intervention have been ruled out (such as an acute herniated disc with neural compromise), treatment is weight loss (easier said than done), exercises, and, in certain cases such as clearly

identified monoradicular pain of recent onset, epidural steroids. Other treatments include facet injections and trigger point injections. The purpose of these blocks is to lay local anesthetic and steroids at an affected spot, interrupt pain and inflammation, and stop the cycle of pain leading to immobility leading to more pain and around and round you go.

3. Ablative procedures, such as celiac plexus destruction, can have a host of complications and are perhaps best reserved for the terminal cancer patient.

There are a million pain syndromes and ten million treatment options, perhaps indicating that we don't have a clear-cut grip on chronic pain, a most nebulous medical problem. At least be able to discuss the major points of chronic pain management, even if you do little pain management yourself.

REGIONAL POSTOP QUESTIONS

After an arm block, a patient complains of persistent radicular pain. On exam, it appears he may have had an intraneural injection. What do you do?

An ounce of prevention is worth a pound of litigation. In the best of all possible worlds, you would jump in a time machine, go back to the injection, and pay close attention *as* you injected. Exquisite pain means you may be going intraneural. STOP!

But, since you can't use a time machine, you are now stuck.

Pain relief with oral analgesics, evaluation by neurology and referral to a pain specialist are the only options. Long-term pain may result from this intraneural injection, that's all there is to it.

Following your epidural for a gyn procedure in lithotomy, the patient has some nerve dysfunction. How do you determine the etiology?

If you or a neurology consult cannot determine the distribution (nerve root versus peripheral nerve), then EMGs can isolate where along the nerve conduction is compromised, pinpointing (more or less) the site of injury.

After a stellate ganglion block, a patient with RSD says she had relief for just a few hours. Do you continue with treatments?

Yes, often a series of blocks are necessary. The first block may provide relief for a few hours, the next for a few days, the following one for a few weeks. It's hard to predict, but the best thing is to persist with treatments. If no relief is forthcoming, try an alternative approach. The key with pain patients is to be persistently there for them. Throwing up your hands and saying, "Tough luck, there's nothing I can do for you" can be devastating, as the pain specialist is often the "last chance" for these patients.

So be it for pain. You may want to grab a cold one before the next chapter.

CHAPTER

19 | Nothin' but Beers

"But doc, I don't drink!"

You look at the SGOT. It's four times normal. "Really Mr. Jones?" You can smell it on his breath; he had some before he came in for his vasectomy reversal. "You never drink?"

"Well," he blushes to disclose, "don't drink nothin' but beer."

HEPATIC PREOP QUESTIONS

A patient presents with "elevated liver function tests." Do you proceed with surgery?

The elevated liver function test is a vexation. First, the term liver function test should apply to PT/PTT, as these test the liver's *function*. SGOT is a liver *marker* test. Do you cancel for a slightly elevated number? Are you crying "Wolf!" when there really is no danger? The answer is a tough one because it all depends on which way the liver is going.

1. The occasional patient may just be starting to go into fulminant hepatic failure. The SGOT is 85 today, tomorrow it will be 200, next week the patient will be ready for a liver transplant. If you happen to anesthetize the patient during the first stage of their liver failure, then you may add insult to injury as all anesthetic techniques decrease hepatic blood flow, and you will certainly get all the blame.
2. More commonly, the patient may have a little bump in SGOT from a weekend partying or from a little liver inflammation from, say a minor flu bug. A few days later, the SGOT is down.
3. Some patients have chronically elevated SGOT. "Oh yeah, it's always up." Then the patient's regular doc faxes you a sheet of paper detailing this chronic elevation. That is just dandy when that happens but you're rarely that lucky. On the boards, no way will you be that lucky.

Holy hepatitis, Batman! What do we do in such a case?

Repeat the SGOT to see the pattern. If it's still elevated, get a GI consult and ask whether further workup or treatment is necessary before proceeding with an elective operation. The GI guys may or may not say anything of use, but at least you won't be labeled derelict in your duties to assure the patient is in optimal condition for surgery.

What if the patient is already in a sorry state, liverically speaking?

Since cirrhosis is a multisystem organ disease, using an organ by organ approach is the only way to remember everything (See Chapter 7 to review organizational principles). CNS—encephalopathy. Pulmonary—restriction from the ascites, A-V shunting (thought to be estrogen related) so check a blood gas. Cardiac—possible high output failure. GI—possible full stomach from ascitic pressure, esophageal varices can bleed, so careful with instrumentation and check hgb. Renal—possible total water and Na overload, intravascular dehydration so check Na and BUN/Cr ratio, and rule out eminent hepato-renal syndrome indicated by a rising Cr. Hematologic—could be anemic from decreased production given folate and B_{12} deficiencies and/or iron, increased loss from bleeding given lack of coags combined with bleeding varices so check PT/PTT and diff, and check protein levels as pharmacodynamic effects of a given dose of drug can be exacerbated with decreased protein binding and increased free fraction. Endocrine—impaired gluconeogenesis, often presenting on the boards as delayed awakening from hypoglycemia in the postop period to be distinguished from anesthetic action from decreased drug metabolism to be distinguished from worsening hepatic encephalopathy. Of particular interest is the blood gas, for cirrhotics can really screw up their chemistry.

What if they ask you to explain what is happening on a cirrhotic's ABG? The typical ABG in a cirrhotic shows a respiratory alkalosis. Hypoxemia may result from ascites decreasing FRC or low oncotic pressure producing capillary leak and pulmonary edema or intrapulmonary shunting from A–V shunts. Arteriovenous shunts around the liver will elevate cardiac output and mixed venous oxygen saturation. That shunting steals blood flow from vital organs such as the kidneys. A metabolic acidosis from regional hypoperfusion may also develop.

A wise consultant tells you, "Your anesthetic is dangerous to the liver. Just do a spinal!" How do you respond to this intellectual giant?

Thank you, Dr. Consultant. The *operation*, particularly if close to the liver or requiring traction on the liver, is dangerous to the liver itself. All anesthetics, spinals included, decrease splanchnic blood flow, so one is not necessarily safer than the other. Furthermore, many a case cannot be done under a spinal. Perhaps Dr. Consultant would like to place the spinal?

Sluggo the medical student suggests, "Drain off that terrible ascites, that will cure him."

Thank you, Sluggo. The patient will reaccumulate the ascites in no time and your volume will get all messed up. Ascites is a marker of, a symptom of the diseased liver. Now, Sluggo, go back to the library and get away from my anesthesia machine. However, if there is significant pulmonary compromise from the ascites (rapid respiratory rate, shallow tidal volumes, desaturation in the supine position), then it is a reasonable course of action to drain it prior to induction, understanding the need for very careful attention to fluid status.

HEPATIC INTRAOP QUESTIONS

How will a cirrhotic respond differently to your anesthetic ministrations and nostrums?

1. Cirrhotics all have increased body water, as reflected in an often low sodium. This altered body water increases water soluble volume of distribution, but decreased metabolism slows elimination of drugs like neuromuscular blockers. So you need a larger initial dose, and then expect a prolonged effect with longer times between administrations.
2. Cirrhotic patients may have a greater hangover effect, but drugs with redistribution (like fentanyl) will not have a prolonged effect when given in moderate doses.
3. For that poor patient who goes on to liver failure and needs a liver transplant, keep in mind that during the anhepatic phase of the operation, there are no, you heard me, *no* clotting factors to be found. You better havum heapum biggum IV accessum. A rapid transfuser is a must. As the blood is pouring in, don't forget the occasional dollop of calcium. The citrate in the blood will bind up all the calcium and drop the blood pressure. A thromboelastograph during the transplant will guide your factor replacement.

Should you avoid halothane in the hepatic patient?

Postoperative liver dysfunction, though often ascribed to the anesthetic, can be traced to other causes if a diligent search is undertaken. Cytomegalovirus, transfusion injury, or just damage from surgical compression is often to blame.

But NOOOOOOO! It *had* to be the anesthetic. That's why in the thesaurus, the synonym given for anesthesia is San Andreas, because anesthesia is always the *fault.*

In a practical sense, halothane hepatitis was most often seen in days of yore, when a patient might be exposed to several halothane anesthetics in a short time. That is rarely seen today, and most anesthesiologists don't use halothane.

The most important things to avoid in the liver patient are hypoperfusion—the routine things that could damage any organ system. Take good care of the patient, and you're taking good care of the liver.

HEPATIC POSTOP QUESTIONS

After a liver transplant with a stormy course, you are asked to evaluate the patient for extubation.

A liver transplant is a high abdominal procedure with great fluid shifts, blood loss, and manipulation right next to the diaphragm. Caution in weaning from the ventilator is a must. But the patient is also now immunosuppressed, and you can't keep them on the ventilator forever. So extubation criteria follow the usual guidelines.

- Does the patient need PEEP?
- Is the patient's upper airway tremendously swollen from volume shifts, that is, could you reintubate if necessary?
- Can the patient maintain adequate ABGs on his own?
- Does the patient's neuro status allow maintenance of an airway and clearance of secretions?
- Are surgical considerations all squared away? Bile production, bleeding stopped. You hate to extubate the patient then right away go back to the OR.

If the usual criteria for extubation are met and the specific concerns of the liver transplant patient are met, then extubate.

A nurse in the PACU sticks herself with a dirty needle from a patient with cirrhosis. What do you advise the nurse?

Clean the wound as best you can now and get to employee health ASAP. Have them contact the ID expert on the latest recommendations for "dirty needle exposure." (The recommendations vary as time passes.) The nurse may need to get treatment for HIV (early polyagent therapy may reduce the risk of seroconverting). The recommendations may include immune globulin. The most important thing is to seek help early, for if any treatment will help, it should be started right away.

OK, this chapter's done. It's Miller time!

CHAPTER

20 | Colloid Is Thicker Than Water

When, oh when, do you transfuse? The occasional horror story makes the rounds of the following oral board scene.

"So, you wouldn't transfuse at a hematocrit of 25, huh? How about 24, or maybe 23? Where is your cutoff, doctor? Where is your cutoff?"

Not to sweat it. Arm yourself for this question with the best possible information, the best physiologic explanation for your reasoning. Where to find it, where to get the latest, greatest info on blood component management? Why, it's free for the asking and available from your friendly neighborhood American Society of Anesthesiologists.

Here's the address. Send for their catalogue of guidelines (they have everything—difficult airway, blood component therapy, guidelines for pain management—and they will send you a copy free if you're an ASA member).

ASA
520 N Northwest Hwy
Park Ridge, IL 60068-2573

For blood component therapy, for example, the ASA sent me a review article from *Anesthesiology*, Mar 1996;84(3):732–747, entitled "Practice Guidelines for Blood Component Therapy."

This is the kind of article you want to read. A review, a summation of the current thinking. What better way to defend your thinking than quoting the latest review?

If you're of the scholastic bent, the extensive bibliography will detail the research and studies that entered into our current thinking. If you're just a mere mortal trying to pass this exam, a few minutes reading such a review article may make the difference between nailing a question versus failing that question.

That said, let's hit the high points of managing fluids and blood in the OR.

BLOOD RELATED PREOP QUESTIONS

A renal failure patient has a hematocrit of 25 and is scheduled for an AV graft revision. Do you OK the patient for surgery?

Base the answer on patient physiology, rather than an arbitrary number, and take into account the proposed operation and anticipated blood loss. If this patient is able to get around, perform his daily activities, and doesn't have another pressing concern for a high hemoglobin (say, heart disease) then this patient is OK for surgery. Get a type and screen, though, in case the surgeon loses a lot of blood redoing the AV graft. If the patient was scheduled for, say, a Dupuytren's release, we wouldn't bother with the type and screen.

A patient with idiopathic thrombocytopenic purpura is scheduled for a splenectomy. Her platelet count is only 30,000. Do you give her platelets preop?

No, the spleen will just gobble them up. Have the platelets in the room and transfuse after the spleen's blood supply is isolated.

BLOOD RELATED INTRAOP QUESTIONS

You have a patient whose blood supply is partly intravascular, and partly running on the OR floor linoleum. When do you transfuse? This is *the* question in this area of the boards.

As always, the answer depends on the patient and the circumstances, here are some examples:

1. Sickle cell patient. In and out of the ER with frequent abdominal pain from sickling crises. Needs frequent transfusions. Now scheduled for a total hip revision. This patient is worth transfusing and it's useful to know the percentage of hemoglobin S. Not for a goal of any arbitrary number (it used to be etched in stone that the Hgb S had to be less than 50%), but because this patient's clinical course and proposed operation dictate that transfusions will be necessary. He's going to lose a lot of blood and he has shown that he is prone to crises.

2. An 83-year-old woman surprised that she needs a CABG. Nonsmoker, no TIAs, good kidneys, two-vessel disease. In spite of her age, you may let her Hct drift down a bit in the post bypass period. Why? Post bypass her heart has good blood flow, and her other organ systems are in good shape.

3. An 83-year-old with carotid stenosis, borderline creatinine, long-time smoker. Scheduled for CABG. Different physiology, different needs. Critical vascular beds are damaged in the cerebral circulation and the kidneys. Post bypass, you would lean toward transfusing this patient up.

Come up with a dozen other examples you see every day. Transfuse *as dictated by patient need.* That is the answer of a consultant.

Defense of hard number answers are under Chapter 7 "Thresholds." When would you transfuse platelets?

Numbered guidelines exist, namely, it's rare to need platelets if the count is greater than 100,000 and often needed when the count is less than 50,000, but again, the whole clinical picture has to enter the picture.

1. Post AVR. Stable patient, bleeding less than 20 cc/hr. The platelet count comes back 75,000. Do you transfuse platelets to treat the number? No. You only give platelets to treat a *patient.*
2. Oozing, oozing, oozing and the PT/PTT are normal. Only abnormality in the labwork is a borderline platelet count. Do you *not* transfuse because the platelet count is just over the "magic number" of 100,000? No. Treat the *patient.* Give the platelets if either a) it's clearly not surgical hemostasis or b) the alternative is reopening the chest since one would hate to reoperate unnecessarily.

When do you transfuse FFP?

Same story as with platelets. The entire clinical picture guides the transfusion. There are a few specific indications for FFP:

1. Acute reversal of Coumadin.
2. Correction of specific deficiencies when other concentrates are not available. (The indication that most of us give it for is the following.)
3. Correction of microvascular bleeding when PT and PTT are more than 1.5 times normal.

Back to thinking like a consultant. Don't give the FFP after a magic number of packed cells have been given. Don't give FFP for volume expansion. Don't give FFP because the big orthopod threatens to kill you if you don't give it. Don't give it as a "poor man's hyperalimentation." Give it for the indicated reason. The only reason for transfusing FFP without a solid reason is ongoing massive blood loss, in which case mathematics dictate it is probably indicated after 10 L of blood loss in healthy individuals, and sooner if the patient was malnourished and had fewer clotting factors around to start with.

When do you transfuse cryoprecipitate?

A little more specific here. The experts say for:

1. Von Willebrand's patients unresponsive to desmopressin.
2. Von Willebrand's patients actively bleeding.
3. Bleeding patients with fibrinogen levels below 80-100 mg/dL.

Back to sounding like a broken record. Treat the patient. Use the guidelines (however imperfect) that we have. The good thing for you, the test taker, is that there aren't that many things we pour into our patients, and if you know the guidelines for the major ones (blood, FFP, cryo), you can't be too far off the mark. Specific laboratory numbers lost in the heat of your exam? No worry, mate, you can always tell the board examiners you would ask your blood bank. (Of course, that's not quite as good as answering their question.)

BLOOD AND FLUID RELATED POSTOP QUESTION

You've finished another tough day, saving lives and stomping out pestilence. You sit down in the doctor's lounge, open a Twinkee, put your feet up, and watch *World's Goriest Videos* on the doctor's lounge TV. Into the doctor's lounge walks Sluggo, the med student. He sits next to you, and asks you to settle—once and for all—the great crystalloid versus colloid debate.

You cut your Twinkee exactly in half (with a certain relish wielding a very sharp knife) and ask Sluggo which half he wants. He replies, "It doesn't matter." You then ask him why he asks you questions he already knows the answers to. After offering young Sluggo half your Twinkee, you tell Sluggo, "Crystalloid versus colloid has generated much in the way of articles and little in the way of clarifying the issue. The bottom line is, give enough of whatever you're giving. The second bottom line is, don't give too much of what you're giving. Whether you believe in your heart of hearts in lactated Ringer's or hespan, don't give so *little* that the kidneys dry up and blow away. And, in the same vein, don't give so *much* that your patient is gurgling pink frothy stuff at the end of the case."

Then make a point of concentrating on the televised mayhem, and hope Sluggo goes away.

One volume guideline is worth mentioning.

Minimize the free water given to patients with cerebral edema. Again, you can debate crystalloid versus colloid on this, but you would have a hard time defending giving D5W to a patient with a cerebral contusion.

Before going on to the next chapter, we suggest a glass of whole milk liberally laced with chocolate and a Krispy Crème donut. You'll need your energy sitting there doing all of that thinking.

The Worst Disease
You Will Ever Face

Imagine for a moment, a plague. This plague affects one-third of the population in the United States and is growing every year. The causes of the plague are many—some say genetic, some say metabolic, some say cultural, and some just say it's the patient's fault! Treatments for the plague outnumber the stars in the sky, and no treatments have proven truly effective. Hucksters, movie actors, TV personalities have all suffered from this plague, then have gone on to proffer their stories of cure and redemption. The worst thing about this plague? It is an anesthesiologist's nightmare.

The plague? Obesity.

First, a systemic review of obesity.

Psychiatric—Obesity is a complex problem, with a million and one psychiatric, psychologic, and societal factors thrown in. All this comes to a head when you meet the obese patient in the holding area.

"What do you mean you can't get an IV? They didn't have any trouble drawing blood! What do you mean you have to put an IV in my neck?"

You may encounter passive aggression, failure of insight ("Why do you say I am at high risk for this operation?"), and any of a number of challenges in the course of the preop.

"Why do you have to put me on a breathing machine after the operation?"

Your concerns for safety—particularly your concern for rapid arterial desaturation—may come head to head with the patient's view of their disease. For example, you may explain to a 450-pound patient that you need to do an awake intubation, and they may resist the idea, insisting that "they never did this before." You are thinking, "To hell with before, this is now, and I don't want to try to intubate this patient while their O_2 saturation is plummeting."

Airway—More accurately put. Airway, airway, airway.

The large tongue, redundant pharyngeal tissue, and thick, unyielding neck of the obese patient can lead to mucho badness in the intubation department. Large breasts can interfere with movement of the laryngoscope handle, hampering intubation efforts.

Lungs—High oxygen demand and small FRC (the lungs compressed by a kind of restrictive defect) lead to rapid and spooky desaturation.

Cardiac—Chronic hypoxemia can lead to cor pulmonale. Even assessing cardiac function in the often sedentary obese patient can be difficult.

GI—Obese patients are at increased risk for increased gastric volume and aspiration. Couple that with their propensity for difficult intubation, and you can see disaster a' coming.

Now let's look at these same considerations in the preop, intraop, and postop format.

OBESITY PREOP QUESTIONS

Describe the implications of obesity for the conduct of an anesthetic?

Desaturation and airway management—Decreased functional residual capacity, high oxygen consumption, and a forbidding upper airway all combine to make obesity the worst disease an anesthesiologist can encounter. Why? You induce. The airway, which may have looked easy in the preop exam, caves in on itself, the saturation plummets, your laryngoscope handle is blocked by large breasts, the tongue is too big to get around or lift, the saturation continues to drop, and now you're in a panic. Even calling for help may not save the day. So you've taken a (often young) patient and pushed them to death's door with a *simple* induction. Unheard of scenario? Ask anyone in our line of work. The scariest episodes for most anesthesiologists have happened with obese patients.

Effects of chronic hypoxemia—Long-standing obesity carries the risk of chronic hypoxemia, with resultant cor pulmonale. What does that mean to us? Say you made it through the case OK, managed the fluids judiciously, maybe even monitored central pressures. Now it's time to extubate. Patient is working a little hard at breathing. Is the patient working against the extra load of their pannus? Is the patient in pulmonary edema? Will your pain relief be enough (so they won't splint), but not too much (so they get respiratory depression)? Obesity paints you into a corner both in the areas of fluid management and pain relief.

Line placement—Peripheral IVs can be daunting. Central lines no easier. An A-line, though not necessary for the case itself, may be necessary if the blood pressure cuff cannot work.

Aspiration—Obesity implies a full stomach, no matter what the NPO status.

Professional conduct challenge—We've all heard it, the snickers, the comments. Not only is this poor professional conduct, but it can land you in court. Any patient, after all, can have recall. And you should conduct every anesthetic as if the patient hears every word you and the OR staff say. (This was mentioned earlier in the trauma chapter.) If you or anyone else makes wisecracks about the patient's habitus and the patient hears and remembers that, you will lose a boatload of money. Preachy as this may sound, view obesity as a serious disease whose cause is poorly understood. Why? Because, truth to tell, it is!

Preop Visit

1. *The preoperative visit itself.* Explanations may have to be longer and more detailed than "normal." Obesity often carries with it a plethora of poorly understood psychological problems such as depression, codependency (whatever that is), anxiety. Blowing through this visit may not be appropriate. Take time to detail the care the patient will get and look for clues that they are not "happy" with the explanation—not looking you in the eye, turning away, curt replies to questions. It is taxing, and difficult, but ultimately worth it, to make sure the patient is satisfied going into the case.

2. *Physical exam.* Airway, airway, airway. If you are going to induce anesthesia on a morbidly obese patient, you are betting their life that you can get that endotracheal tube in. And you are betting that you can get it in *fast* before they desaturate. Look from the side. How big are the teeth? Is the tongue filling up the whole mouth, affording you no view of the posterior pharynx? The airway exam is important in every patient, of course, but in the obese patient, it is of utmost importance. Remember, when they start to desaturate, you start running out of options fast. This is about the only time the board examiners will ask you to detail how you are going to evaluate this patient's airway. Be prepared to say something other than "well I'd see how it looks." There's a lot of actual experience in that statement that you get *no* credit for on the boards.

3. *Labs.* At the least, the very least, put that pulse oximeter on them in the holding area. Baseline sat 91%? Hmm. Better start thinking about where this patient is going postop. A blood gas is a pain, especially in this day of outpatient everything, but if you suspect the patient is a CO_2 retainer, it's good to have one. Pickwickian perhaps? Sleep apnea perhaps? EKG? Yes. If for no other reason, in case disaster strikes and they do go into pulmonary edema postop. At least you'll have a baseline to look at. You would hate to be sitting there in the ICU afterwards when the cardiologist asks, "Were these T waves flipped preop?" and you say, "Duh."

4. *Lines.* May need an A-line in case the cuff won't work. Great to have an A-line for a postop gas or two, to assure that the patient is doing well from a respiratory standpoint. CVP? A triple lumen can be quite handy in the postop care of an inpatient

because the nurses on the floor can get their blood sample from it. Intraop, it is great to have a central line that can reliably deliver the fluids and the drugs. Peripheral IVs in the obese are hard to get in. Rather than end up with some positional, small gauge IV that keeps you nervous the whole case, it's often better to stick that central line and have a good line.

5. *Aspiration prophylaxis with antacid or other pharmacotherapy?* Good idea. Never been proven to make a difference in outcome, but it makes physiologic sense.

OBESITY INTRAOP QUESTIONS

What special considerations do you consider in the obese versus the nonobese patient.

1. Awake intubation. Darn good idea if you are the *least bit* concerned about that airway. If they have a perfect and I mean *perfect* airway, then induce using cricoid pressure to avoid aspiration. But, *caution is the byword*, especially on the boards, and don't hesitate for a second to secure that airway awake.

2. *If you do, induce general anesthesia.* A little reverse Trendelenburg takes some weight off the diaphragm, buys you some FRC, and makes mask ventilation (maybe just a few teeny weenie puffs through the cricoid pressure to keep the patient saturated) easier. Have stuff handy, such as intubating stylets, extra hands, an LMA as an imperfect but helpful fallback, just in case you get in trouble. ENT standing by to do a trach? If you're *that* worried, maybe you should have intubated them awake.

3. *Conduct of the anesthetic.* More than a lot of cases, think about how you will handle emergence. The obese patient's tendency to desaturate will happen at the end of the case just as it happened at the beginning of the case. The patient's small FRC, fleshy upper airway, big tongue, and pannus didn't disappear during the operation. Keep the patient intubated until they are major league awake. I mean *awake* awake. Writing letters to friends awake. Logging on to the Internet with their laptop computer awake. However you choose to manage this, keep in mind that the end of the case in an obese patient can be just as much of a disaster as induction, so keep your vigilance up. Having successfully intubated the patient awake in a controlled induction, don't be surprised if the board examiners now make you do it emergently.

OBESITY POSTOP QUESTIONS

In the PACU, the patient has a sore throat. Intubation was difficult secondary to the patient's obesity. How do you evaluate?

Inspect the oropharynx. If the tissue is gashed to bloody awful ribbons, seek ENT consultation. If not, Cepacol throat lozenges (assuming an awake patient who will not aspirate the lozenge) provide good relief. As oral mucosa heals quickly, time should heal this malady. Also, take this opportunity to inform the patient of the difficulty in intubation. Inform the patient that the next operation may require an awake intubation. A good strategy in this case is to write a letter addressed to the next anesthesiologist.

In that letter, detail the troubles you had and have the patient carry that letter with them to give to the next anesthesiologist. That may avoid a later catastrophe.

And with any luck, this mechanic's manual will help you avoid catastrophes when you take your exam.

A caveat worth repeating. Entire books are written about the areas that we have covered in just a few pages. The mechanic's manual was intended to give you a look at major issues and how they might be used in the exam. The mechanic's manual is not comprehensive, just illustrative. Do your comprehensive reviews elsewhere.

And now you have some guideposts and some review under your belt. Time to quit dilly-dallying. Time to jump into the test track. Time to do some tests.

Just do it.

PART

III | Test Track

PRACTICE QUESTIONS

Part I of this book gave you some study tips, time proven methods that help people pass the boards.

Part II of this book gave a sketch, just a sketch, of some high points that might appear on the exam.

Part III is your time to work, to apply what you've learned. The questions are a mix, in no particular order. Sometimes the problems have long detailed explanations after them, sometimes short.

Certain things will recur, airway management, for example.

Certain complications will recur, such as rhythm disturbances. It is the authors' hope that by the end of these practice questions, you will be sick to death of saying the same answers to the same questions. We hope that by the end of these questions there is nothing you will not be ready to handle.

As previously mentioned, any disagreement or alternative explanation you come up with is *good*! Think it through yourself; don't take our word on it. *You* will be taking the test, not us. Look it up, talk it over with friends or colleagues. Get on the Internet and run the problems past someone in an anesthesia chat room. Maybe we got it wrong and you've got it right.

Where did we get these questions, these scenarios? Some we made up. Others we lived. We did these cases ourselves. And yes, we sweated bullets during the worst of them.

To most accurately reflect the karma of the test, this sample test section will follow the format of the real oral boards.

Chapter 22 comes from David and Steve's academic practice. Their approach to analyzing problems and answering questions is more detailed, analytical, and up-to-date. (This is Chris writing—David and Steve have better answers, to be brutally honest.) These questions will be a mixture of short- and long-stem questions. They will have extensive answers that outline the case preparation as well as detail the major aspects of each question and hopefully mimic the thought processes of a board examiner. This section will concentrate on preparing for the stem question. If you ace the stem, it's tough to fail the exam.

Chapter 23 comes from Chris's perspective and private practice. If there is a "systemic fault" in Chris's answers, that fault will be the "systemic fault" of the private practice world.

"Oh hell, let's just do the case."

The truth is not always pretty.

Session 1 will be a long question with all the preop stuff done. The questions will be intraop and postop. Following that question will be three shorter, grab bag questions.

Session 2 will be a shorter stem question followed by preop and intraop questions. After that will be another three grab bag questions.

Not enough, you say? OK, just for you, make that four grab bag questions.

Answers follow right away, so you don't have to flip to the back of the book. Don't cheat and look before you try to answer them yourselves! This is *your* time to answer the test, *your* time to shine. Our answers might not even be any good.

As a matter of fact, one of our answer sections will be completely wrong, and we're not even going to tell you which one! (Sort of a "Where's Waldo?" only you have to spot the bogus answers.) Why do we do this? To emphasize a point we've made again and again, this is a *guide book*, not a *textbook*.

Don't *read* this book; *work* this book.

There will be overlap. (There is no getting around the failed intubation question, for example.) You will see different "takes" on things. Is one right and one wrong?

Ah, you tell us, grasshopper.

We will approach each stem question using our suggested technique for outlining the stem and preparing for the exam. With practice, you will be able to effectively outline the stem question in 5 minutes or less, leaving the remaining 5 minutes of your preparation time to contemplate potential problems and their solutions based upon hints provided by the stem question.

Because the oral exam now has two formats, your preparation after receiving the stem question should concentrate upon the phases of the anesthetic targeted by the stem type. Regardless of the format, we recommend that you organize your thoughts in a uniform fashion with our systematic outline. However, because most of the preoperative workup information is already provided in the extended stem question format, your outline can be rapid with the main question being, "Have I been denied a crucial piece of information that precludes me from performing the anesthetic?"

Once you have answered this question, you should rapidly move on to the intraoperative and postoperative phases and anticipate the problems you are likely to encounter. Always remember that the examiners have a predetermined script, which is designed to provide a thorough and unbiased evaluation of your clinical abilities. Therefore, the problems encountered should be logical complications closely related to the clinical scenario provided. If you wind up discussing clinically irrelevant scientific minutiae, chances are that you missed the point of the question and need to rapidly refocus on the patient in your scenario.

Using only a general knowledge of anesthesia and our familiarity with the oral board mode of questioning, we have constructed a comprehensive review of the most likely points to be touched on during the exam. The majority will be familiar to you. Each case provides you a stem question. After reading the stem, stop and outline the scenario yourself using the techniques discussed earlier in the book. Then review our outline (with comments inserted in parentheses) for comparison. A list of questions similar to those the board examiners might ask is provided and then our responses. Practice writing (*and saying aloud*) your own answers. Then look at our answers and compare. Your answers may be different. They may be better. In any case, be able to defend what you say. We can.

CASE #1

An 85-year-old, 68 kg male sustains minor head trauma after falling from a swing set. He has a transient syncopal episode after the fall. Three days later he presents in the ER with a history of vomiting and confusion. An emergency craniotomy is scheduled. BP 170/90; HR 48; T 38°C; BUN 55.

***
Your Outline
(Don't be lazy. Do it yourself before reviewing ours!)
***

Our Outline

Urgency: This case is urgent. Although vital signs are strongly suggestive of elevated ICP that will require surgical treatment, the surgeon will request an emergent CT scan unless the patient's neurologic status is deteriorating rapidly. Therefore, some time is available for optimizing the patient's medical condition.

Reason for exam: Differential diagnosis of signs and symptoms in a life-threatening scenario. (Conflicting therapies are possible, as are signs and symptoms of multiple organ system disease. However, protecting the brain and managing complications are likely to be the major focus of this question.)

Problem List by System (Head-to-Toe Approach)

Head and neck: Possible cervical trauma (fall with head injury).

Neurologic: Status post head trauma (head injury was not "minor" if followed by syncope).

Increased ICP (vomiting, confusion, hypertension, bradycardia), possible impending herniation.

Airway: Possible C-spine injury

Cardiovascular:
1. Elderly male (increased sensitivity to pentothal, decreased drug clearance, decreased reserve in all organ systems)
2. Potential hemodynamic compromise (major surgery)
3. Hypertension and bradycardia (from increased ICP)

Respiratory: Possible aspiration (vomiting, altered mental status and elevated temp)

Gastrointestinal:
1. Vomiting due to increased ICP
2. At risk for gastric ulceration following head injury (Curling's ulcers)
3. Full stomach

Renal and electrolytes:
1. Elevated BUN
2. Vomiting and decreased intake

Hematopoietic: None
Other: None

Desired history and physical exam information:
- Exercise tolerance preinjury
- Medication and allergy history
- Brief neurologic exam (rule out preoperative neurologic deficits)
- Pupillary exam (R/O dilated pupils on one side suggesting herniation)
- Neck exam (tenderness along posterior spinous processes indicating injury)
- Airway exam
- Lung exam (rule out consolidation from aspiration)
- Neck veins, mucous membranes, urine output (clinically assess volume status)

Desired laboratory data:
- Serum K, Na, Cr
- Urine Na
- ABG
- Hematocrit

Desired tests:
- Head CT
- C-spine films
- Baseline EKG
- Chest x-ray (rule out pneumonia)

Preoperative therapy and monitoring:
- Large bore IV
- Arterial line
- Foley
- Routine ASA monitors (including ET CO_2)
- Multiorifice CVP line
- Precordial doppler
- Colloid infusion if oliguric
- Correct K and Na if dangerously low

Induction:
- Preoxygenate with 100% O_2
- Assuming normal airway, RSI with pentothal and rocuronium, in-line traction if C-spine is not cleared

Maintenance: Oxygen, isoflurane, fentanyl, rocuronium or cisatra-curium

Emergence: Extubate awake

Postoperative: ICU

Examiner's Questions

Preoperative

1. What are the signs and symptoms of increased intracranial pressure?
2. What is the fundoscopic finding diagnostic of increased ICP?
3. What is the significance of pupillary dilation in a patient with head trauma?
4. Would you delay the operation for C-spine films in this patient? Why or why not?
5. The patient becomes somewhat agitated and the surgeon asks your recommendation for sedation in the CT scanner. What would be your response?
6. What is the significance of the elevated blood pressure? Should the BP be treated? Why or why not? What is the definition of cerebral perfusion pressure?
7. Is your management altered by the temperature of 38°C? Why or why not?
8. Why is the BUN elevated? What is the difference between prerenal azotemia and intrinsic renal disease? How do you make the diagnosis? Assuming a FeNa of less than one, how would your therapy be altered? How do you calculate FeNa? What is the significance of a urine Na less than 10?
9. An arterial blood gas reveals the following: pH 7.54/pCO_2 34/pO_2 85. Please interpret the result for this patient. What would you expect the serum Cl level to be?
10. Should you place a nasogastric tube preoperatively to drain the stomach?

Intraoperative

11. How would you induce this patient? Why? Is the risk of uncal herniation increased with RSI? Is succinylcholine contraindicated in this scenario? Why or why not?
12. What monitors would you place? Why? What IV fluid would you select for maintenance? Why? Would you add dextrose to the IV fluid to offset the poor PO intake over the last 3 days?
13. As you prepare the patient in the preop holding area, the patient develops grand mal seizure activity. What would you do? The patient develops an elliptical pupil on the right side. Why? How can you acutely decrease ICP? The pupils become symmetric. What is your target $ETCO_2$ in this patient?
14. A right craniotomy is performed. During the operation, the patient acutely develops severe hypotension and tachycardia?

What is the diagnosis? What is your management? How do you make the diagnosis of venous air embolism? What is the management of venous air embolism?

15. Is invasive ICP monitoring necessary in this patient? Why or why not? What techniques are available to monitor ICP? What are the advantages of a ventriculostomy over a subdural bolt? What are the risks of ICP monitoring?

Answers to Questions

1. The signs and symptoms of increased ICP are headache, vomiting without nausea, altered mental status (lethargy, confusion), and papilledema. Hypertension and bradycardia are the classic "Cushing's response" to dangerously elevated ICP. Obtundation, focal neurologic findings and hemodynamic instabilty are late findings that indicate pending uncal herniation.

2. Papilledema is swelling and obliteration of the normal optic disc as back pressure and swelling of the optic nerve occurs from increased ICP.

3. Unilateral then bilateral pupillary dilation (classically in an elliptical shape) are focal neurologic findings that signal downward herniation of the uncus through the tentorium of the brain with pressure exerted on cranial nerve III.

4. Assuming the patient is able to respond appropriately to pain and has a normal airway (make the patient healthy!), lack of tenderness along the posterior spinous processes of the neck makes a cervical fracture extremely unlikely and we would proceed without the x-ray if it had not already been done. If the examiners make the patient's exam unreliable, a lateral C-spine x-ray done at the same time as the chest x-ray will not significantly delay the operation and will rule out the vast majority of significant neck fractures. As long as the patient's neurologic exam is not deteriorating, we would obtain this film. If the patient deteriorates, we would proceed with intubation with in-line traction. Awake fiberoptic intubation with potential for coughing and gagging would significantly raise ICP. (Remember, adaptation to a changing clinical scenario is one of the major aptitudes the examiners are looking for in the oral exam.)

5. Red flags, alarms, and flashing lights should go off in your head when a question is phrased this way. This is a trap. If you recommend sedation without accompanying the patient to the CT scanner, you better hope your frequent flyer miles are adequate for another round-trip ticket to next year's boards. Agitation can be a sign of deteriorating neurologic status, hypoxemia, or hemodynamic instability. Sedation obscures the neurologic exam. Surgical intervention may be necessary without the CT scan.

6. You may simply be asked if you want to treat the patient's hypertension. Don't be fooled, the blood pressure is up for a reason; the patient has increased ICP with a reflex bradycardia. If you lower the blood pressure, you will *decrease the cerebral perfusion pressure* (examiners love to hear that). Cerebral perfusion pressure = mean arterial pressure – intracranial pressure. Don't lower the blood pressure in this scenario.

7. The patient's temperature is elevated, increasing his cerebral metabolic rate. Cool the patient—acetaminophen, don't warm the IV fluids or the room—to decrease the cerebral metabolic rate of oxygen consumption ($CMRO_2$). Also, the temperature may be elevated from an infection, such as pneumonia secondary to aspiration during the loss of consciousness. Check the chest x-ray.

8. You won't get lots of lab data on this type of stem question, but the examiners will ask you about the lab data you do get. Why the high BUN? Dehydration from vomiting, preexisting intrinsic renal disease, obstructive uropathy, or reabsorption of a hematoma (or blood in the gut) are all possible. Is this a new abnormality? Old lab values as a baseline would be helpful. How should you actually answer the question? Don't waste time pecking around for more information if it is not readily available. Get on with the answer (time used without scoring points is time wasted). Control the exam and say, "I would try to get old labs as a baseline. Assuming that this is a new abnormality, my most likely diagnosis would be dehydration secondary to vomiting. I would then look to see if further lab tests—such as an arterial blood gas, potassium chloride, and creatinine—confirmed that diagnosis." The examiners will then ask you what you expect those further lab tests to show. You say, "Hypochloremic, hypokalemic metabolic alkalosis with a BUN/creatinine ratio >20/1." (The examiners then check off bonus points on your score sheet and you move on. This is kind of fun, isn't it?) Prerenal azotemia is inadequate renal perfusion (from any cause) that results in inadequate glomerular filtration to allow adequate clearance of BUN. If severe and allowed to persist, prerenal azotemia will progress to renal tubular damage and nonfunctional nephrons (intrinsic renal disease). The diagnosis is made by the patient's clinical condition (dehydration, hypotension, low cardiac output suggest prerenal), absence of obstuctive uropathy (place a Foley), BUN/Cr ratio (>20/1 is consistent with prerenal), fractional excretion of Na (less than 1 is consistent with prerenal), and urine sodium less than 10 (as the kidney attempts to conserve Na in a prerenal state). FeNa is calculated as urine/plasma Na ratio divided by urine over plasma Cr ratio. Vital signs are vital, they are all given to you for a reason.

9. When you are given blood gas results, write them down. This ABG represents a mixed metabolic and respiratory alkalosis. Spontaneous hyperventilation is likely as a response to increased ICP. The metabolic component is a combination of dehydration and loss of potassium and hydrogen ions in the vomitus. The Cl level will be low as a result of excess bicarbonate.

10. We would not place a nasogastric tube. The risk of coughing and gagging with acute elevation of ICP would outweigh the benefit. A nasogastric tube does not preclude vomiting and aspiration. Placing an NG tube also tends to decrease the effectiveness of the esophagogastric junction. We are planning a rapid sequence induction with cricoid pressure.

11. Assuming the airway was normal, we would use a rapid sequence induction with preoxygenation, lidocaine preinduction to blunt the response to intubation, pentothal, and rocuronium. We would intubate with the head fixed in neutral position if the C-spine had not been cleared. Pentothal is effective at decreasing $CMRO_2$. Rocuronium is fast-acting and hemodynamically neutral. Coughing and gagging increase ICP. Therefore, care must be taken during a RSI to administer adequate muscle relaxant and wait long enough before laryngoscopy. Fentanyl would be nice to blunt the hemodynamic response to laryngoscopy but may not be advisable for a true RSI—it would have to be administered by titration to an already lethargic patient with possible loss of consciousness at first dosing. Therefore, we selected IV lidocaine for this purpose. Succinylcholine does raise ICP—maybe. Some of the increased ICP in old studies was thought due to hyperextension of the neck and subsequent compromise of venous outflow during the RSI. However, even if true, the rise is not drastic and is short-lived. Therefore, if there was concern over a potential difficult airway, we would use succinylcholine in this scenario.

12. In addition to routine ASA monitors including $ETCO_2$ (capnography is now considered routine by most practitioners but we would mention it anyway because of its importance in this case), we would place a Foley catheter, an arterial line, a multiorifice CVP line, and a precordial doppler if the head is higher than the heart. Assuming no evidence of cardiac disease, a PA catheter is not necessary. The arterial line is necessary for tight BP control during the operation. The CVP is optional with the rationale being a potential for large fluid shifts in this procedure and for potential aspiration of venous air. Crystalloid or colloid is not important (we would likely use a combination of lactated Ringer's and hetastarch). However, the fluid should not be hypotonic or contain dextrose in order to prevent elevation of intracranial free water.

13. If grand mal seizure activity occurs, bad things are happening in the brain that will worsen with prolonged seizures (markedly increased $CMRO_2$). Anesthesia should be induced at once with whatever monitoring is readily available. If medications are given to stop the seizure activity, the patient will hypoventilate and drive up the ICP. We would do a RSI with an IV and a NIBP cuff. The elliptical pupil is a harbinger of uncal herniation. After assuring correct ETT placement and adequate ventilation, we would hyperventilate to a pCO_2 of 25 to 30 mm Hg, raise the head of the bed 30°, administer Lasix and mannitol, and encourage the surgeon to decompress the brain expeditiously. Steroids are of little benefit in head trauma (cytotoxic versus vasogenic edema—remember? OK, maybe you don't, not to worry.). Target $ETCO_2$ is 25 mm Hg. $ETCO_2$ runs about 4 to 7 mm Hg below pCO_2 in a patient with normal ventilation.

14. The most likely diagnosis for acute hypotension and tachycardia in this patient is venous air embolism. Anesthetic overdose, hypovolemia and anaphylaxis are certainly possible, but give the most likely diagnosis first. An acute change without an obvious acute blood loss in an otherwise stable anesthetic is likely air embolism during craniotomy (you almost can't fail if you slam-dunk the question on venous air embolism). The diagnosis of venous air embolus is made with the following—best to worst (decreasing order of sensitivity): transesophageal echo, precordial doppler, end-tidal nitrogen, acute drop in $ETCO_2$, increase in arterial to $ETCO_2$ gradient, increased PA pressures, ECG pattern of right heart strain, hemodynamic collapse. Treatment of air embolus is as follows: supportive measures, 100% oxygen while flooding the field, call for help, position the patient head down and tilt the table so that the right side is up (takes air away from pulmonary outflow track and relieves obstruction) and aspirate through your multiorifice CVP line. Raise CVP by fluid loading. Avoid PEEP as you might risk sending a paradoxical air embolus through a patent foramen ovale. Get ready for CPR if necessary. Have epinephrine ready. Congratulations! Your patient just survived the intraoperative critical event in this case.

15. ICP monitoring would be very helpful in this case. The ICP is elevated preoperatively and postoperative edema will not help the situation. A ventriculostomy has the advantage of allowing the sampling of CSF and can be therapeutic in drainage of CSF if the ICP becomes dangerously high. A subdural bolt is a pressure monitor only. The risks of ICP monitoring are mainly the risks of cerebral tissue damage during placement and infection. We would prefer a ventriculostomy for postoperative management in this case, given the subtentorial herniation that was beginning to occur at the start of the anesthetic.

(I told you that Steve and David had good answers.)

CASE #2

A 67-year-old male is scheduled for elective AAA repair. Past medical history is significant for hypertension and coronary artery disease status post subendocardial myocardial infarction 4 months ago. The patient has been pain-free on medical management since his myocardial infarction. Patient smokes two packs of cigarettes per day and is attempting to cut down. His local physician detected a left carotid bruit on a recent physical exam. He has a history of an allergy to penicillin, which causes a rash. He leads a sedentary lifestyle. No history of orthopnea, PND, peripheral edema, syncope, or near-syncope.

Medications:
- Atenolol, 100 mg qAM
- Lisinopril, 10 mg bid

- Hydrochlorothiazide, 25 mg qAM
- Digoxin, 0.25 mg qAM
- Sublingual NTG prn

Physical Exam: Height—71 inches, weight—215 pounds, BP 160/95, HR 64, R 18, T 37°C

Head and neck: Left carotid bruit, normal carotid upstroke bilaterally

Airway: Malampati class III, full range of motion of the neck, normal thyromental distance, large tongue

Cardiac: Regular rate and rhythm, 3/6 midsystolic crescendo/decrescendo murmur over right upper sternal border without radiation

Pulmonary: Distant breath sounds, barrel chest, bibasilar crackles with deep inspiration, no wheezing

Abdomen: Pulsatile abdominal mass

Extremities: Decreased pulses in the feet; thinned shiny skin with loss of hair over shins bilaterally

Laboratory values: Hematocrit 51%, K 3.1, BUN 32, Cr 1.8

Chest x-ray: Flattened hemidiaphragms, lower lobe plate-like atelectasis bilaterally, calcified aortic knob and tortuous aorta, no acute infiltrates

ECG: Normal sinus rhythm, LVH with flattened T wave in lateral leads

Exercise treadmill test 1 month ago on current medications: Maximum heart rate 106, no chest pain, no ECG changes, test stopped at 6 minutes and 47 seconds secondary to claudication

Abdominal CT scan: 6-cm AAA extending from above the renal arteries to the aortic bifurcation

***
Your Outline
***

Our Outline

This case is representative of the newer type of format. You are provided with extensive preoperative information, not necessarily complete information. Avoid the urge to let the examiners place you in the middle of an anesthetic, which you would never have performed in the first place. You will not be able to avoid performing the anesthetic, but at least make the examiners aware of your preoperative concerns. If possible, attempt to make the patient healthy by assuming that the workup information not provided is normal. Do not dwell on the preoperative outline. Identify any crucial information that is missing from the workup. Then concentrate on the problem list and plan formulation.

Urgency: This case is elective. If crucial information is missing, opportunity exists to complete the workup.

Reason for exam: Ramifications of multisystem disease. The problems you are likely to encounter should be predictable from the stem question.

Problem List

Head and neck: None

Neurologic: None

Airway: Potential for difficult airway with Malampati Class III

Cardiovascular:

- Abdominal aortic aneurysm
- Major surgery requiring aortic cross-clamp
- Peripheral vascular disease with claudication
- Poor distal perfusion of the legs
- Known coronary artery disease with recent MI
- Increased risk for perioperative MI
- Possible myocardium at risk with nondiagnostic TMST (treadmill stress test)
- Poorly controlled hypertension
- Cerebrovascular disease with carotid bruit
- Possible aortic stenosis with systolic murmur
- Digoxin therapy
- Possible history of atrial dysrhythmias
- Potential for digoxin-induced dysrhythmias with low K

Pulmonary:

1. COPD
2. Heavy tobacco use
3. Elevated hematocrit possibly due to chronic hypoxemia

Gastrointestinal: None

Renal and electrolytes:

1. Renal insufficiency with elevated creatinine and BUN/Cr ratio less than 20/1
2. Hypokalemia secondary to diuretic use
3. Potential acute renal failure from suprarenal cross-clamp

Hematologic: Polycythemia likely secondary to tobacco abuse

Other: None

Physical examination information desired but not supplied: None

Laboratory values desired but not supplied:

- Arterial blood gas
- Screening spirometry with and without bronchodilators

Tests required: Dobutamine stress echocardiogram. With the recent MI and elective aortic surgery, the risk from the coronary artery disease may be prohibitive. A persantine thallium would identify myocardium at risk and a MUGA would evaluate LV function. A dobutamine echo would evaluate myocardium at risk and LV function as well as rule out significant aortic stenosis. The results would alter therapy because we would cancel the elective case for cardiac catheterization and possible primary heart surgery if significant myocardium at risk or valvular disease is present.

Preoperative therapy and monitoring:
- Large bore IV access
- Replace K to a level above 3.5 mEq/L
- Control hypertension prior to induction with esmolol or metoprolol (Beta 1 blockers, leave airways mostly alone) and/or infusions of nitroglycerin and nitroprusside; have phenylephrine available for titration
- Routine ASA monitors
- Five-lead ECG
- Six units of type and cross-matched blood in the OR
- Foley
- Arterial line
- Epidural catheter
- Pulmonary artery catheter
- Consider transesophageal echocardiography

Induction:
- Premedicate with midazolam
- Preoxygenate with 100% oxygen; have #4 and #5 LMA in the room for potential difficult intubation
- Assuming patient is NPO for surgery and LV function is OK (again make the patient *HEALTHY*), induce with fentanyl, pentothal, and succinylcholine

Maintenance: Oxygen, isoflurane, fentanyl, vecuronium

Emergence: Extubate only if surgery is uncomplicated and patient is optimized

Postoperative care: ICU

Anticipated problems:
- Hemodynamic instability
- Myocardial ischemia
- Bleeding
- Oliguria
- Dysrhythmias
- Complications from epidural catheter

Examiner's Questions

Intraoperative

1. What monitoring would you use for this case? Why? If a PA catheter is used, should it be placed before or after induction? Why? Would continuous mixed venous saturation be helpful? Why or why not? What is the differential diagnosis of an acute drop in SvO_2? What causes a high SvO_2? Would transesophageal echocardiography be helpful in this case? Why or why not? Would you use TEE?

2. Would you place an epidural catheter prior to induction in this patient? Why or why not? Would a thoracic epidural be better than a lumbar epidural in this case? What medications would you administer via the epidural? If you aspirated blood through the catheter immediately following placement, what would you do? Would you cancel the case? Would you replace the catheter?

3. How would you monitor for myocardial ischemia in this patient? How about dysrhythmias? If you only had a three-lead ECG, what is the best way to monitor for ischemia? Is a PA catheter a sensitive monitor of ischemia? How about TEE?

4. What vasoactive agents would you prepare for use in this case? Why? What fluids would you use? Is colloid better that crystalloid in this case? Why?

5. How would you induce this patient? During induction, the patient develops hypertension and tachycardia with acute ST segment elevation in lead V5. What would you do? If bigeminy developed, what would appropriate action be? Why?

6. During dissection, the aneurysm ruptures. What are the appropriate actions on your part? What is the surgeon likely to do? What are the consequences of supradiaphragmatic cross-clamp?

7. Following repair of the aorta, as the cross-clamp is removed, severe systemic hypotension develops. What would you do? You note acute elevation of your pulmonary artery pressure. What is the differential diagnosis? What is the appropriate intervention?

Postoperative

8. Two hours after arriving in the ICU, hypotension develops. What is the most likely etiology? What would you do? The surgeon suggests that the hypotension is due to the epidural. How would you respond?

9. The patient develops oliguria in the ICU. What is the differential diagnosis? How would you determine the etiology of the oliguria? Assuming a urine Na of <10, a PCWP of 24, a MAP

of 72, heart rate of 67 and a SvO_2 of 55%, what is the most likely etiology of the oliguria?

10. Following extubation, the patient is hemodynamically stable and pain-free, but complains of inability to move his legs. You are called for advice. What is the most likely diagnosis? How would you evaluate?

Our Answers

   1. What monitoring would we use? The works. This case is brimming with opportunities to excel. It is also a prime example of multisystem disease with which an experienced examiner could fail almost anyone. Fortunately, the examiners are not there to fail qualified candidates. The object is to make consultants in anesthesiology out of qualified candidates. You simply have to display what you know. This question is also one in which you must control the environment of the exam. If you jump right in and administer pentothal and succinylcholine, you waste your rather pricey examination fee. Tactfully let the examiners know up front that you have reservations about performing elective major surgery on a patient following a recent MI without a complete cardiac evaluation. When asked about monitoring, you have an opportunity to express your concerns. An appropriate answer might be, "I am extremely concerned about this patient's ability to tolerate the scheduled procedure. In an elective case, I need more information about myocardium at risk and the ability of the heart to respond to the stress which is inevitable for this procedure." The examiners may stop you at this point and ask if you would cancel the case. We would. They also might concede that elective surgery is not recommended and change the scenario to one of a rapidly enlarging aneurysm, which is no longer elective. If they do not stop you, then make the patient healthy with assumptions, "Assuming that there is no further myocardium at risk and that the patient has good LV function, I would proceed with routine ASA monitors, 5-lead ECG, arterial line, PA catheter, and Foley catheter." The examiners should not dwell on the preoperative evaluation in this format and neither should you. However, express your concerns if you are asked to perform an anesthetic that you think is ill-advised. Then move on. Even though this case is complicated, the problems you will face are predictable. Mixed venous oxygen saturation may be helpful in this case. One of the body's earliest responses to a stress is to extract more oxygen from the red blood cells as they go by, resulting in a decreased SvO_2. We think of SvO_2 as a tool that allows us 20 to 30 minutes head start on a cardiac arrest. If you are likely to need this head start, then use the information. An acute drop in SvO_2 results from inadequate oxygen delivery to meet tissue demand. This can be due to low oxygen content of the blood (anemia or hypoxemia), low cardiac output or excessive demand. High SvO_2 results from decreased off-loading of oxygen in the tissue (arteriovenous shunts, abnormal oxygen affinity for hemoglobin, carbon monoxide poisoning, misdirection of blood flow as in sepsis or liver failure, or inability of the cell to utilize oxygen as in cell death or cyanide poisoning), excessive cardiac output (volume overload or drugs), or decreased demand. Transesophageal echocardiography may be helpful in this case. It provides one of the earliest markers of ischemic myocardium (if you are one of those rare experts who really knows how to use it) and is excellent in assessing adequacy of preload in a situation where elevated PCWP may not correlate with increased LVEDV. Avoid the trap of agreeing to TEE placement if you are not comfortable with performing and interpreting the exam. If you do not use TEE regularly, either acknowledge that the information may be valuable, but that the case can be performed safely without it (no outcome studies have ever been done), or else consult a cardiologist to perform and interpret the exam. If the exam is performed, the examiners will certainly expect you to use the information.

2. Assuming no history of bleeding and no preoperative anticoagulant therapy other than aspirin or mini-dose subcutaneous heparin, we would place an epidural in this case. Low molecular weight heparin is another story—no epidural then. Optimal epidural pain control may enhance postoperative pulmonary function without excess sedation, especially in a patient with a heavy history of tobacco use and COPD. However, there is no conclusive data that outcome is improved over PCA narcotics. Although the incision extends above the umbilicus, there is no outcome evidence that a thoracic epidural is superior to lumbar for this case. As a matter of fact, in anesthesia, given the proclivity of our academic brethren to produce and publish rat studies, "There is no outcome evidence to support that," can be your mantra. After giving a test dose of lidocaine with epinephrine, we would use epidural narcotic to avoid potentiating hypotension that is likely to occur during the procedure. You could argue that the sympathectomy induced with local anesthetic is protective against myocardial ischemia, especially in the postoperative period. True, but we would rather not deal with the dilemma of irreversible sympathectomy during a case with the possibility of massive blood loss, or with postoperative hypotension possibly related to our catheter. If blood aspirates from the catheter after placement, we would remove it and repeat the placement at a different level. We would not cancel the case. Heparin administration is more than 1 hour away and we would not have placed the catheter in the first place if the patient were at excessive risk of an epidural hematoma. If frank blood is obtained through the catheter, some would argue for a couple hours of delay to allow appropriate clotting. Some could suggest cancellation as that is "proven" safe in one study. Pick a position and defend it, even while acknowledging the merits of the other side's argument.

3. Assuming there is no myocardium at risk, we would use a 5-lead ECG and a PA catheter to monitor for ischemia in this case. If the examiners did not allow us to assume lack of myocardium at risk, the cardiac anesthesiologists among us would add TEE. Lead II is best for monitoring dysrhythmias. The unavailable 5-lead system is a classic exam question. You can move the left arm lead to the V5 position and monitor Lead I to create a V5 lead. Elevation of pulmonary artery pressure or a V wave on PCWP are late findings in ischemia. Other things

(like fluid loading conditions) can mimic these changes as well. Lead V5 is more sensitive. TEE is a sensitive and early monitor for ischemia, but on-line interpretation has been shown to be pretty abysmal so be prepared for some challenge if you select TEE.

4. The vasoactive medications we would select are nitroglycerin, nitroprusside, and phenylephrine infusion. We would have labetolol or esmolol as well as dilute nitroprusside, phenylephrine, and epinephrine for bolus dosing. Rapid-acting agents are necessary to control the inevitable blood pressure swings in this case. If the debate over crystalloid versus colloid did not exist, scientific meetings would be a lot shorter. This tells you that the correct answer is unknown. We would use a combination of crystalloid and blood when necessary. The only outcome studies out there suggest adequate resuscitation is more important than choice of fluid. Pick a stance and defend it.

5. Assuming the patient is NPO for at least 6 hours, we would premedicate with midazolam and preoxygenate with 100% oxygen. We are concerned about a possible difficult airway. However, we feel the risk of hemodynamic instability upon awake fiberoptic intubation or rapid sequence induction outweighs the benefit. Although starting with a fiberoptic with careful attention to hemodynamics and great topicalization is an option if you like. However, we will choose succinylcholine and have an appropriate sized LMA in the room because of the Mallampati-3 exam. Given the complexity of this case, difficulty intubating is unlikely to be in the examiners' script. Exercise due care and you are unlikely to be challenged. *Remember, you are always concerned.* We would induce with fentanyl, pentothal, and succinylcholine. Hypertension, tachycardia, and ST changes in V5 demand immediate attention. Assure adequate oxygenation and ventilation with 100% oxygen (airway is always first, followed by breathing), deepen the anesthetic, administer esmolol, start a nitroglycerin infusion. If not a preexisting stable rhythm, bigeminy is a marker for ischemia, hypercarbia, light anesthesia, or acidosis. If the measures just listed do not resolve the bigeminy, then check an ABG and optimize ventilation and acid-base status. Lidocaine is indicated if multifocal PVCs or couplets develop. Remember, even unifocal PVCs can be a harbinger of badness if they are being caused by new ischemia.

6. If the aneurysm ruptures, open up the IVs, turn off any inhaled agents, assure 100% O_2, call for help, temporize with phenylephrine and possibly epinephrine, and start transfusing. The surgeon should apply direct pressure. He may have to clamp the aorta above the diaphragm. If so, the risk of splanchnic ischemia and spinal cord ischemia is increased and added to the predicted renal ischemia.

7. Hypotension on cross-clamp removal is common. It should be transient and secondary to an acute decrease in SVR, hyperemic dilation of the venous system, as well as negative inotropic effects of washout of lactic acid and potassium from the ischemic lower extremities. The patient is likely to be intravascularly volume depleted. Temporize with phenylephrine, turn on 100% O_2, turn off inhaled agents, and administer IV fluids. Acute pulmonary hypertension can be due to metabolic acidosis, hypoventilation, hypoxemia, LV failure, over-aggressive volume resuscitation, or pulmonary embolus. Assure adequate ventilation and oxygenation, draw an ABG, turn on or increase the nitroglycerin infusion, check PA pressures and pulmonary capillary wedge pressure to differentiate LV failure from pulmonary arterial vasoconstriction, and measure cardiac output. Consider pulmonary vasodilation and right heart support with a phosphodiesterase inhibitor such as milrinone, if indicated.

8. Hypotension in the ICU following AAA repair is most likely relative hypovolemia as "third-space" fluid accumulates. If the examiners ask you for the most likely diagnosis, do not provide a list. They want to know if you are able to use clinical judgement to prioritize your treatment. You could just mention that you would consider "preload, contractility, afterload, rate and rhythm with the most likely cause being…." Assuming the PA catheter pressures confirm your diagnosis and the hematocrit is acceptable, administer IV fluid. If the surgeon blames the epidural for the hypotension and you have no local anesthetic infusing, "Deny, deny, deny!" (tactfully, of course). If local anesthetic is infusing and the cardiac filling pressures are adequate, hold the infusion to prevent clouding the clinical picture. You can always change to bolus narcotic or infusion hydromorphone.

9. Classic question. Oliguria is due to prerenal, intrinsic renal, or post-renal causes. Flush the Foley to rule out obstruction then differentiate between the other two. Differential diagnosis includes intravascular volume depletion, low cardiac output, inadequate renal artery perfusion pressure, atherosclerotic emboli to the kidneys from suprarenal cross-clamp, and renal ischemia from prolonged cross-clamp. After assuring Foley patency, we would evaluate the hemodynamic status with the PA catheter, collect urine for creatinine clearance, measure urine sodium, administer a fluid bolus, and observe over the next hour. With a low urine Na, the oliguria is likely prerenal. High PCWP, adequate MAP, and low SvO_2 argue that the prerenal state is secondary to LV failure with low cardiac output.

10. Painless lower extremity weakness postoperatively is either due to the epidural or spinal cord ischemia from the aortic cross-clamp (especially if the clamp was emergently placed above the diaphragm), although one must always be concerned about a potential epidural hematoma (most likely associated with breakthrough pain in the back). *Examine the patient!* Do not treat anything over the telephone on the oral boards. Assuming lower extremity weakness is present, turn off any local anesthetic infusion running in your epidural. Observation for

2 to 4 hours following discontinuation of the local anesthetic is risky, but can be defended based upon the half-life of the anesthetic. If no local anesthetic is running, the concentration is low enough to be unlikely to produce lower extremity weakness or the weakness persists following discontinuation of the local anesthetic infusion, obtain a CT scan or MRI emergently. Spinal cord ischemia is a diagnosis of exclusion. Epidural hematoma must be treated with emergent decompressive surgery.

CASE #3

A 47-year-old female status post left nephrectomy and chemotherapy for renal cell carcinoma 3 years ago is admitted with a large pericardial effusion. Attempted pericardiocentesis was unsuccessful on two occasions secondary to loculation of the effusion. The patient did not tolerate the procedure well and demands to be put to sleep before any further diagnostic or therapeutic intervention. She is scheduled for emergent subxiphoid pericardial window under general anesthesia. She has a history of gastroesophageal reflux controlled with medication.

> *Medications:*
> - Furosemide, 20 mg PO bid
> - KCl, 40 mEq PO qAM
> - Omeprazole, 20 mg PO qhs
> - Mylanta, prn

> *Physical exam:* Ill-appearing, anxious female in moderate respiratory distress
> *Vital signs:* BP 86/64, pulse 128, resp rate 32, temp 37.2°C, SaO$_2$ 98% on 3 L O$_2$ per nasal cannula, height 64 inches, weight 157 pounds.
> *Head and neck:* Palpable bulky tumor from clavicle to angle of the mandible bilaterally; tumor bulk more prominent on left than right; no neck veins visible or palpable
> *Airway:* Mallampati II, small mouth, unable to extend neck due to tumor, short chin
> *Cardiovascular:* Muffled heart sounds, regular rate and rhythm, rapid thready pulse that disappears on inspiration, slow capillary refill in nail beds, 4+ pitting edema in upper and lower extremities bilaterally
> *Pulmonary:* Clear to auscultation
> *Abdomen:* Enlarged liver with tender edge, fluid wave present
> *Extremities:* Infiltrated 22-gauge IV in left antecubital vein, no visible or palpable peripheral venous access
> *ECG:* Sinus tachycardia with electrical alternans, no significant ST wave changes

Chest x-ray: Enlarged "waterbag" cardiac silhouette with clear lung fields

Head CT: Done 1 month ago, negative for metastatic disease

Laboratory: HCT 32; Creatinine 1.2; BUN 46; SGOT 96; SGPT 116; bilirubin 1.2; sodium 128; potassium 3.2; WBC 13.2; pH 7.28, pCO_2 32, pO_2 72, BE −12, PT 13.2, urine output 20 cc/hr; urine sodium <10

Echocardiogram: Large pericardial effusion, right ventricular diastolic collapse, small D-shaped left ventricular cavity, no wall motion abnormalities

***
Your Outline
***

Our Outline

Urgency: Emergent. Vital signs are unstable. Attempts at nonsurgical therapy unsuccessful.

Reason for exam: Conflicting therapies. Sure you have multiple system organ disease, but the real emphasis on this exam is how to deal with a life-threatening scenario in an uncooperative patient with a difficult airway, no IV access and a sick heart. The diagnosis is handed to you with ample information in the stem question. Therefore, move quickly through the outline and prepare for what is likely to be a challenging anesthetic.

Problem List

Head and neck: Bulky tumor
- Potential airway compromise
- Venous obstruction with upper extremity edema

Neurologic: None

Airway: Difficult airway
- Laryngoscopy likely unsuccessful
- Patient refuses awake intubation

Cardiovascular: Cardiogenic shock
- Pericardial effusion with tamponade physiology
- Right ventricular diastolic collapse
- Pulsus paradoxus
- Electrical alternans
- D-shaped LV
- No pulmonary congestion
- Right heart failure
- Hepatic congestion
- Lower extremity edema
- Low cardiac output syndrome
- Peripheral hypoperfusion
- Metabolic acidosis
- Oliguria

Pulmonary: None

Gastrointestinal:
- Passive hepatic congestion
- Elevated LFTs
- Ascites
- Gastroesophageal reflux

Renal:
- Prerenal azotemia
- Elevated BUN
- Oliguria
- Una <10
- Metabolic acidosis

Hematopoietic: None

Extremities: Poor IV access
- Peripheral edema
- History of chemotherapy

Other: Ethical dilemma
- Likely to refuse recommended therapy
- Emergent situation
- Capacity to decide?

Desired physical exam findings: None
Desired laboratory values: None
Desired tests: None
Consults: Discuss plan with surgeon

Preoperative therapy and monitoring:
- IV access
- Arterial line
- Routine ASA
- CVP
- Foley
- #3 and #4 LMA in room
- Fiberoptic bronchoscope in room
- Surgeon in room
- Prep before induction
- Phenylephrine, Na bicarbonate, epinephrine, and norepinephrine

Induction: Premed with glycopyrrolate and midazolam, 100% O_2 preoxygenation, $NaHCO_3$ to reverse acidosis, ketamine sedation with spontaneous ventilation

Maintenance: NO_2/O_2, ketamine boluses, local anesthetic at incision site

Emergence: Extubate awake, if intubation is required

Postop: ICU

Anticipated problems:
- Ethics
- IV access
- Loss of airway
- Hemodynamic instability on induction

Examiners' Questions

Intraoperative

1. What options are available to you for anesthesia in this case? Which would you prefer?

2. The patient refuses any procedures before being "knocked out." How do you counsel the patient? Does this patient have the "capacity to decide" her treatment? What are the components of capacity to decide? When would you be forced to "act on her behalf?" Does the presence of next-of-kin alter a decision to "act on her behalf?" How about a living will? How about a power of attorney for medical decisions? Assuming the patient has capacity to decide and accepts arterial and central line placement, but continues to demand to be asleep for the procedure, what would you do?

3. How would you obtain IV access in this patient? Why? What monitoring would you use? If you chose femoral venous access, how would your CVP correlate with right heart filling in this patient? What are the risks of internal jugular vein cannulation in this patient? How about subclavian? Is a PA catheter of any benefit in this case?

4. Are you concerned about the risk of regurgitation and aspiration in this patient? Would a rapid sequence induction be indicated? Why or why not? Upon induction (or sedation or skin prep), but before securing an airway, the patient's BP falls to 45/30 and heart rate increases to 170 with frequent irregular complexes. What would you do? Why? You are unable to visualize the epiglottis on laryngoscopy and unable to mask ventilate. What would you do? Why? The patient develops severe bradycardia with no palpable pulse. What would you do?

5. After surgical release of the tamponade, the patient stabilizes. You note yellow fluid in your airway. What would you do? Is bronchoscopy indicated? Why? Is intratracheal HCO_3 indicated? Why? Assuming you are ventilating through a LMA, how would you secure the airway before transfer to the ICU?

Postoperative

6. Upon arrival in the ICU, the patient is intubated with high airway pressures. She has bilateral breath sounds and diffuse rhonchi. ABG on 100% O_2 and PEEP5 shows pH 7.31, pCO_2 45, pO_2 53. How do you interpret this blood gas? What is your differential diagnosis? What is the difference between shunt and dead space ventilation? What is V/Q mismatch? How do you calculate A-a gradient? How do you make the diagnosis of ARDS? What is the pathophysiology of ARDS? Could this patient have ARDS from aspiration? How would you ventilate this patient? Why?

7. Is a PA catheter indicated at this point? Why or why not? If you were to place a PA catheter, how would you do it? What would you expect the PA catheter to show?

8. The patient is unarousable on POD #1. What are the possible etiologies? How would you evaluate?

9. What are the diagnostic criteria for brain death? If the patient meets the initial criteria for brain death, but the family "wants everything possible done," what would be the next step? The family refuses further testing for cerebral blood flow. What would you do? The patient meets all criteria for brain death upon reexamination on POD #2. What do you tell the family?

Our Answers

Caution! This series of questions and answers was developed by a cardiac anesthesiologist who was first an internist then a critical care specialist. Therefore, any references to Rho and La antibodies and their interaction with the Krebs cycle must be excused. The good news is that we will try to keep him from wandering into the land of medical esoterica. The bad news is that the people who write and administer oral board questions also tend to be boarded in way too many specialties. So...enjoy!

1. You have several options in this case, but be aware that pent/sux/tube is unlikely to be the correct choice. There may not be a correct choice. You could do the subxiphoid window under local anesthesia alone, which would most likely be the safest approach. The problem is that your patient won't cooperate. We would suggest this possibility and use it if the board examiner lets us (fat chance!). You could do an inhalation induction and attempt laryngoscopy with spontaneous ventilation, but you are unlikely to be able to intubate. Your patient may also crash with the inhaled agent due to vasodilation. Your patient will definitely crash with pent/sux/tube plus the tube part is unlikely to be successful. If you give a muscle relaxant, you will have another opportunity to take the orals next year. Tracheostomy is not an option with a bulky tumor. Positive pressure ventilation will compromise right heart filling and result in hemodynamic compromise. Assuming that intravenous and arterial access had been obtained, and given the fact that the heart needs to be maintained "fast, full, and tight" in this scenario, we would pretreat with a small dose of midazolam and glycopyrrolate (to prevent excess secretions) as well as give $NaHCO_3$ to offset the acidosis prior to induction. We induce with ketamine (remember that evil PCP derivative that causes flashbacks?). Ketamine maintains ventilation, heart rate, and vascular tone and a small dose of midazolam should be adequate to prevent the flashbacks. We would then support the airway (with a face mask or LMA depending on patency of the upper airway) and maintain with nitrous oxide and oxygen. We would use local anesthetic in the incision and intermittent ketamine as needed. Things are sure to go wrong, but we can defend our choices.

2. We would counsel the patient about the risks of general anesthesia or even sedation in her case and do our best to safely minimize discomfort. Capacity to decide has four components: 1) the patient understands her disease process, 2) the patient understands the natural history of the disease, 3) the patient understands the treatment options available, and 4) the patient understands the ramifications of her decision. Forget competency. Competency comes in handy when you are writing your will or establishing guardianship for financial affairs of an elderly parent, but is a legal determination that has little to do with medicine in a critical situation. Capacity to decide is a determination made by a patient's physician concerning his or her ability to make a decision taking into account the impact of the current disease process. Capacity to decide is extremely relevant in this case. You would be forced to act on her behalf if you determine that she lacks the capacity to decide because the hypotension or acidosis precludes her from thinking clearly and no surrogate decision-maker is available with a power of attorney for medical decisions. Next-of-kin can be helpful if they can tell you that she has voiced desires in the past which apply to the current situation. However, the desires of the next-of-kin are secondary to the patient's desire and are not binding if you have any doubt about whether they are acting in the patient's best interest. A living will usually does not apply in an acute, life-threatening event and only kicks in if the "attending physician and one other physician involved in the patient's care" agree that the current situation is terminal. Draining the effusion may resolve a life-threatening scenario. A medical power of attorney is different. This document selects an individual to make the tough choices if the patient lacks the capacity to decide. That individual becomes the patient's voice if the patient is unable to choose for themselves. Remember, in spite of all the legal mumbo-jumbo, you are never required to perform an anesthetic that, in your opinion, will harm the patient. If the patient accepted the IV and arterial line, we would counsel the patient that we are not performing a deep general anesthetic and the possibility exists that she might recall some of the events in the operating room, but that we would do our very best to ensure her safety and unconsciousness during the procedure. Then we would do the procedure as outlined above.

3. We would attempt right subclavian access on this patient. The tumor cannot be felt below the clavicle and venous pressures should be elevated. The tumor is less bulky on the right. We would not persist if unsuccessful because the vein may be completely obstructed by the tumor. Femoral venous access would be our second choice. We would monitor with routine ASA monitors, arterial line, CVP, and a Foley catheter. Femoral venous pressure may not correlate with CVP due to ascites with increased abdominal pressure. The trend may still be helpful. IJ cannulation will be next to impossible in this case due to the bulky tumor distorting the anatomy and will risk carotid puncture, pneumothorax, and uncontrolled bleeding from a vascular tumor. Subclavian cannulation has a higher risk of pneumothorax, risk of subclavian artery puncture, and vein laceration if the vein is obstucted. In our opinion, PA catheterization will be time-consuming and will not provide much additional information in this case. The diagnosis of tamponade is already confirmed.

4. Any time you are asked if you are concerned about something, the answer is, "Yes, I am concerned. However, because of _____, I would do _____." "Yes, we are very concerned about aspiration. However, the risk of hemodynamic compromise and losing the airway with a rapid sequence induction are much greater than the risk of aspiration pneumonia in this case." (Then ready your mind for aspiration pneumonia.) Surprise, surprise! The patient crashes on induction. Here we go! "Assuming the subxiphoid region had been prepped before induction as we had planned, we would apply 100% oxygen by mask to the spontaneously breathing patient and tell the surgeon to cut into the pericardium. We would call for help and administer phenylephrine to support the blood pressure. If the patient stops spontaneously ventilating we would attempt laryngoscopy and intubation. If we can't intubate or ventilate, we would use a LMA as in the airway algorithm (memorize it!). Chances are that the examiners will allow the LMA to work as emergent tracheostomy is not really a viable choice. If not, you might have your peer attempt intubation or try fiberoptic. Bradycardic arrest...classic hypoxemia. ABC, ABC, ABC.... Assure 100% O_2, check breath sounds, start CPR, communicate with the surgeon. The effusion has to be drained and direct cardiac massage will be much more effective even if they have to split the sternum. Administer drugs according to the ACLS algorithm for asystole (memorize it!).

5. The patient aspirated. Endotracheal suction should be immediately performed. Bronchoscopy with a large bronchoscope is only helpful acutely if particulate matter is present. Sterile sodium bicarbonate as a lavage fluid may be helpful if gastric acid is aspirated. Assuming the LMA is in place, we would load a #6 ETT over an intubating bronchoscpe, pass the scope through the LMA into the airway, slide the tube over the scope and slide the LMA off the tube. This is similar to the technique of a "fast-track LMA."

6. ICUs and ventilators—they go together like turkey and dressing. The blood gas shows a mild mixed respiratory and metabolic acidosis with severe hypoxemia. The main differential diagnosis *in this patient* includes oxygen disconnect, acute lung injury from aspiration and/or shock, acute cardiogenic pulmonary edema following cardiac arrest, previously undiagnosed pneumonia, hypoventilation with atelectasis, right mainstem intubation (unlikely with bilateral breath sounds). Shunt is perfusion through nonventilated lung, which produces arterial hemoglobin desaturation unresponsive to oxygen. Dead space ventilation is ventilated lung without perfusion, which produces arterial hemoglobin desaturation responsive to oxygen. V/Q mismatch is somewhere between shunt and dead space ventilation. Part of the lung is ventilated but inadequately perfused; part is perfused but inadequately ventilated. This produces (you guessed it) arterial hemoglobin desaturation somewhat responsive to oxygen. A-a gradient is calculated by subtracting water vapor pressure (47 mm Hg at sea level) from 760 mm Hg (atmospheric pressure), then multiplying the result (713) by the FIO_2, and subtracting 5/4 of the pCO_2 to obtain the alveolar pO_2

(PaO_2). Then simply subtract the PaO_2 (arterial pO_2 from the ABG) to get the A-a gradient. This is a marker of the severity of the V/Q mismatch. The diagnostic criteria for ARDS vary somewhat. Generally, they require severe hypoxemia ($pO_2 < 55$ on $FIO_2 > 0.5$ and at least 5 cm H_2O PEEP, for instance), bilateral pulmonary infiltrates on chest x-ray and a pulmonary edema without cardiogenic etiology (PCWP < 18). A simplistic approach to the pathophysiology of ARDS is to think of the syndrome as a pulmonary capillary leak phenomenon that occurs as a response to a stress (infection, aspiration, shock, cardiopulmonary bypass, watching prominent political figures waste your tax dollars and simultaneously lie to you over the past eight years, etc.). The stressor can be either a direct chemical irritant to the endothelial cell such as fat emboli or an insult such as shock that results in a systemic inflammatory response with release of all sorts of nasty mediators that attack the endothelial cell. This patient certainly could have early ARDS from aspiration. Because of the risk of barotrauma in acute lung injury, we would ventilate the patient with pressure ventilation sufficient to provide a tidal volume of 5–7 cc/kg, minimum rate of 15–18 to start, and PEEP titrated to optimize oxygenation without compromising hemodynamics.

7. A PA catheter would be helpful in this patient if the pulmonary defect does not rapidly reverse in order to optimize fluid administration and assure adequate oxygen delivery. In the setting of ARDS, we would use mixed venous oxygen saturation to optimize oxygen delivery. If the PA catheter did not float easily, we would use fluoroscopy to float it from either the subclavian or the femoral. Assuming the heart recovered from the resuscitated arrest and the problem is predominately acute lung injury, we would expect the PA catheter to show normal to low filling pressures, normal to high cardiac output and a decreased arterial to venous oxygen difference due to a systemic inflammatory response and peripheral arterial to venous shunting.

8. The etiologies of altered mental status are either neurologic, metabolic, or pharmacologic. After ruling out life-threatening problems such as hypotension, hypoxemia, or hypoglycemia, we would proceed to search for causes in each of the three categories. In this patient on POD #1 following a cardiac arrest, the most likely etiology is ischemic neurologic injury. However, we would look closely at the medications administered and possible electrolyte abnormalities that could explain the problem. We would assure muscle relaxant reversal and perform a neurologic exam to identify gross neurologic deficits. We would consult neurology. If no other etiology is identified and the patient is stable, a head CT may be indicated.

9. Diagnostic criteria for brain death are well established. First, all sedative and anesthetic agents must be cleared from the system. The etiology of the patient's neurologic deterioration must be known (for example, prolonged ischemic arrest in this patient). The patient must be hemodynamically stable and free of metabolic disturbances such as severe uremia or hypothermia that can alter neurologic function. The patient must be unarousable to voice and pain. The patient must have no brainstem reflexes; absent pupillary reflexes, absent corneal reflexes, negative cold-water calorics, no gag reflex, apnea. Apnea is confirmed by instilling 100% O_2 into the trachea and confirming that there is no respiratory effort in spite of a rise in arterial pCO_2 to ≥ 60 mm Hg. The next step in evaluation is confirmatory tests such as EEG and cerebral blood flow. If the family refused further tests, repeating the neurologic exam including the apnea test after 12 hours of observation in an adult confirms the diagnosis. With confirmatory testing, the observation time is shortened to 6 hours. Once brain death is clinically declared, the patient is dead and must be removed from life support after the family has had the opportunity to pay their last respects (unless the patient is an organ donor awaiting operating room availability).

CASE #4

A 54-year-old, 80-kg man is scheduled for a thoracotomy for carcinoma of the right lung. Three months ago he had a myocardial infarction and he currently takes atenolol, 100 mg/day. You detect a unilateral carotid bruit and end-expiratory wheezing on physical exam. BP 140/80; P 60; R18; T 37°C; Hgb 17.

***
Your Outline
***

Our Outline

Urgency: Elective (sort of). This is the type of case that can be delayed for workup, but cannot be put off indefinitely because of the risk of metastasis.

Reason for Exam: Differential diagnosis of signs and symptoms. This is a classic short-stem format. The emphasis is on preoperative evaluation. Rest assured that the intraoperative phase will have ample problems to deal with. However, if you nail the preoperative workup and preparation for surgery, the remainder of the exam should flow smoothly.

Problem List

Head and neck: Unilateral carotid bruit
Neurologic: None
Airway: None

Pulmonary:
1. Right lung mass
2. Wheezing on physical exam
3. Elevated hemoglobin suggestive of chronic hypoxemia

Cardiovascular: Coronary artery disease with recent MI
Gastrointestinal: None
Renal: None
Hematologic: Polycythemia
Other: None

History and physical:
- History of symptoms of stroke or TIA?
- Airway exam to assess ease of dual-lumen ETT
- History of treatment for reactive airways?
- Lung exam to localize wheezing
- History of workup following MI?
- History of recurrent chest pain?
- Current exercise tolerance
- DOE, orthopnea, PND, edema?
- History of tobacco use?
- History of bleeding (contemplating epidural)?

Labs: ABG

Tests:
- Old and new ECG
- Treadmill stress test (to assess myocardium at risk)
- MUGA or echocardiogram to assess LV function if evidence of CHF
- Chest x-ray (confirm lesion location and rule out infiltrates)
- Pulmonary function tests with and without bronchodilators
- Further pulmonary testing as indicated by ABG/PFTs

Consults:
- Surgeon—Discuss planned extent of resection
- Cardiologist—"Does this patient have myocardium at risk following his MI?"
- Pulmonologist (maybe)—"Can pulmonary function be further optimized prior to this procedure?" We would not get this consult, but many would and it can be defended. You should be comfortable interpreting PFTs (if not, study them). Do not expect this consult to be much help. The consultant will likely recommend a spinal.

Preoperative therapy and monitoring:
- Preoperative atenolol (good evidence that periop MI is decreased)
- Delay surgery for treatment of wheezing if reversible with bronchodilators
- Routine ASA monitors
- Five-lead ECG
- Arterial line

- CVP
- Consider PA cath based on study results
- Epidural
- Fiberoptic bronchoscope
- Foley

Premed: Midazolam, albuterol inhaler, epidural test dose, preoxygenate with 100% O_2

Induction: Assuming normal airway and NPO status, fentanyl/pentothal/1 mg vecuronium, establish mask ventilation, succinylcholine

Maintenance: Isoflurane/O_2, vecuronium, lidocaine, and narcotic via epidural, esmolol for tachycardia or hypertension

Emergence: Neostigmine/glycopyrrolate, esmolol as needed, epidural infusion

Postop care: ICU

Anticipated problems: There are few things in life that are certain; except death, taxes, and dual-lumen endotracheal tubes that don't work on the oral boards.

Also, this patient is likely to develop:

- Myocardial ischemia
- Bronchospasm
- Bleeding
- Postoperative respiratory insufficiency
- Epidural complications
- Delayed awakening

Common things are common and the exam is designed to follow a logical progression during a complicated anesthetic. If you keep the exam in perspective and apply what you know to the patient in your exam scenario, you will significantly reduce the board-certification-expense column of your itemized business expenses.

Examiners' Questions

Preoperative Evaluation

1. How would you evaluate this patient's pulmonary status? Why? What additional information is necessary to evaluate the patient's wheezing? If bronchodilators produced a 25% improvement in FEV1, what would be your recommendation? Why?
2. Is the patient able to tolerate the anticipated procedure without remaining ventilator dependent? Why? The patient's pCO_2 is 49 on room air and the FEV1 is 1.3 L. The surgeon tells you that because of the hilar position of the tumor, pneumonectomy is a distinct possibility. What would you do?

Why? If split lung function testing revealed marginal reserve for pneumonectomy, what further studies could you do?

3. What evaluation is necessary for the carotid bruit? Should the patient undergo carotid endarterectomy prior to his pulmonary resection? Why or why not?

4. Are you concerned about the patient's MI 3 months ago? How would you evaluate the patient's cardiac disease? Is a cardiac cath necessary?

5. The surgeon tells you that further cardiac evaluation is not necessary because the patient has a malignancy and will die of cancer if it is allowed to metastasize. How would you respond? If the patient had significant coronary artery disease with progressive angina, would you perform a CABG on a patient with a malignancy? Would you remove the malignancy at the same time as CABG? Why or why not?

Intraoperative

6. What monitoring would you select for this procedure? Is a PA catheter necessary?

7. What sort of postoperative pain control would you use for this patient? Assuming you are considering epidural analgesia, are PT and PTT results necessary prior to placement? After placing an epidural and giving a 3-cc test dose of 1.5% lidocaine with epinephrine, the pulse rate rises 20 beats per minute within 60 seconds of injection. What would you do?

8. Is a double-lumen endotracheal tube mandatory for this case? What are the absolute indications for a double-lumen ETT? Is fiberoptic bronchoscopy necessary for safe positioning of a double-lumen ETT? Why or why not? How would you clinically check for correct placement?

9. During induction, the patient develops occasional unifocal and then multifocal PVCs. What is your differential diagnosis? Prior to positioning, you note ST segment elevation in lead V5. What is the appropriate action?

10. During one-lung ventilation, the surgeon reports inflation of the operative lung. What are the appropriate actions? The patient becomes hypoxemic on one lung. What do you do? Pneumonectomy is necessary for complete resection, but the surgeon desires further evidence of the patient's ability to tolerate the pneumonectomy. How?

Our Answers

1. Evaluation of the patient's pulmonary status encompasses two separate but related issues. First, the patient has evidence of chronic pulmonary disease with wheezing on exam, as well as an elevated hematocrit suggestive of chronic hypoxemia. Second, the patient must be evaluated for his ability to tolerate the planned resection. Initially, we would start with a more extensive pulmonary history, a room air ABG and measurement of FVC, FEV1, and MMEF25-75% (maximum midexpiratory flow) with and without bronchodilators. (THEN STOP! The examiners have given you an open-ended question and may let you ramble on until you say something stupid. Then they will pounce on the mistake and waste valuable time. The suggested answer shows that you are considering all aspects of this patient's pulmonary status and provides a start to a workup. Remember, the examiners have a script. If they want a more detailed answer, they will coax you.) A history of hospitalizations or intubations for respiratory distress, recurrent pneumonia, or aggressive ongoing treatment such as steroids for reactive airways disease would alert you to severe pulmonary dysfunction that must be optimized before considering pulmonary resection. The reason we would start with an ABG and simple spirometry is that these tests provide an excellent screen for untreated, but reversible, reactive airways disease as well as screening parameters for safe extent of pulmonary resection. Improvement in FEV1 or MMEF25-75% with bronchodilators and a chest x-ray would provide additional useful information. Improvement of at least 20% in FEV1 or MMEF is considered significant. We would delay the case for at least 72 hours of optimization with bronchodilators to decrease the risk of acute bronchospasm in the perioperative period.

2. This question is a classic oral board ploy. Ask you a question about the procedure when you don't even know what the procedure will be. Don't expect to be handed an abundance of useful information. They may never give you the information you need. Yet, you must make the examiner aware that you know precisely what information is necessary. You can address such a question with two strategies. First, you can discuss the nature of the procedure with your surgical colleague. Then the examiners should at least provide you with the planned procedure. Second, you can assume the best scenario for you, such as, "Assuming the FEV1 is greater than 2 liters and the pCO_2 is normal, then the patient should be able to tolerate any unilateral pulmonary procedure." With an assumption like this, the examiners must either let you get away with a healthy patient or else provide you the needed data upon which to base your decision. FEV1 < 2 L and elevated pCO_2 on RA ABG are both flags that the patient may not tolerate pneumonectomy. You must test further. It is possible that the diseased lung is nonfunctional, leaving the patient with an adequate postoperative FEV1. The test of choice is differential lung function testing which involves testing for ventilation and perfusion. The ventilation portion

of the test provides an estimate of FEV1 postresection. The perfusion should roughly match the ventilation. If not, the right heart may not tolerate the increase in pulmonary vascular resistance that will result from resection of a portion of the lung tissue with a large percentage of the total pulmonary perfusion. It is recommended that the predicted postoperative FEV1 is at least 800 cc. A postoperative FEV1 of 600 cc or less is almost certain to cause ventilator dependence. If more than 70% of the blood flow is to the diseased lung, the right heart is unlikely to tolerate a pneumonectomy. If split-lung function testing is marginal, balloon occlusion of the pulmonary artery to the diseased lung could be performed. If mean PA pressure remains less than 40 mm Hg, MAP does not plummet and room air ABG reveals adequate gas exchange, then the patient will likely tolerate a pneumonectomy.

3. *Make the patient healthy!* "Assuming that the patient has no signs or symptoms suggestive of stroke or transient ischemic attack, no further evaluation is necessary. Carotid endarterectomy is not indicated." If the examiners create symptoms suggestive of TIA, then carotid duplex or angiography is necessary to rule out a critical stenosis that will require surgical repair prior to a thoracotomy.

4. You are always concerned about the patient's condition. "Of course I am concerned about the recent myocardial infarction. The patient may have additional myocardium at risk or have compromised ventricular function from the recent MI." You can't assume that there is no further myocardium at risk in this scenario because the risk of reinfarction with a major operation is unacceptable in a patient only 3 months post MI. You have to prove that the condition of the heart is optimized. We would seek additional history from the patient concerning his exercise tolerance, any symptoms of recurrent angina or symptoms of congestive heart failure such as orthopnea, PND, or peripheral edema. We would also obtain old and new ECGs and chest x-rays for comparison to identify any evidence of ongoing ischemia or pulmonary vascular congestion. We would consult the patient's cardiologist to find out the results of post-MI stress testing or catheterization. If a stress test had not been performed, we would order one to identify myocardium at risk. If the exercise tolerance were poor or the patient had any symptoms of CHF, then a test such as a MUGA or an echocardiogram is indicated to assess LV function. A cardiac cath is indicated if there is myocardium at risk.

5. The risk of death from progression of the patient's natural disease is not a license to assassinate the patient with a surgical procedure. We would tactfully inform the surgeon that, "The risk of the procedure outweighs the benefit without further evaluation." Performing a CABG on a patient with a malignancy is the type of dilemma that oral boards thrive upon. There is no correct answer. Removing the malignancy first without CABG may kill the patient. Performing the

CABG without resecting the tumor may put a patient with already unresectable disease through a painful and dangerous procedure with no survival benefit. A combined procedure compounds risk. Discuss the situation with your surgical colleague and the patient after obtaining as much helpful data as possible, consider the options, and select a logical course of action with the patient's best interests and desires at heart.

6. We would use the following monitors in this case: routine ASA, 5-lead ECG, Foley catheter, arterial line (frequent blood gases), CVP (large operation with significant volume shifts). Assuming there is normal left ventricular function, we would not use a PA catheter. Stop your answer here. If the examiners overrule your assumption and give you a patient with poor LV function, we would use a PA catheter, realizing that the absolute value of the pulmonary artery pressures may be compromised in the lateral position with the chest open. However, the trends in the pressures would be valuable as would the ability to monitor cardiac output (especially postoperatively). If the patient had significant myocardium at risk but PTCA or CABG was not an option, we would monitor for ischemia with TEE. New wall motion abnormalities are a very sensitive indicator of ischemia, even in the lateral position. PA pressures and 5-lead ECG may not be as sensitive in this scenario. If you do not use TEE regularly but feel you need it, get a cardiology consult for intraoperative TEE.

6. We would use epidural narcotic infusion for postoperative pain control. Local anesthetic infusion is certainly acceptable, but we would rather not deal with the postoperative hypotension questions that are inevitable with this technique. PCA is also an easily defendable choice but the examiners are unlikely to let you off that easily. PT/PTT results are frequently ordered preoperatively for patients receiving epidurals. Assuming a negative history of bleeding, liver disease, renal disease, or anticoagulant therapy, there is no definitive data that screening PT/PTT decreases the likelihood of epidural hematoma. The false-positive rate will deny patients of epidural analgesia. We would not order them unless we clinically suspected an abnormality. A pulse rate rise greater than 10 beats per minute with a test dose signifies intravascular injection. We would remove the catheter and replace it at a different level.

8. Assuming no active pneumonia that is likely to contaminate the good lung, a double-lumen ETT is not mandatory. It would be desirable for this procedure. Absolute indications for a double-lumen ETT include 1) alveolar proteinosis where you lavage one lung, 2) hemorrhage where you bleed into one lung, 3) purulence where you gross out one lung, and 4) bronchopleural fistula where you blow out one lung. Benumof uses a fiberoptic bronchoscope to position double-lumen ETTs. Benumof writes the textbook on thoracic anesthesia. Board examiners read textbooks on thoracic anesthesia. Therefore, we recommend using a bronchoscope to position your double-lumen ETT on the oral boards.

We know you are great at placing them and have done it a million times. We know it slows you down. We also know that you may be slowed to a halt on the exam if you have ambivalent clinical findings while checking tube position and do not have a bronchoscope handy. The rationale for using a fiberoptic scope to position the ETT is that the margin for error is small. Too far in and you can occlude the upper lobe takeoff, traumatize the carina, or obstruct ventilation through your tracheal lumen. Too far out and you will have poor lung isolation or the balloon may herniate across the carina and again obstruct ventilation through your tracheal lumen. To clinically check position of the dual-lumen ETT, first assure gas exchange to both lungs with only the tracheal balloon inflated. Then inflate the bronchial balloon and listen for breath sounds on the side of the tracheal lumen. Clamp the tracheal lumen. The breath sounds should disappear on that side. Assure continued gas exchange on the contralateral side. Unclamp the tracheal lumen and breath sounds should return on the ipsilateral side. This proves that your bronchial tip is in the side it should be, the bronchial cuff is occluding the contralateral bronchus, and that the tracheal lumen is not obstructed. Then listen on the side of the bronchial cuff and assure breath sounds are present with the balloon up. Clamp the bronchial lumen and breath sounds should disappear. Assure breath sounds on the contralateral side. This double-checks that the bronchial cuff is adequately occluding the bronchus, resulting in good lung isolation.

9. The main differential diagnosis of multifocal PVCs at induction *in this patient* includes coronary ischemia, hypoxemia, or hypercarbia. Less likely culprits would include electrolyte disturbances, metabolic acidosis from malignant hyperthermia, baseline ectopy not previously diagnosed, or ectopy related to inhaled anesthetics such as halothane. ST segment elevation in V5 is ischemia until proven otherwise. Decrease myocardial oxygen consumption by slowing heart rate and offloading the left ventricle to decrease wall tension (nitroglycerin for venodilation, morphine and/or furosemide for pulmonary vasodilation). Optimize myocardial oxygen delivery by maximizing SaO_2 (100% O_2 if necessary), assuring adequate aortic diastolic pressure (the driving pressure for coronary perfusion), dilating the coronary arteries with nitroglycerin, slowing heart rate (increase diastolic perfusion time), and offloading the left ventricle with furosemide to decrease LVEDP (increase the pressure drop for coronary perfusion). After resolution of the ischemia but before proceeding, we would place both a PA catheter and a TEE probe.

10. If lung isolation is poor, you must 1) check to make sure you deflated the correct lung, 2) reconfirm the position of the dual-lumen ETT, and 3) assure that the bronchial cuff is adequately inflated. By bronchoscopy, only the very top of the bronchial balloon should be visible at the level of the carina. The proper amount of air in the bronchial cuff is the minimal amount necessary to make the air movement cease in the deflated lung. Hypoxemia on one lung not only occurs on the oral boards, but in real life as well. Therefore, your answer should be slick. First, we would listen to breath sounds and check EtCO$_2$ to assure ventilation of the nonoperative lung. Then we would confirm that we were delivering 100% oxygen and an adequate tidal volume to prevent atelectasis in the ventilated lung (5–10 cc/kg). Next, we would deliver 5 cm H$_2$O of CPAP to the nonventilated lung. Then we would deliver up to 10 cm H$_2$O of PEEP to the ventilated lung. Then we would inform the surgeon that we are forced to intermittently expand the non-ventilated lung. Never mind that the surgeon should already know whether the patient will be able to tolerate a pneumonectomy. Answer the question. At this stage, a pulmonary artery catheter is necessary to measure PA pressures and measure cardiac output during a test clamp of the artery to the lung to be removed. If PA mean pressure exceeds 40 mm Hg, systemic mean arterial pressure falls significantly, or cardiac output plummets during test clamping, the procedure must be aborted.

CASE #5

A 48-year-old male is scheduled for emergent thoracotomy for closure of a bronchopleural fistula and drainage of an empyema.

HPI: The patient underwent right upper lobectomy for squamous cell carcinoma of the lung one week ago. Since that time he has had a progressive air leak from the chest tubes and has failed attempts to wean the ventilator. The patient was started on broad spectrum antibiotics on POD#5 for fever and elevated WBC count. ETT suctioning returned purulent material. Dopamine was started on POD#6 for hypotension and oliguria. Cultures are pending.

PMH: Significant only for hypertension controlled with medication for the past 8 years and a 60-pack-year history of cigarette smoking. No known drug allergies.

Medications:
- Imipenem, 500 mg IV q8hrs
- Gentamicin, 80 mg IV q12hrs
- Dopamine infusion @ 5 mcg/kg/min
- Fentanyl infusion @ 100 mcg/hr
- Heparin 5000 units SQ bid
- Furosemide, 40mg IV q6hrs
- High nitrogen tube feeds @ 60 cc/hr
- Lorazepam and Tylenol, prn

Physical exam: Ill-appearing, cachectic male, older than stated age, sedated on ventilator.

VS: BP 80/40, P 110, R 40, Temp 40°C, height 175 cm, weight 62 kg

Head and neck: Poor oral hygiene, 18 Fr nasogastric tube in right nare, feeding tube in left nare, purulent drainage from right nare, pinpoint pupils, neck veins flat

Airway: Intubated with 8.5 mm oral ETT positioned 22 cm at the teeth, copious purulent secretions from ETT, normal thyromental distance, uncooperative with oral exam

Chest: Triple-lumen catheter present in right subclavian vein, coarse breath sounds in right chest more prominent with inspiration, basilar rales in left chest, chest tube ×2 on right connected to 20 cm H_2O wall suction

Cardiovascular: Regular rate and rhythm, II/VI SEM over LUSB, brisk cap refill, 2+ edema of extremities

Abdomen: Unremarkable, Foley catheter in place with 15 cc/hr of urine output

Chest x-ray: Subcutaneous air on right, chest tube ×2 in right pleural space, pleural effusion obscuring lower right lung field, atelectasis versus infiltrate in left base

ECG: Sinus tachycardia, no acute ischemia

Ventilator settings: A/C with backup rate of 18, TV 800, FiO_2 100%, PEEP 5, PS 10, insp TV 810 cc, exp TV 430, RR 40 ABG, pH 7.28, PaO_2 62, pCO_2 36

Laboratory data: HCT 29%, WBC 18K, plts 92K, BUN 54, Cr 1.6, Na 131, K 3.7, glucose 147, PT 14.1, PTT 36

You are asked to transport the patient to the operating room.

***
Your Outline
***

Our Outline
This is another example of the newer oral exam format. You are given a large amount of information to sift through and asked to start the case. Focus on identifying any necessary information not provided and proceed to considering your technique and potential problems.

Urgency: Even though the case is scheduled as an emergency, you have time to optimize prior to surgery. The patient has been hypotensive and oliguric for at least 1 day. Rushing to the OR without appropriate monitoring and needed therapy would be unwise.

Reason for exam: Multisystem disease and its ramifications.

Problem List
Head and neck: Sinusitis

Neurologic: None

Airway: Potentially difficult double-lumen ETT due to secretions

Pulmonary:
1. Bronchopleural fistula:
    - Marginal CO_2 elimination in spite of high minute ventilation
    - Almost 50% of each breath out chest tubes

2. Empyema:
   - Persistent effusion unresponsive to chest tube
   - Fever, elevated WBC count
   - Purulent secretions
3. Infiltrate versus atelectasis in left lung:
   - V/Q mismatch with increased A-a gradient
   - Inadequate expansion of left lung due to high flow through BPF

Cardiovascular:
- Septic shock
- Low systemic resistance
- Metabolic acidosis
- Oliguria
- Fever, leukocytosis
- Unknown cardiac function; conflicting exam data
- Cardiac murmur, likely flow murmur

Gastrointestinal:
1. Full stomach
2. Unknown feeding tube location

Renal:
1. Oliguria
2. Prerenal azotemia with elevated BUN/Cr ratio

Hematologic:
1. Anemia
2. Thrombocytopenia

Other: None

Essential Additional Data Required
History and physical: None
Labs: None
Tests: Left ventricular function
Consults: None

Preoperative therapy and monitoring:
- Pulmonary artery catheter to optimize cardiac function. Possible LV dysfunction with septic shock. May require volume loading as well as inotropic support prior to surgery.
- Portable suction
- Portable monitor
- Pressure ventilator for OR
- Routine ASA monitors

- Arterial line
- Foley in place

Induction: O_2, fentanyl, midazolam, pancuronium
Maintenance: O_2, fentanyl, midazolam, pancuronium
Emergence: N/A
Postop: ICU

Anticipated problems:
- Instability during transport
- Difficult lung isolation
- Hemodynamic instability due to sepsis
- Desaturation during one-lung ventilation
- Possible pneumonectomy with marginal reserve
- Acute renal failure

Examiners' Questions

Intraoperative

1. Why is the patient hypotensive? Is the patient optimized for transport to the OR? How do you differentiate between septic shock and hypovolemia? What monitors would you use for this case? Would you place them before or after transport?

2. Pulmonary artery catheter values return as follows: CVP 12; PA 32/18; PCWP 15; BP 70/40 (mean 52); cardiac output 8 L/min. How do you calculate SVR? What is your diagnosis? How would you treat?

3. What special anesthetic considerations must be considered in a patient with a BPF (That's bronchopleural fistula to the uninitiated)? Would you use a double-lumen ETT in this case? Why or why not? What are the absolute indications for a double-lumen ETT?

4. While in the elevator on the way to the OR, the patient's arterial line reads 40/22, HR 155 in sinus tachycardia, and pulse oximetry no longer tracks. What would you do? What is your differential diagnosis?

5. Upon arrival in the operating room, the surgeon states that he must have good lung isolation. How do you obtain isolation? You place a double-lumen ETT and confirm breath sounds and $EtCO_2$. After turning on his left side and initiating one-lung ventilation, the patient becomes cyanotic. FIO_2 is 1.0, PaO_2 is 46 and $PaCO_2$ is 60. How do you evaluate? How do you treat?

Postoperative

6. After successful closure of the BPF and drainage of the empyema, the patient is brought to the ICU with a single-

lumen ETT in place. ABG on a T-piece is as follows: FIO_2 0.5; PaO_2 48; $PaCO_2$ 42; pH 7.32; RR 32. Would you extubate? If continued mechanical ventilation were necessary, what settings would you use? Would you use PEEP? How does PEEP impact A-a gradient? Does PEEP increase the risk of BPF recurrence?

7. The patient remained oliguric through the case. How do you evaluate? What is the etiology of the renal dysfunction? How can prerenal azotemia occur with a cardiac output of 8 L/min? What are the indications for dialysis?

8. What are the hemodynamic goals for a septic patient in the perioperative period?

Our Answers

1. The components of blood pressure are cardiac output (flow) and systemic vascular resistance (resistance). Cardiac output is elevated, so the peripheral resistance must be decreased. With fever, leukocytosis, purulent secretions, and empyema, the most likely diagnosis for the decreased SVR is sepsis. The patient is not optimized for transport. Clinical findings are conflicting regarding the patient's volume status. While peripheral edema, rales, elevated cardiac output, and brisk capillary refill argue for adequate intravascular volume, flat neck veins and oliguria suggest that volume loading may be needed. This is a trick question. The patient may have septic shock (inadequate oxygen delivery to meet tissue demands) and intravascular volume depletion while being total body fluid overloaded. We would place a pulmonary artery catheter to optimize intravascular volume and cardiac output prior to transport of a hypotensive, tachycardic, febrile, oliguric patient with a metabolic acidosis. Other monitors would include routine ASA monitors, arterial line, CVP, and Foley catheter (in place). We would transport this patient with ECG, arterial pressure, and SaO_2, as well as portable suction for the rapid air leak.

2. SVR (dyne·sec/cm^5) is calculated as the difference between MAP and right atrial pressure multiplied by 80 and divided by the cardiac output in L/min. This is a calculated resistance and is influenced by altering the individual variables of the equation. The diagnosis is sepsis (systemic inflammatory response syndrome) which is a form of high output cardiac failure (plenty of blood flow, just not to the right spots). With elevated filling pressure, we will likely need inotropic support and vasoconstriction with a drug such as norepinephrine to maintain an adequate perfusion pressure. If volume were needed, we would choose red blood cells to increase oxygen carrying capacity.

3. Bronchopleural fistula presents several challenges to the anesthesiologist. Without adequate chest tube drainage, tension pneumothorax develops rapidly. Ventilation is inefficient with a large portion of the minute ventilation escaping through the fistula. Work of breathing is markedly increased. If ventilated with positive pressure, the airflow seeks the path of least resistance, which is out the chest tubes, with resultant hypoventilation of the unaffected side. Ventilation-perfusion matching is disturbed with an increase in the A-a gradient and hypoxemia. This case has two of the four absolute indications for a double-lumen ETT, bronchopleural fistula, and unilateral empyema/pneumonia with risk of infectious spread to the other lung. However, ETT exchange is not without risk in this critically ill patient and consideration should be given to alternative forms of lung isolation such as a bronchial blocker. Absolute indications for a double-lumen ETT include 1) unilateral hemoptysis, 2) unilateral purulence, 3) bronchopleural fistula, and 4) alveolar proteinosis with planned lung lavage.

4. Transport catastrophe…think ABC. Ventilate the patient and listen to breath sounds. Assure 100% O_2 delivery (check pressure in tank, connections intact, flow on), palpate a pulse, administer temporizing drugs to support the circulation. If no pulse, start CPR. In this case, when you listen to breath sounds, the patient will be hard to ventilate, there will be no breath sounds on the right, the trachea will be deviated to the left and the chest will be tympanitic to percussion on the right. Need any more clues? The patient has a tension pneumothorax. Inspection of the chest tubes will reveal that the tubing has been caught under the transport monitor and occluded. Acute events during transport almost always are related to malfunction of your equipment, such as kinked or dislodged tubes, infusions that become disconnected, or monitors that malfunction. In a patient with a bronchopleural fistula, anything that prevents evacuation of pleural air will result in a tension pneumothorax within a few breaths. We would use a portable suction device attached to the chest tubes for transport of this patient as long as the capacity of the device is adequate to accommodate the brisk air leak. If the chest tubes are left to water seal, you must be sure that the egress of air is adequate to prevent a tension pneumothorax prior to movement. A simple kink of the chest tubes during movement will produce this scenario.

5. Airway, airway! Don't lose the airway. If you simply pull the old ETT out (because you can intubate anyone), you will be met with a continuous stream of copious secretions obstructing your view, regurgitation of tube feeding will occur, or you will be unable to reintubate. This patient has no reserve and will not do well in that situation. A double-lumen tube is desirable but should be placed over a tube exchanger for safety. You can also obtain lung isolation with a bronchial blocker in the right mainstem. This is not as desirable because you would have to let the blocker down to re-expand the right lung if unacceptable hypoxemia develops, but it would avoid the risk of exchanging the ETT. If using a blocker, a test period of single lung ventilation before incision is indicated to assure adequate oxygenation on one lung. Letting the blocker down during surgery allows purulent secretions to pour into the dependent (relatively healthy) lung. First assure delivery of 100% oxygen and adequate ventilation of the dependent lung by listening to breath sounds in the ventilated lung. Next, confirm position of the ETT with fiberoptic bronchoscopy. If SaO_2 is still inadequate, add CPAP to the nonventilated lung. A low level of CPAP (5 cm H_2O) in a motionless lung should not make surgical exposure unacceptable. If still hypoxemic, add 5 to 10 cm H_2O PEEP to the ventilated lung. This may help or hurt depending on the effect of PEEP on blood flow distribution between the ventilated and nonventilated lung. Finally, inform the surgeon that you are forced to intermittently hand-ventilate the operative lung and work with your surgical colleague to provide both a surgical field and hemoglobin saturation that are acceptable.

6. This patient does not meet extubation criteria. Extubation criteria we use include: PaO_2 >60 mm Hg on $FIO_2 \leq 0.5$ and PEEP ≤ 5 cm H_2O, TV > 5 cc/kg IBW, FVC > 10 cc/kg IBW, RR < 30, MIF < −25 cm H_2O, pH ≥ 7.30. These criteria are only guidelines, but are defendable based upon the literature. This patient fails two of the criteria without even checking respiratory mechanics. Because of the fresh BPF repair, high peak airway pressures must be avoided. Therefore, initially we would use pressure control ventilation with an initial FIO_2 of 1.0, RR 18, inspiratory pressure adequate to maintain a TV of 5–7 cc/kg, PEEP 5, I:E ratio of 1:2. We are using a low TV and a high rate to decrease the required inspiratory pressure. After the first ABG on the ventilator, we will wean the FIO_2 as tolerated. We would use PEEP titrated to maintain PaO_2 of 60 on nontoxic FIO_2. PEEP decreases A-a gradient by increasing FRC (functional residual capacity) with a resultant improvement in ventilation/perfusion matching and PaO_2. PEEP raises mean airway pressure and may slightly increase the risk of bronchial stump breakdown. However, so will chronic hypoxemia. Because of a favorable impact on pulmonary compliance (optimizing FRC), the peak airway pressure may actually fall with the addition of PEEP and lower the risk of BPF recurrence.

7. Oliguria is either due to prerenal azotemia, intrinsic renal disease, or obstructive uropathy. The easiest fix is to correct urinary tract obstruction. Assuming a Foley catheter is in place, assure continuous drainage and irrigate the Foley with sterile technique, if indicated. Elevated BUN/Cr ratio (>20:1) and decreased urine Na (<10) suggest prerenal causes of oliguria. In a patient with systemic infection, adequate filling pressures, and an elevated cardiac output, sepsis (or systemic inflammatory response syndrome) is the most likely etiology. In the septic state, cardiac output is elevated but the blood flow is misdirected, so that the fingertips may be well perfused but the kidneys are not. Treatment is supportive with optimization of oxygen delivery and elimination of the source of the infection. Indications for dialysis include clinically significant hyperkalemia, clinically significant metabolic acidosis, uremic encephalopathy, uremic coagulopathy, and refractory volume overload. The decision to dialyze should be based upon clinical indications, not preset numbers for BUN or creatinine.

8. While there are no definitive studies which identify specific hemodynamic management strategies that significantly improve outcome, analysis of hemodynamic data in patients who survive sepsis reveals that survivors increase cardiac output significantly while maintaining adequate filling pressures and mean arterial pressures to prevent the development of lactic acidosis. In one such analysis, norepinephrine was the drug that maintained the hemodynamic parameters of the septic patients closest to the characteristics observed in the surviving patients. Unfortunately, this does not prove that norepinephrine improves survival.

CASE #6

A 58-year-old, 80 kg male is scheduled for CABG. He developed recurrent angina following an inferior myocardial infarction 8 months ago. Bronchial asthma has been present since childhood. Nonsmoker. Ventriculogram shows moderate inferior wall hypokinesis, ejection fraction 60%. Exam reveals a systolic murmur along the sternal border. Medications include hydrochlorothiazide, isosorbide dinitrate, metoprolol, albuterol/atrovent inhalers, and theophylline. BP 160/90, HR 62, RR 14, temp 37.0°C, Hgb 12.

***
Your Outline
***

Our Outline

Urgency: Urgent. Recurrent angina following MI suggests myocardium at risk

Reason for exam: Differential diagnosis of signs and symptoms as well as conflicting therapies

Problem List

Head and neck: None
Airway: None
Pulmonary: Reactive airways disease

Cardiovascular:
* Myocardium at risk
* Hypertensive heart disease
* Possible valvular disease

Gastrointestinal: None
Renal: Diuretic therapy
Hematologic: Anemia
Other: None

Additional history and physical desired:
* History of intubation, hospitalization or steroid use for asthma
* Exam evidence of wheezing?
* Recent pattern of angina
* Syncope or near-syncope?
* JVD, PND, orthopnea, or edema?
* Coronary anatomy and pull-back pressures across the aortic valve from recent catheterization, mitral regurgitation on LVgram?
* Exam evidence of hematoma or pseudoaneurysm from recent catheter which would explain anemia
* Stool guaiac

Additional labs:
- Serum K
- Theophylline level
- Room air ABG
- Reticulocyte count

Additional tests:
1. FEV1, FVC, MMEF25-75 with and without bronchodilators
2. New and old ECG
3. New and old chest x-ray
4. Echocardiogram for evaluation of murmur if cardiac catheter data inconclusive or unavailable

Consults: Cardiology

Preoperative therapy and monitoring:
1. Preoperative respiratory therapy for 48–72 hours, if PFTs show reversible disease or patient wheezing
2. Preoperative theophylline and inhalers, consider steroids if required in past
3. Routine ASA monitor
4. Foley catheter
5. Arterial line-frequent blood draws
6. Pulmonary artery catheter-optimize fluid therapy for condition in which right and left ventricular pressures may not correlate

Premedication: Lorazepam, metoprolol, theophylline, albuterol, O_2
Induction: O_2, fentanyl, midazolam, pancuronium
Maintenance: O_2, isoflurane, fentanyl, midazolam, pancuronium
Emergence: N/A
Postop: ICU

Examiners' Questions

Preoperative
1. What additional information about the patient's cardiac status do you require before proceeding with surgery? Would the coronary anatomy data alter your management of this case? How? Are you concerned about the systolic murmur in this patient? Why?
2. How would you evaluate the patient's asthma preoperatively? If the patient had diffuse wheezing on exam and a 25% improvement in FEV1 with bronchodilators, would you delay the case? What if the patient had left main disease? How would the diagnosis of moderate aortic stenosis alter preoperative management of reactive airways disease in this patient? What are the hemodynamic effects of beta-2 agonists?

3. What premedication would you give this patient preoperatively? What are the advantages of morphine/scopolamine premed? What are the disadvantages? Would you continue the metoprolol preoperatively? If the patient had required 3 weeks of steroid therapy for an asthma flare 3 months previously, would you alter your perioperative medical therapy? Why or why not?

4. Serum K returns 2.9. Would you delay the case? Why or why not?

Intraoperative

5. What monitors would you select for this patient? Is a pulmonary artery catheter indicated? Why or why not? When would you use transesophageal echo for a CABG case? Is the PA catheter a sensitive indicator of ischemia? What are the causes of a "giant V-wave" on your PCWP trace?

6. On induction the patient cannot be ventilated after the fentanyl is given. What are the most likely etiologies? What is your treatment?

7. Following intubation, you note 2 mm ST segment elevation in the anterior leads with multifocal PVCs. BP 85/50, HR 110. Cardiac catheter data revealed >95% proximal stenoses of both the LAD and LCx arteries. What do you do? What are the determinants of myocardial oxygen delivery? Myocardial oxygen consumption? The patient develops pulseless V-tach. What are the appropriate actions?

8. The patient is unable to be weaned from CPB. What are possible reasons? How do you treat? How does an IABP work? How is inflation timed? How is deflation timed?

Our Answers

1. Additional helpful information would include the pattern of angina and coronary anatomy data from the cardiac catheterization. Assessment of the murmur would include historical data for syncope/near-syncope, orthopnea, PND, or worsening edema. Physical exam would identify JVD, hepatic congestion, rales, or peripheral edema suggestive of heart failure. Careful evaluation of the cardiac murmur may differentiate between MV, AV, or PV origin. With an ejection fraction of 60%, signs or symptoms of heart failure would suggest significant valvular disease. Differential pressures between the LV and the aortic root would help assess the extent of any aortic stenosis and MV regurgitation can be seen if present on the LV-gram. Old and new ECG and chest x-ray would help assess progression of cardiac disease. Echocardiography would be the test of choice for valvular lesions. Identification of critical left main or left main equivalent disease would make optimization of coronary perfusion pressure and heart rate essential at induction. Are you concerned about the murmur? On the oral exam, you are always concerned about issues raised. An answer like, "No dude, I can handle it," will not score points with the examiners. The systolic murmur is likely aortic stenosis, mitral regurgitation, aortic sclerosis, or a benign pulmonary flow murmur. Other lesions are possible but not likely. Aortic sclerosis is thickening of the valve leaflets and loss of pliability of the annulus, but no true flow obstruction. Pulmonary flow murmurs usually occur in young, athletic patients who have high cardiac outputs. The main concern is the presence of either significant AS or MR that may require surgical treatment at the time of bypass.

2. Physical exam will identify active wheezing which should be treated prior to any major surgery, if possible. FEV1, FVC, and MMEF25-75, with and without bronchodilators, are the tests of choice for obstructive lung disease. Room air ABG and a theophylline level are also indicated. Moderate obstruction that responds to bronchodilators should be treated prior to surgery for 48–72 hours if feasible. Left main disease with angina at rest should not be delayed in our opinion, even if the patient is wheezing. The risk to benefit ratio argues for expeditious surgical therapy. The presence of aortic stenosis (or left main disease) makes tachycardia and hypotension extremely hazardous. Beta-2-agonists as well as theophylline can induce tachycardia and systemic vasodilation with decreased coronary perfusion pressure and shortened diastolic perfusion time for the myocardium. These agents should be used with caution.

3. We would premed this patient with a benzodiazepine with or without a narcotic, metoprolol, and nasal cannula O_2. If the patient were actively wheezing, we would likely give him regularly scheduled inhalers. To avoid tachycardia, we would likely avoid theophylline/aminophylline unless actively bronchospastic and a low theophylline level. Morphine/scopolamine provides excellent premedication for cardiac surgery. Morphine is antianginal and scopolamine provides amnesia and anticholinergic effects such as limited secretions and bronchodilation. Disadvantages include confusion, dysphoria, and post-operative sedation and/or disorientation. Scopolamine has much less effect on heart rate than atropine. Data is amassing that beta-blockers improve outcome for cardiac surgery if continued in the perioperative period. Metoprolol is B1-selective and should not induce broncho-spasm. We would definitely give it as a premed. Conventional wisdom (a.k.a. anecdotal medicine) suggests use of perioperative steroid supple-ments if a patient has required treatment with steroids for more that 2 weeks in the past year to avoid perioperative adrenal insufficiency. While widely practiced, supporting data is extremely limited and we tend to observe the patient for evidence of adrenal insufficiency and only treat as clinically indicated. However, if there is evidence of reversible obstructive airways disease, perioperative steroid therapy may be a way of avoiding dangerous bronchospasm without using large doses of beta-2-agonists or phosphodiesterase inhibitors.

4. We would not delay the case for a K of 2.9. We will supplement the K after central line placement. In a patient receiving chronic diuretic therapy, the low K is unlikely to be acute and therefore is less dangerous. The surgery is urgent.

5. Recommended monitors would include routine ASA monitors, 5-lead ECG, arterial line, Foley catheter, core and nasal temperature, and CVP. A pulmonary artery catheter is a logical choice and can be defended because left and right ventricular function may not be related in the presence of myocardial ischemia. For the oral boards, we would consider a PA catheter, the conservative choice. We can deal with the complications if they occur and the information gained may be invalu-able. TEE is helpful in a CABG case if there is possible undiagnosed valvular disease or a weak left ventricle with poor targets. It is not nec-essary in this case as long as the patient's heart murmur was adequately evaluated preoperatively. A PA catheter is not the most sensitive indi-cator of ischemia. Five-lead ECG monitoring is easier to interpret and wall motion abnormalities on TEE are more sensitive. A large V-wave on the PCWP trace signifies back flow from the left atrium and is most frequently a marker for mitral regurgitation. A new V-wave suggests acute myocardial ischemia with papillary muscle dysfunction and new MR. A stiff left atrium can enhance normal V-wave traces.

6. In *this patient*, the most likely etiologies of difficulty ventilat-ing are bronchospasm or fentanyl rigidity. *Assuming a normal airway*, we would give a rapid acting muscle relaxant such as succinylcholine (K 2.9) and perform laryngoscopy after fasciculation.

7. They floated a slow curve over the middle of the plate. Hit it out of the park. Proximal LAD and LCx lesions that are critical are hemodynamically equivalent to left main disease. The patient is tachycardic and relatively hypotensive. Therefore, raise aortic diastolic pressure with phenylephrine and slow heart rate with a beta-blocker. Slowing heart rate reduces myocardial oxygen consumption and prolongs diastolic myocardial perfusion time. Raising aortic diastolic pressure enhances coronary perfusion pressure. IV nitroglycerin will enhance coronary vasodilation and venodilate to decrease preload to the ischemic ventricle. The determinants of myocardial oxygen consumption are heart rate, contractility, wall tension, and afterload. The determinants of myocardial oxygen delivery are coronary perfusion pressure (aortic diastolic pressure—LV diastolic pressure), hemoglobin concentration, hemoglobin saturation, and diastolic myocardial perfusion time. Pulseless V-tach requires immediate defibrillation ×3 per ACLS protocol. Check your airway and ventilate with 100% O_2. Then CPR, epi, lido, shock, etc. You may not be able to resuscitate the patient, so heparinize and have the surgeon cannulate as quickly as possible.

8. Failure to wean from cardiopulmonary bypass is usually due to poor starting LV function, inadequate myocardial protection during bypass, refractory dysrhythmias, inadequate heart rate, electrolyte abnormalities, inadequate revascularization with persistent ischemia, air in the coronary arteries, metabolic acidosis, or hypothermia. Appropriate therapy is to optimize what can be corrected, start inotropic support, apply pacing wires, if not already in place, and have the surgeon recheck the grafts. It may be necessary to provide mechanical support with an IABP or a ventricular assist device. An IABP is placed in the descending aorta just distal to the left subclavian artery. By inflating during diastole and deflating prior to systole, it enhances proximal aortic diastolic blood pressure (improves coronary perfusion) and decreases afterload (improves stroke volume and cardiac output) by deflating just prior to systole. Inflation and deflation are timed either to the aortic pulse wave or the ECG. During electrocautery, timing with the aortic pressure wave is more reliable. ECG timing is less subject to mechanical failure in the ICU. The balloon should start inflation at the dicrotic notch of the aortic pressure wave. It should deflate prior to ejection through the aortic valve (upstroke of the aortic pressure wave).

CASE #7

A 66-year-old, 105 kg male is scheduled for TURP for benign prostatic hypertrophy. He desires to be asleep for the procedure.

HPI: Patient has had progressive frequency and hesitancy as well as diminished urinary stream for several months. He has no hematuria and his PSA is normal. Last week he was seen in the emergency room with acute urinary obstruction and had a Foley catheter placed, which drained 1200 cc of urine. The Foley remains in place.

PMH: The patient has chronic obstructive pulmonary disease. His last workup included PFTs as follows FEV1 0.95 L, FVC 1.8 L, MMEF 25-75 60% pred. RA ABG 7.44/pCO_2 46/pO_2 60. He has dyspnea on exertion at about 50 feet. This has been stable. He has a 70-pack-year smoking history and continues to smoke. He snores so loudly at night that his wife sleeps in another room. He frequently gets up in the middle of the night to take a liquid antacid for indigestion.

He also has had hypertension, for many years. There is no history of angina or MI. He has noninsulin dependent diabetes. No known drug allergies. He admits to drinking three beers per day.

Meds: Atrovent and albuterol inhalers, glyburide, extended-release nifedipine

Physical exam: HR 85, BP 160/90, RR 20, afebrile

Airway: Edentulous, appears normal

Chest: Mild diffuse expiratory wheezes

Cardiac: WNL, no organomegaly or peripheral edema

Chest x-ray: No acute disease, cardiomegaly, and flat diaphragms are present

ECG: Normal sinus rhythm, LVH, nonspecific ST-T wave changes

Labs: Hgb 17, normal electrolytes, normal coags

He arrives in the OR and has taken all of his medications today.

***
Your Outline
***

Our Outline
Urgency: Urgent due to indwelling Foley
Reason for exam: Multisystem disease

Problem List
Head and neck: None
Airway: None

Pulmonary:
- Obstructive lung disease
- Decreased FEV1/FVC ratio and MMEF
- Expiratory wheezing on exam
- Hypercarbia on room air ABG
- Tobacco abuse
- Flat diaphragms on chest x-ray
- Possible sleep apnea
- Nighttime snoring
- Elevated hemoglobin
- Marginal room air pO_2

Cardiovascular:
- Hypertensive heart disease
- Diabetes

Gastrointestinal:
- Significant ethanol consumption
- Gastroesophageal reflux at night

Renal: Obstructive uropathy for TURP
Hematologic: None
Other: None
Additional history and physical data desired: Confirm NPO status
Additional lab data desired: Preoperative glucose
Additional tests desired: PFT response to bronchodilators
Consults: None

Preoperative therapy and monitoring:
- Check fingerstick glucose
- Albuterol inhaler
- Routine ASA
- Five-lead ECG
- Arterial line

Anesthetic plan: Confirm NPO status and check fingerstick glucose preop; premedicate with O_2, metoclopramide, ranitidine; bupivicaine spinal with minimal midazolam sedation

Anticipated problems:
- Spinal unlikely to work
- TURP syndrome
- Respiratory failure
- Possible coronary ischemia
- Mental status changes postoperatively

Examiners' Questions

Intraoperative

1. What is your anesthetic plan? What are the advantages of spinal anesthesia in this case? What are the advantages of general anesthesia? How do you counsel the patient?
2. What are the physiologic abnormalities associated with sleep apnea? How would a diagnosis of sleep apnea alter your anesthetic plan in this case?
3. Assume a spinal anesthetic is selected. Local anesthetic is administered and within 60 seconds the patient complains of inability to breathe. He is unable to talk above a whisper. What is the appropriate action to take? What agents would you select for intubation? Why? You are unable to intubate or mask ventilate the patient and the oxygen saturation is falling into the 80s. What is your next step? SaO_2 is falling into the 60s and PVCs are present on the monitor. What do you do?

4. The case proceeds after successfully securing an airway. After 90 minutes of surgery, the patient's SaO_2 again begins to fall. How do you evaluate? What is the differential diagnosis?

Postoperative

5. The remainder of the surgery is uncomplicated but prolonged. You extubate the patient at the end of the case. You are called by the recovery room nurse because the patient is confused. What is the differential diagnosis at this point? What tests would you order? What is TURP syndrome? What is the treatment?

6. The patient has persistent hematuria postoperatively. Hematocrit returns 24%. Would you transfuse? Why or why not? What are the acceptable indications for red blood cell transfusion?

7. You are called on POD#2 because of a persistent headache. How do you evaluate? How is an epidural blood patch performed?

Our Answers

   1. We would choose spinal anesthesia for this procedure, realizing fully that the spinal will not work or will be fraught with difficulties on the oral exam. However, it is the technique most practitioners would select. *In this patient,* the advantages of spinal include the ability to monitor for mental status changes during the procedure, avoidance of intubation/mechanical ventilation in a patient with significant pulmonary disease, and the ability to minimize sedatives, anesthetics, and analgesics in a patient with possible obstructive sleep apnea. General anesthesia has the advantages of controlling a potentially difficult mask airway, having less potentially deleterious hemodynamic effects than spinal anesthesia and complying with the patient's wishes. We would counsel the patient that given his lung disease with increased risk for prolonged mechanical ventilation, spinal anesthesia is the safest technique for him and that we will keep him as comfortable as possible throughout the procedure.

   2. Obstructive sleep apnea results in chronic hypoxemia with secondary polycythemia and disturbed sleep patterns with daytime somnolence. If severe enough, pulmonary hypertension and malignant dysrhythmias can result. Not to mention alienation of your significant other. These patients can be exquisitely sensitive to narcotics and sedatives with resultant apnea. The sleep apnea patient should be monitored with telemetry and continuous pulse oximetry overnight following a general anesthetic.

   3. What a surprise! The patient has developed a high spinal. Respiratory arrest is imminent. The patient must be intubated. We would perform a rapid sequence induction with cricoid pressure. We would administer face mask oxygen, etomidate, and succinylcholine. Hypotension is inevitable with a high spinal, so etomidate would be our agent of choice. Although the respiratory muscles are blocked by the high spinal, laryngeal muscles may not be and succinylcholine is indicated. If we are unable to intubate, we would mask ventilate through cricoid pressure. If we are unable to ventilate, we use the ASA emergency airway algorithm (memorize it!). The next step would be to call for help, notify the surgeon that a surgical airway might be necessary and place a laryngeal mask airway. LMA is relatively contraindicated in gastroesophageal reflux disease, but is the quickest alternative for a hypoxemic, paralyzed patient. We can deal with aspiration if it occurs. Prolonged hypoxemia wrecks the whole system. Once the LMA is placed and ventilation with 100% oxygen is possible, we would intubate with a 6.0 mm ETT over an intubating bronchoscope through the LMA. If ventilation is not possible with the LMA, then perform needle cricothyroidotomy and jet insufflation. Get the surgeon in on the act. He or she will need to perform an emergent tracheostomy to obtain a more secure airway. The cricothyroidotomy is just a bridge to buy more time while you secure the more definitive tracheostomy.

4. Falling oxygen saturation. Back to basics. ABC. Turn to 100% oxygen. Check your oxygen pressure and inspired O_2 monitor. Check your airway and listen to bilateral breath sounds to rule out a disconnected, clogged, or kinked endotracheal tube, right mainstem intubation, esophageal intubation, bronchospasm, or pneumothorax. Check your pulse oximeter to assure good pulse tracking. Measure an ABG. The differential diagnosis of hypoxemia is extensive. After ruling out mechanical failure of your equipment, move on to likely causes *in this patient*. Assuming bilateral breath sounds are present and 100% oxygen is being delivered, likely causes include hypoventilation with atelectasis, unrecognized aspiration, mucous plugging with shunt, pulmonary edema from absorption of irrigant, or heart failure. Less likely causes include pulmonary embolus and preexisting pneumonia.

5. Postoperative mental status changes. With the increased emphasis on postoperative management incorporated into the oral exam in the past few years, it is highly likely that you will encounter this scenario. As usual, you need to approach the answer systematically and tailor the answer to the most likely etiologies *in this patient*. Oral board examiners hate memorized lists. They want logical thought process. So...away we go. "I would go and evaluate the patient. (A call from the nurse is a trap. We recommend that you manage nothing over the telephone on the oral boards.) First, I would rule out life-threatening causes of mental status changes such as hypotension, hypoxemia, and hypoglycemia. The patient is a diabetic and took his glyburide in spite of being NPO. Assuming an acceptable MAP, SaO_2, and fingerstick glucose, the most likely cause is hyponatremia from excessive absorption of the irrigant into the bloodstream with resulting dilution of serum sodium. Other etiologies can be divided into neurologic, metabolic, or pharmacologic causes of CNS malfunction. The patient could have neurologic injury from a stroke or hypoxemia during the difficult intubation. He could also be postictal from an unrecognized seizure. Possible metabolic causes include hypercarbia, severe anemia, alcohol withdrawal, hypocalcemia, or hypothermia. Pharmacologic causes might include residual anesthetic, pain medication, sedative medication, or inadequate muscle relaxant reversal. Unlikely causes include hypothyroidism, adrenal insufficiency, malignant hyperthermia, hypermagnesemia, or preexisting dementia." We would order a serum sodium, ABG, bedside glucose, calcium, magnesium, hematocrit, and an ECG. We would test muscle strength, perform a brief neurologic exam to identify gross neurologic deficits, and listen to the lungs. TURP syndrome is a hypervolemic hyponatremia, which results from excessive absorption of free water from the irrigant used at surgery. Mental status changes can develop in patients with acute drop of their serum sodium into the 120s, but are more common below 120. Seizures and dysrhythmias develop with very low sodium (~110). The syndrome is frequently associated with hypervolemia from excess free water that can result in congestive heart failure and pulmonary edema. Treatment for hyponatremia without symptoms is free water restriction. If the patient is symptomatic with either volume overload or mental status changes, furosemide therapy is indicated with partial replacement of the urine output with normal saline. The object is to bring the serum sodium up gradually. Too rapid a rise can result in CNS damage, such as central pontine myelinolysis. If seizures or dysrhythmias occur, hypertonic saline (3%) is indicated to get the sodium concentration up above 120.

We would transfuse this patient. He has ongoing blood loss with diabetic and hypertensive vascular disease. The indications would be to replace ongoing blood loss and *increase oxygen carrying capacity* in a patient with marginal reserve. Transfusion at a hematocrit above 21% is not supported by the blood bank gurus without clinical indication to *increase oxygen carrying capacity*. If you are stuck for an indication to transfuse on the oral exam, you might consider transfusing to *increase oxygen carrying capacity*.

7. Postoperative headache following dural puncture is due to the dural puncture until proven otherwise. *Go evaluate the patient!* Dural puncture headaches tend to be positional and develop with decreasing frequency up to 7 days following the procedure. They tend to be bilateral and severe, and without a throbbing component. Initial therapy includes enhanced fluid intake and caffeine. If the headache persists, the risk of epidural blood patch is far outweighed by the benefit. An epidural blood patch is best performed by two people. The anesthesiologist obtains epidural access with a Tuohy needle in the vicinity of the prior dural puncture using sterile technique. Also using sterile technique, the helper simultaneously obtains 20 cc of venous blood. The blood is injected into the epidural space until gone or the patient complains of an uncomfortable fullness in the back. The headache should lessen or disappear within an hour. If the diagnosis of post-dural puncture headache is correct, the success rate is high.

CASE #8

A 67-year-old, 65 kg female presents for resection of a cecal carcinoma.

HPI: Patient was in her usual state of health until 4 weeks ago when she presented with fatigue, crampy abdominal pain, and dark stool which tested guaiac positive. Colonoscopy revealed a large cecal mass with partial obstruction. Biopsy was positive for adenocarcinoma. She was scheduled for surgical resection but showed up inebriated to the same day surgery clinic. Surgery was rescheduled for today.

PMH: Long history of alcoholism with history of upper GI bleed from esophageal varices two years ago. Sclerotherapy was performed. UGI bleeding has not recurred. Liver biopsy revealed alcoholic cirrhosis.

She has been followed for elevated liver enzymes and ascites. SGOT fluctuates with alcohol intake and was 398 on the day surgery was cancelled. She was placed on multivitamins including thiamine/folate and was counseled to decrease her ethanol intake. Last reported alcohol intake was 2 days ago. She denies orthopnea, PND, or dyspnea at rest. She sleeps on two pillows because of indigestion and leads a sedentary lifestyle. No known drug allergies. Average daily alcohol consumption depends on availability.

Medications: Aldactone, multivitamin, folate, omeprazole

Exam: Pale, elderly female with truncal obesity in no apparent distress, nervous but coherent

Vital signs: BP 95/60, HR 102 and regular, RR 20, afebrile

Airway: Poor dentition, full motion of the neck, small mouth, short chin, Mallampati 2

Chest: Decreased breath sounds in bases, systolic crescendo/decrescendo murmur at LUSB

Abdomen: Enlarged liver, caput medusae and fluid wave are present, active bowel sounds

Extremities: Thin skin, bruising present at several locations, 2+ ankle edema, normal reflexes

Chest x-ray: Low lung volumes, normal cardiac silhouette, no acute infiltrates

ECG: Sinus tachycardia, no acute ischemia

Echocardiogram: Hyperdynamic LV without wall motion abnormalities or valvular pathology

Labs: Na 129, K 4.2, Cr 1.4, total protein 5.4, albumin 2.1, SGOT 278, SGPT 190, bili 1.2, WBC 3.2, Hematocrit 29, platelet count 85, prothrombin time 15.6(1.4x ULN), glucose 65

She has been NPO and is not inebriated, but wishes she could have a shot of whiskey.

***
Your Outline
(Don't be a slug—work it!)
***

Our Outline

Urgency: Elective (sort of). She has been postponed and has a partially obstructing mass.

Reason for exam: Multisystem disease

Problem List

Head and neck: None

Neurologic:
- Alcohol withdrawal
- Not acutely intoxicated
- Nervous but not hyperreflexic
- No known history of DTs

Airway: Potentially difficult airway with small mouth and short chin
Pulmonary: Restrictive lung disease from ascites
Cardiac: Hyperdynamic heart with benign flow murmur

Gastrointestinal:
- Alcoholic cirrhosis
- Portal hypertension with ascites
- Hypoalbuminemia
- Elevated prothrombin time
- History of bleeding varices
- GE reflux

Renal: Potential hepatorenal syndrome

Hematologic:
- Anemia
- Thombocytopenia

Other: None
Additional history and physical: None
Additional labs: Baseline ABG
Additional tests: None
Consults: Gastroenterology

Preoperative therapy and monitoring:
- Baseline ABG
- Vitamin K, folate, and thiamine IM
- Sodium citrate
- Routine ASA monitors
- Foley catheter
- Arterial line
- CVP

Premedication: O_2, H_2 antagonist, benzodiazepine, thiamine, vitamin K
Induction: Preoxygenate, awake fiberoptic oral intubation with topical anesthesia, and midazolam followed by propofol and *cis*-atracurium once the airway is secured
Maintenance: O_2/forane, fentanyl, midazolam, *cis*-atracurium
Emergence: Extubate awake
Postoperative: ICU

Anticipated problems:
- Uncooperative for awake intubation
- Aspiration
- Coagulopathy with surgical and/or upper GI bleeding
- Hepatorenal syndrome

207

- Delayed awakening
- High output cardiac failure
- Alcohol withdrawal/DTs

Examiners' Questions

Intraoperative

1. Are you concerned about the patient's elevated liver enzymes? Should you cancel the case? What implications does ascites have for general anesthesia? Room air ABG reveals pH 7.38, pCO_2 30, pO_2 72. Should you drain the ascites before induction?

2. Would you expect altered pharmacokinetics of medication in this patient? How? What premedication would you administer to this patient? Why? How would you manage postoperative pain in this patient?

3. What monitors would you place prior to induction? Why? How would you induce anesthesia in this patient? You are unable to intubate. What is your back-up plan for securing an airway?

4. Following induction, the patient becomes hypotensive and tachycardic. What do you do? What is the differential diagnosis? Is additional monitoring required?

5. During the case, the surgeon reports excessive oozing of venous blood. What is the etiology? Hematocrit returns 26%. Would you transfuse? What products would you give?

Postoperative

6. The case proceeds without further incident. Would you extubate at the end of the case? If not, what weaning parameters would you consider acceptable for exubation?

7. Following extubation, you are called because of tachycardia, agitation, and hallucinations. How do you evaluate? What lab tests would you order?

8. What is delirium tremens? What is Wernicke-Korsakoff encephalopathy? How do you distinguish between the two? What is your treatment?

9. Oliguria develops in the postoperative period. What is the diagnosis? How do you evaluate? How do you treat? Should you use crystalloid or colloid for this patient?

Our Answers

1. Yes, you are concerned. You are concerned about everything on the oral exam. Proceeding on an elective case with an acute elevation of SGOT/SGPT is folly. Worsening hepatocellular inflammation will not be helped by anesthesia. General, spinal, and epidural anesthesia all decrease hepatic blood flow and could turn an active hepatitis into a fulminant, necrotizing hepatitis. However, the SGOT has fallen since the case was last cancelled and the patient's condition may be as good as it's going to get. Delaying the case further may lead to complete bowel obstruction and make the surgery emergent with attendant elevation of perioperative risk. Obtaining a gastroenterology consult is reasonable, but it will be unlikely to help. Interventions that will optimize the patient's liver function are limited unless the patient was to become miraculously abstinent from alcohol. Fat chance! This is a judgement question. As long as you can defend your decision, go for it and prepare to deal with the consequences. Ascites is a ramification of severe hepatic disease with portal hypertension. The fluid may exert so much pressure on the abdomen that excursion of the diaphragm is impaired. The functional residual capacity then decreases and hypoxemia results, especially in the supine position. The ABG reveals a respiratory alkalosis, which is common in severe liver disease. Oxygenation is adequate which argues that drainage of the ascitic fluid will not have much impact on pulmonary function. Draining ascites can be dangerous if too much is removed. Hepatic failure patients already have low plasma oncotic pressure from hypoalbuminemia and tend to be intravascularly volume depleted. Rapid removal of ascitic fluid will cause a net fluid movement into the peritoneal space from the intravascular space and induce severe hypotension.

2. The decreased total protein, albumin, and sodium along with ankle edema all tell you that the patient has an excess of total body water. The response to protein-bound drugs will be increased. Neuromuscular blockers need to be given in larger doses initially to overcome the increased volume of distribution associated with an excess of total body water. These patients then need lower subsequent doses due to decreased hepatic clearance. Succinylcholine action will be slightly prolonged due to decreased pseudocholinestase made by the liver. Atracurium and *cis*-atracurium doses will not need to be decreased since they utilize nonhepatic elimination pathways (pH-mediated Hoffman degradation and enzymatic destruction by nonspecific plasma esterases that tend to be abundant even in severe liver disease). The patient may be tolerant of sedatives yet have markedly prolonged elimination of barbiturates and benzodiazepines. If not already done on admission, we would administer thiamine, folate, and vitamin K. We would give an H-2 antagonist IV and sodium citrate PO to neutralize stomach acid. We would administer nasal cannula O_2 and midazolam after an IV is started to decrease anxiety and prevent alcohol withdrawal. We would manage postoperative pain with patient-controlled analgesia. Epidural analgesia is contraindicated with easy bruising, thrombocytopenia, and an elevated prothrombin time.

3. We would use routine ASA monitors, Foley catheter, arterial line, and CVP for this case. The CVP could be placed following induction and is indicated to monitor anticipated fluid shifts. We would perform an awake, oral fiberoptic intubation in this patient because of a full stomach (ascites) and potentially difficult airway. Nasal intubation is not recommended because of the patient's coagulopathy. If the patient were unable to tolerate awake intubation, we would assure availability of an appropriately sized LMA to use in a failed intubation scenario and perform a rapid sequence induction with propofol and succinylcholine.

4. Blood pressure is a function of vascular resistance and cardiac output. Assuming the tachycardia is a sinus tachycardia and is not rapid enough to compromise ventricular filling, it is likely a physiologic response to increase cardiac output in a hypotensive patient. Given that the heart is functionally normal by echo and that general anesthesia produces a fall in systemic vascular tone, the hypotension is likely a combination of inadequate preload and decreased vascular resistance. We would turn to 100% oxygen and assure adequate ventilation. Then we would temporize with phenylephrine and deliver intravenous volume. If not already in place, we would obtain central venous access. A pulmonary artery catheter is unlikely to be helpful at this point as long as the patient responds to therapy and urine output is maintained.

5. Bleeding in this case is multifactorial. Assuming adequate surgical hemostasis, decreased levels of hepatically synthesized clotting proteins such as Factor VII will induce a coagulopathy. Splenic sequestration of platelets in a patient with portal hypertension causes thrombocytopenia. Malnutrition produces fragile tissue that may be difficult to suture. We would transfuse this patient below a hematocrit of 30% to *optimize oxygen carrying capacity.* While data is inconclusive, the optimal hematocrit for oxygen delivery may be 35% because this level provides adequate oxygen content of the blood as well as optimal rheology to enhance tissue perfusion. We would give packed red blood cells to *optimize oxygen carrying capacity* and fresh frozen plasma to provide depleted clotting proteins. If oozing continued, we would check a platelet count and give platelets if the count were falling.

6. *Make the patient healthy!* Assuming hemodynamic stability, normothermia, normal electrolyte and acid-base status, adequate reversal of neuromuscular blockers, adequate hemostasis, purposeful response to voice, adequate respiratory rate/tidal volume and SaO_2 >95%, we would extubate at the end of the case. Extubation criteria we use are: $PaO_2 > 60$ mm Hg on $FIO_2 \leq 0.5$ and $PEEP \leq 5$ cm H_2O, $TV > 5$ cc/kg IBW, FVC >10 cc/kg IBW, RR < 30, MIF < −25 cm H_2O, pH ≥ 7.30. These criteria are only guidelines but are defendable based upon the literature.

7. Tachycardia, agitation, and hallucinations in this patient. Well, let's see. What could be wrong? Alcohol withdrawal, ya think? Duh! However, we still must be systematic. *Go and see the patient!* Rule out immediately life-threatening causes. Check ABC (airway, breathing, circulation). Check pulse oximetry and administer supplemental oxygen. Check blood pressure, heart rate, and rhythm to assure adequate brain perfusion. Do a finger stick for glucose (glycogen stores are depleted in hepatic disease and hypoglycemia can develop at any time) and send an ABG. Mention that you consider alcohol withdrawal the most likely diagnosis. Then start down the differential in an organized fashion; drugs, metabolic, neurologic. For this patient, list the most likely causes in each category first. All preop, intraop, and postop drugs can be responsible, especially given the expectation of reduced metabolism of anesthetics and narcotics. Consider if the patient has been prophylactically treated for alcohol withdrawal with too much benzodiazepine. Hallucinations make the diagnosis of overtreatment with benzodiazepines less likely. Check muscle strength to rule out residual neuromuscular blockade. Metabolic causes include hypoglycemia, hypoxia, hypercarbia, and metabolic acidosis. Hyponatremia, hepatic encephalopathy with elevated serum ammonia, and severe anemia are secondary possibilities. Adrenal and thyroid problems, malignant hyperthermia, hypocalcemia, and hypermagnesemia are possible, but much less likely in this patient. Neurologic causes include delirium tremens, Wernicke-Korsakoff encephalopathy, or previously undiagnosed subdural hematoma (in an alcoholic). Intraoperative insults to the brain such as stroke, prolonged hypotension, hemorrhage, or hypoxia are possible.

8. Delirium tremens are manifestations of acute alcohol withdrawal. High sympathetic tone and "emergence delirium" with hallucinations in an alcoholic are classic for DTs. If not treated, seizure activity and/or myocardial damage with ischemia and malignant dysrhythmias can develop. Even if treated, the mortality rate of full-blown DTs is 15%. Treatment is CNS sedation with benzodiazepines or high-dose barbiturates, if necessary. Wernicke-Korsakoff encephalopathy results from the administration of high-dextrose content IV fluids to an alcoholic with thiamine deficiency. Without thiamine as a substrate of carbohydrate metabolism, the body's energy plant gets all revved up with no place to go and neurologic damage occurs (You might consider a slightly more technical description for the purpose of the oral boards. Look it up. We had to!). Wernicke-Korsakoff syndrome produces a psychosis and sometimes focal neurologic findings, but does not tend to have a markedly elevated sympathetic tone or seizure activity. Treatment is tough—thiamine and supportive care. Prevention with preoperative thiamine is the best treatment and should not be forgotten.

9. *In this patient*, oliguria is an ominous finding which may indicate onset of hepatorenal syndrome. BUN, creatinine, urine sodium, urine osmolality, and FeNa should be sent but will likely be consistent with prerenal azotemia, regardless of whether the diagnosis is simple intravascular hypovolemia or hepatorenal syndrome. Response to a fluid challenge argues for hypovolemia as the diagnosis. Hepatorenal syndrome is a condition that develops in end-stage liver disease in which the kidneys are underperfused and develop first a prerenal azotemia and then damage to the nephrons with the development of acute renal failure. The prognosis is not good for this condition. Unless the patient responds in a gratifying manner to a volume challenge, we would place a pulmonary artery catheter to determine the effect of preload on enhancing cardiac output. Maintenance of intravascular fluid volume and optimizing oxygen delivery to the tissues is the mainstay of both prevention and treatment. Dialysis may be necessary. If the crystalloid versus colloid debate did not exist, critical care meetings would also be a lot shorter. As with most highly debated topics in medicine, there is no definitive answer to the debate. Either answer can be defended. We would use a combination of crystalloid and colloid as guided by invasive monitoring in this scenario. In the presence of low oncotic pressure due to hypoalbuminemia, a greater percentage of the crystalloid will exit the vascular space and add to "third space" fluid. Colloid will stay intravascular for a longer period of time, but will also eventually find its way into the tissues and cannot be removed by diuretics or dialysis in the volume-overloaded patient. If the hematocrit is less than 30%, we would use packed red blood cells as our fluid of choice. As always, therapy in moderation is the key.

CASE #9

A 20-year-old, 5'0" tall, 95 kg, G1P0 female is admitted in transfer from an outside hospital for an elective C-section. The last trimester has been complicated by hypertension and proteinuria. Current therapy includes magnesium sulfate and hydralazine. BP 145/95; HR 85; RR 16; afebrile.

***
Your Outline
***

Our Outline
>*Urgency:* Elective
>*Reason for exam:* Multisystem organ disease

Problem List
>*Head and neck:* None
>*Neurologic:* At risk for seizure or intracranial hemorrhage

Airway:
- Difficult airway
- Laryngeal edema of pregnancy
- Short and obese
- Full stomach

Pulmonary:
- Pregnancy
- Decreased FRC
- Decreased reserve for hypoxia

Obesity
1. Enhances decreased FRC (I love that semantic twist—enhancing a decrease)
2. Possible chronic hypoxemia
3. Increased oxygen consumption

Cardiovascular:
- Preeclampsia
- Decreased intravascular volume
- Hypertension
- Increased adrenergic tone
- Possible congestive failure

Gastrointestinal: Possible HELLP syndrome
Renal: Possible acute renal failure
Hematologic: Possible thrombocytopenia
Other: Possible passive-aggressive personality

History and physical:
- Why was patient transferred?
- Visual changes?
- Hyperreflexia?
- Difficult airway?
- History of prior intubations?
- Rales on lung exam?
- Serial blood pressures?
- Enlarged, tender liver?

Laboratory evaluation:
- Hematocrit
- ABG
- BUN, Cr, K, glucose
- SGOT/SGPT
- Platelet count
- Urine for protein and urine output

Tests: Fetal heart tones

Consults: Referring physician and obstetrical colleagues to discuss plan

Preoperative therapy and monitoring:
- Sodium citrate
- Oxygen
- IV hydration
- Fetal heart tones
- Tocodynamometer
- Foley catheter
- Routine ASA
- Arterial line
- CVP, if oliguric
- PA catheter, if pulmonary edema

Anesthetic plan: Assuming platelet count >100K and normal airway, administer supplemental oxygen and epidural bupivacaine with incremental bolus dosing to a T6 level. Prepare for difficult intubation with LMA and fiberoptic scope. Blood pressure control with labetolol/hydralazine.

Postoperative: Recovery area with IV $MgSO_4$ × 24 hours.

Anticipated difficulties:
- Failed epidural with difficult intubation
- Eclampsia
- Hypertensive crisis with CHF/mental status changes
- Renal failure
- Neonatal resuscitation

Examiners' Questions

Preoperative

1. What effects does pregnancy have on pulmonary function? How about morbid obesity? What concerns do you have about pulmonary function in this patient?
2. How do you distinguish mild preeclampsia from more severe forms of the illness? What are the cardiovascular implications of preeclampsia?
3. What additional history, physical, and laboratory data would you require prior to anesthesia? Why?
4. What is the significance of decreased variability of the fetal heart rate? What do variable decelerations of the fetal heart rate imply? Late decelerations?

Intraoperative

5. What monitors would you choose for this case? When would you use a CVP? A PA catheter?

6. What is your anesthetic plan? Why? The old chart arrives from the other hospital. The patient was referred from the outside hospital because of a failed intubation on induction of general anesthesia. How do you proceed? During preparation for the anesthetic, the patient has a grand mal seizure. What is your treatment? The maternal SaO_2 is 72%, you are unable to intubate, and the fetal heart rate is 60. What do you do?

7. The patient stabilizes and C-section is performed. The baby is stained with meconium. No one is available to care for the mother. What is the appropriate action? The mother develops acute oxygen desaturation. What is the differential diagnosis? How would you evaluate?

8. The patient is slow to awaken. What are the likely etiologies? Is an emergent head CT scan indicated? Why or why not?

Our Answers

1. During the third trimester of pregnancy, minute ventilation increases due mainly to an increase in tidal volume. However, functional residual capacity decreases due to the enlarging uterus causing upward pressure on the diaphragms. Oxygen consumption is increased by term pregnancy. Obesity also decreases FRC and increases oxygen consumption. Chronic hypoxemia with pulmonary hypertension may also be present with morbid obesity. Both obese and pregnant patients have an increased risk of aspiration. With induction of anesthesia, this patient will have very little oxygen reserve and will desaturate quickly. The risk of aspiration makes a rapid sequence mandatory if general anesthesia is induced. Laryngeal edema of pregnancy along with redundant oropharyngeal tissue in an obese patient increase the risk of failed intubation and difficult mask ventilation.

2. Mild preeclampsia is heralded by elevated diastolic blood pressure and proteinuria. Severe forms of the disease show evidence of end-organ damage, such as oliguria with prerenal azotemia and marked proteinuria, thrombocytopenia, coagulopathy, elevated liver enzymes, congestive heart failure, visual changes, hyperreflexia, and fetal distress. Acute renal failure, DIC and intracranial hemorrhage can develop. Seizure activity heralds onset of eclampsia. Preeclamptic patients have increased vascular tone with significant afterload elevation that can induce ventricular failure. Yet, they have a relative deficiency of intravascular fluid volume.

3. What a great opportunity to use your outline! We would ask why the patient was transferred as well as seek a history of visual changes that would classify the preeclampsia as severe. We would ask about prior general anesthetics and any history of difficult intubation. Exam findings we would seek include serial blood pressures and evidence of a difficult airway, hyperreflexia, hepatomegaly or rales. Preoperative laboratory evaluation would include hematocrit, platelet count, ABG, BUN, Cr, K, glucose, SGOT/SGPT, urinalysis for protein and urine output. All of this information would help us identify problems which can be treated prior to an elective C-section or help us anticipate problems which might develop and allow preparation for dealing with the problems.

4. Decreased fetal heart rate variability can be a normal finding which occurs while the fetus is sleeping or, if prolonged, can signify limited fetal reserve and be an early warning for possible development of fetal distress. Variable decelerations are likely the result of transient umbilical cord compression during uterine contraction. Changing the maternal position will likely eliminate the problem. Late decelerations signify fetal hypoxemia and convert an elective delivery into an emergency.

5. *Make the patient healthy!* "Assuming that urine output is good and that the lungs are clear, I would use the following monitors in this case: fetal heart tones, tocodynamometer, Foley catheter, routine ASA monitors, and arterial line." *Then stop!* The examiners may not let you get away with your assumptions, but at least they must level the playing field with additional information about the patient if they want her to be sicker. If they accept your assumptions, great! If the patient is oliguric, we would add CVP. If pulmonary edema is present, then a pulmonary artery catheter is indicated.

6. *Make the patient healthy!* "Assuming a normal airway, normal platelet count, and a healthy fetus, I would place an epidural and give incremental doses of bupivacaine to gradually attain a T6 sensory level. I would be prepared for a failed epidural and potential difficult intubation with an LMA, a fiberoptic bronchoscope and a tracheostomy tray in the room. I would control BP with labetolol and hydralazine." *Then stop!* We have shown appropriate concern for the airway and hypertension issues. If you keep talking, you will say something you wish you hadn't. When they ask why, then respond. "General anesthesia carries the risk of postoperative pulmonary complications in this significantly obese female. While a spinal anesthetic would be appropriate for this patient, I am concerned about emergent intubation in the event of a high spinal and would use a well-tested epidural to obtain surgical anesthesia in a spontaneously breathing patient." Wait, not so fast! There's trouble a'brewin'. The patient can't be intubated according to the old chart. Tough problem. If you assume you can intubate anyone, your patient is unlikely to do well and you will have plenty of time to reconsider your response over the next year of board preparation. "While a risk of hypertensive crisis and intracranial hemorrhage exists with awake fiberoptic intubation in this patient, given the history of failed intubation, the risk of hypoxemia to the patient and fetus outweigh the benefit of a rapid sequence induction. I would counsel the patient thoroughly and obtain patient approval of the plan, then I would use topical anesthesia in the oropharynx and secure an airway with a 6.5 mm ETT over an intubating bronchoscope. I would control BP with labetolol and hydralazine." Grand mal seizure and eclampsia—great! "I would support the airway and administer 100% O_2 by mask. I would give 5 mg of IV diazepam and then small doses of pentothal to stop the seizure activity. I would assure left lateral decubitus position and administer labetolol for BP control." Desaturation and can't intubate. It just keeps getting better! *Remember the airway algorithm.* "I would call for help and place a LMA. I would call for the surgeon to prepare for a surgical airway and the obstetrician to prepare for C-section. If unable to ventilate through the LMA, I would place a needle cricothyroidotomy and jet ventilate with 100% O_2 until a surgical airway can be obtained."

7. Meconium staining. Your first responsibility is to the mother. If she is unstable, you cannot tend to the baby. It would then be up to the obstetrician, the pediatrician, or the respiratory therapist to intubate and suction any meconium out of the airway prior to ventilation with 100% O_2. Differential diagnosis of acute oxygen desaturation in the mother includes airway problems, oxygen disconnect, atelectasis with shunting, pulmonary edema, bronchospasm, amniotic fluid embolus, pulmonary thromboembolus, or pneumothorax. ABCs. "I would deliver 100% O_2, check my inspired oxygen monitor to assure oxygen delivery, listen to bilateral breath sounds to assure ventilation, and exclude pneumothorax, bronchospam, or pulmonary edema. I would then add PEEP to increase FRC and improve ventilation/perfusion matching."

8. "The causes of delayed awakening are metabolic, pharmacologic, or neurologic. This patient is at increased risk of intracranial hemorrhage or hypoxic encephalopathy following the complicated delivery. Assuming hypoxemia, hypotension and hypoglycemia have been ruled out, I would confirm reversal of any muscle relaxant, check the pupils and respiratory rate for evidence of narcotic effect and perform a thorough neurologic exam looking for evidence of a focal neurologic deficit. If a focal deficit is found or awakening is delayed after pharmacologic causes have either worn off or been reversed, then a head CT is indicated to rule out an acute CNS event."

CASE #10

A 5-hour-old, 2500 gram infant born at 34 weeks is scheduled for emergency repair of a congenital diaphragmatic hernia. P 175; R 54; temp 35°C; Hgb 12.

***
Your Outline
***

Our Outline
Urgency: Emergent
Reason for Exam: Differential diagnosis of signs and symptoms

Problem List
Head and neck: Retrolental fibroplasia may develop
Neurologic: Prematurity, increased sensitivity to centrally acting agents, and at risk for intraventricular hemorrhage
Airway: Cephalad larynx with prominent epiglottis compared with adults

Pulmonary:
- Hypoplastic left lung
- Stomach and intestines in left chest

- Possible associated esophageal malformations
- Immature respiratory drive

Cardiovascular:
- Patent PDA
- Possible associated cardiac abnormalities
- Patent foramen ovale
- Tachycardic and hypothermic

Gastrointestinal:
- Congenital diaphragmatic hernia
- Poor glucose metabolism

Renal: None
Hematologic: Anemia
Other: None

History and physical:
- History of associated anomalies
- Skin turgor
- Fontanelle fullness
- Breath sounds
- Cardiac exam

Labs: Glucose
Tests: Review chest x-ray
Consults: Pediatric pulmonologist for postoperative ventilation

Preoperative therapy and monitoring:
- Warm the room
- Warm IV fluids
- Type and cross RBCs
- Decompress with orogastric tube before induction
- Right-sided pulse oximeter
- Routine ASA monitors
- Foley catheter

Anticipated problems:
- Pneumothorax
- Hypoxemia
- Hypothermia and acidosis
- Hypovolemia
- Hypoglycemia
- IV access

Examiners' Questions

Preoperative

1. How do you interpret this patient's vital signs? Why is the patient hypothermic? How would you treat the hypothermia? Is the weight appropriate for gestational age? Is this a normal hemoglobin concentration? Would you transfuse?

2. The patient's skin has poor turgor and the fontanelles are sunken. How would you obtain IV access? What is an appropriate fluid bolus for this patient? What is an appropriate maintenance rate? How much additional fluid would you give per hour to match anticipated intraoperative losses?

3. What are the differences between this patient's circulation and that of an adult? How do the differences alter your anesthetic management? Are cardiac anomalies associated with this condition? Which ones?

4. What pulmonary condition is associated with this condition? How does this alter management?

Intraoperative

5. What monitors would you place prior to induction? Is an arterial catheter required? Why or why not? How would you induce this patient? Why?

6. Following induction and intubation, the patient becomes cyanotic. What are the most likely causes? The pulse oximeter on the right hand reads 99%. How do you manage the cyanosis?

7. During the diaphragmatic repair, the oxygen saturation by pulse oximetry drops accompanied by hypotension and elevated peak airway pressures. How would you evaluate? How would you treat?

8. Would you extubate this patient at the end of the case? If not, how would you ventilate the patient postoperatively?

Our Answers

1. Memorize your pediatric vital signs. This neonate's vital signs are abnormal. The pulse and respiratory rate are elevated due to respiratory distress in the neonate. The temperature is low. Due to their relatively large surface area and poor shivering mechanism, children of this age are prone to hypothermia. Hypothermic babies develop acidosis and respiratory depression. Warm the room, warm the fluids and keep the baby wrapped during the case (in plastic if available). The weight is reasonable for gestational age. The hemoglobin concentration is not. Oxygen consumption per kilogram is twice as high in neonates as in adults. However, persistent fetal hemoglobin causes the neonate to offload less oxygen per gram of hemoglobin at the tissue level. Therefore, the average hemoglobin level in a neonate is around 17 gm/dl. This hemoglobin level is low enough to compromise oxygen delivery. Given that we are about to perform major surgery on this premature infant, we would transfuse up front.

2. Poor skin turgor, tachycardia, and sunken fontanelles. This kid needs fluid. If no peripheral or scalp veins are accessible, an umbilical vein catheter can be used. An appropriate fluid bolus for this child would be 25 mL/kg of lactated Ringer's. The maintenance fluid should contain dextrose as well as lactated Ringer's because a sick neonate may not have any glucose reserve. An appropriate maintenance rate for this neonate would be 10 mL/hr (4 mL/kg/hr). During a major operation like this, you should add 6 mL/kg/hr to the maintenance rate (total of 25 mL/hr).

3. Assuming no cardiac anomalies, neonates have a patent ductus arteriosus and a patent foramen ovale. Increases in pulmonary arterial pressure relative to systemic pressure will result in increased blood flow through the PDA with systemic arterial desaturation. The pulse oximeter is placed on the right hand to avoid fluctuations in saturation around the connection of the PDA and give a better estimate of the saturation of blood flow to the brain. Avoiding hypoxia, hypercapnia, hypothermia, acidosis, and light anesthesia will all help lower pulmonary vascular resistance and reduce shunting.

4. Hypoplasia of the lung on the side of the hernia is common due to abdominal contents in the chest. Positive pressure ventilation by mask may overdistend the stomach, shift the mediastinum toward the unaffected lung and make adequate ventilation impossible. After repair of the diaphragm, attempts to expand the lung on the operative side should be avoided as elevations of peak airway pressure may cause a pneumothorax in the good lung.

5. We would place routine ASA monitors with a right-sided pulse oximeter and a Foley catheter. While not absolutely required for the case, an umbilical artery catheter would be helpful for frequent blood sampling. Any inhaled agent may depress the myocardium too much in a premature baby. Nitrous oxide is not acceptable if the patient has abdominal viscera in his chest. After decompressing the stomach with an orogastric tube and preoxygenating with O_2, we would use ketamine for induction with spontaneous ventilation. We would intubate the spontaneously breathing child to avoid desaturation or gastric distention. We would use fentanyl combined with a muscle relaxant for maintenance. Postoperative ventilation is indicated, so apnea associated with prematurity is not an issue. Therefore, IV narcotics are not problematic. There is absolutely no right answer to this question, so we propose a reasonable approach to the anesthetic.

6. Cyanosis in this neonate is either due to hypoxia (inadequate oxygen delivery to the lungs) or shunt-induced hypoxemia (mixing of saturated and desaturated blood through the PDA). The SaO_2 of 99% in the right hand confirms shunting through the PDA as the etiology. Management consists of lowering pulmonary vascular resistance. We would increase the minute ventilation to lower pCO_2, administer 100% oxygen, warm the patient, administer fentanyl and administer sodium bicarbonate to offset metabolic acidosis as guided by ABG.

7. "Desaturation, hypotension, and elevated airway pressures in this patient are due to a tension pneumothorax until proven otherwise. I would administer 100% oxygen, hand ventilate, and check breath sounds. If breath sounds are diminished on the nonoperative side, I would ask the surgeons to place an emergent chest tube. If they cannot do so immediately, I would pass a 14 g angiocatheter over the top of the third rib on the nonoperative side and then follow that with a chest tube."

8. "The abdomen is usually scaphoid in these patients and ventilation may be very difficult when muscle relaxation wears off. Incomplete closure or continued paralysis may be necessary. In any event, the work of breathing will initially be unacceptable for this critically ill neonate and continued mechanical ventilation is indicated postoperatively. I would use a pressure ventilator with peak inspiratory pressures less than 25–30 cm H_2O to prevent further barotrauma to the normal lung. I would use ABG measurements to wean the oxygen as quickly as possible to avoid retrolental fibroplasia."

23 | Sample Test Batch Number Two

Sample Batch Number One came from Dave and Steve's kitchen. And no matter how you slice it or dice it, you just can't eat the same cooking all the time. Plus, you got exposed to one way of looking at things. That's why we have Sample Batch Number Two from Chris's kitchen. Many of the questions will be similar. Note that the first question involves falling off something and konking your head. But now you'll see a different approach to the questions, a different approach to the answers, and with any luck, you'll see some contradictions! But wait, David said *this*, but Chris said *that*! Which one's right?

That's the point. The same question can have different answers, the key is explaining your reasoning.

Is there a "Waldo" in these answers? You tell us.

SAMPLE TEST #1

Session 1

A 68-year-old, 75 kg, 5'8" tall male is coming to your OR for a craniotomy for drainage of a subdural hematoma.

HPI: Patient recently started on Viagra and was on a trapeze at a local house of ill repute when he fell off, striking his head on a statue of Priapus. His paramour stated he lost consciousness immediately. Paramedics arrived to find the patient obtunded. Jaw thrust relieved his airway obstruction and he was brought to East Bumblebee Memorial Hospital. Pulse was 45 with a blood pressure of 180/100. Cervical spine showed no fracture or dislocation, but was only visualized to C-6. No other injuries were apparent.

PMH: Unobtainable, though his...uh...friend stated, "He told me no way to give him his nitro tablets when he was in flagrante delicto. Said that would kill him with his new Viagra medicine."

Physical Exam: Neck in a collar. Won't open his mouth to command. Breath sounds normal. Heart sounds normal. Has a median sternotomy scar consistent with heart surgery. Loosely applied and well-padded handcuffs dangle from his left wrist. The patient's friend (from the house of ill repute) has the keys and removes the handcuffs, blushes, then hands you her card.

Chest x-ray: Status post–open-heart surgery with markers for bypass grafts.

Lab studies: Normal except for a K of 2.9 and an EKG that shows a left bundle branch block.

He arrives in the OR with two 18-gauge IVs and has received a liter of LR. He has a Foley with 300 cc of urine in it. The surgeon states the hematoma is large enough that the evacuation should proceed pronto.

Examiners' Questions

Intraoperative

1. Should an intracranial bolt be placed under local before induction? After? Not at all? Why?
2. Given the cardiac history, which invasive monitors will you place?
3. Any special induction considerations with Viagra on board?
4. The C-spine is not cleared, how will you secure the airway? If awake, how will you sedate given his state of consciousness? If you induce first, will you keep the collar on? How will you prevent further injury to the spinal cord, if indeed it is injured?
5. You induce and can't intubate, go through the techniques to assure oxygenation while protecting the spinal cord and preventing increased ICP.
6. What is Cushing's triad?
7. The case has begun, what are your goals for blood pressure?
8. What is cerebral perfusion pressure, how will you "protect" that?
9. Halfway into the case, profuse and generalized bleeding occurs in the operative field. The surgeon says, "Hang cryo." Your response?
10. Ventricular ectopy occurs as closing is occurring. What do you do?

Answers to Intraoperative Questions

No peeking until you do it yourself! Remember, *you're* taking the test. You get zippo out of this if you just look at the answers. And remember the "Where's Waldo?" warning. Somewhere in here is a bogus answer. Maybe here, maybe later. Maybe there's more than one "Waldo" in the answers. Who knows? Maybe each set of questions has one wrong answer in there, you never know.

1. No. Don't hold up things to place an intracranial bolt. Although the bolt provides useful information on intracranial pressure, the surgeon says the hematoma is big and you have to get a move on. Delay could lead to herniation, and that's that. Even with the bolt info, you're going to do the same maneuvers to decrease ICP (hyperventilation, head positioning, diuresis), plus you're going to get going on to *the* procedure to decrease ICP—draining the hematoma! How's that for a good therapeutic maneuver. At the end of the case, a bolt is a good idea to help in the unit. An increase in the measured ICP may be the earliest sign of a rebleed, particularly if "Lover Boy" is still on the ventilator and is unable to participate in a neuro exam.

2. The scar and the nitro tell you there's a cardiac history; however, the gymnastics (he did fall off a trapeze) tell you that he must not have terrible CHF. Place an A-line (a given with a big neuro case) and a Swan. Although his sprightly romantic behavior suggests good pump function, you will be facing volume shifts as you try to "dry out" his brain, and in the postoperative period, you'll be trying to manage his fluids carefully in an attempt to prevent spasm in his cerebral circulation. That's a lot of tricky fluid juggling. An alternative to the Swan is a TEE (great look at volume and contractility). But you can't exactly keep the TEE in the patient the whole time he's in the ICU, so stick with the Swan.

3. "Viagra is a great drug!" according to Elizabeth Dole, and who are we to disagree? It functions as a vasodilator, and in conjunction with other vasodilators—nitro, anesthetic induction agents—Viagra can drop the blood pressure. In this case, where cerebral perfusion pressure (mean arterial pressure minus intracranial pressure) is a crucial consideration, you must consider Viagra's potential to "let you down," so to speak. With your arterial line in place, your volume lines at the ready, your Swan to guide your volume, and your Neo ever ready to raise the blood pressure and maintain cerebral perfusion pressure, you should be able to fight off the evil genies of excessive vasodilation.

4. Thorny dilemma, the uncleared C-spine in the unconscious patient. Examine the airway as best you can, ask if he has dentures. (Perhaps his special friend would have some insight.) If his neuro condition is deteriorating and aspiration, respiratory insufficiency, and hypoxemia are staring you in the face, then you must move without delay to secure the airway. Hypoxemia will exacerbate everything in general, and cerebral injury in specific. Have a trach kit ready (as in the Maryland Shock Trauma protocol when they have a cerebral injury plus an unclear C-spine), induce with pentathol and Sux (yes, Sux can raise the ICP, but complete relaxation, and quick wearing off if you get in airway trouble are its advantages).

5. Hyperventilate through cricoid pressure, and intubate without hyperextending the neck. Have someone maintain axial traction (pulling the hair works, unless "Lover Boy" has a toupee). If no go, then go right to trach. Messy, but the alternative is death, and there's no time to try a fiberoptic if the patient is deteriorating. Remember to treat the patient with steroids, the only therapeutic regimen shown to improve the "secondary injury" picture in cases of spinal cord injury. If you don't remember to give the steroids, the plaintiff's attorney will remind you later on that you should have given it.

6. First, increased intracranial pressure. The body, in an attempt to maintain cerebral perfusion pressure, increases the blood pressure. The heart, in a reflex response to the increased blood pressure, slows down. So the triad is increased ICP, hypertension, and bradycardia. Recall, in any neuro case discussion, cerebral perfusion pressure and the physiology of what's going on in the brain are important points to emphasize, understand, and mention to the examiners.

7. Duh! Maintain cerebral perfusion pressure. (We advise you not to say "Duh!" during your exam.)

8. Mean arterial pressure minus intracranial pressure. The goal is to perfuse the brain. Once the dura is opened, the increased ICP is taken care of, but you still have swollen, damaged neurons with possibly a tenuous blood supply. So keeping the pressure at least normal (keep the transducer at the level of the head, remember) should provide adequate perfusion. What is his normal pressure? That's a toughie, unless you have his old records. In all likelihood, they didn't take his blood pressure at the…uh…place of his accident.

9. Disseminated intravascular coagulation can result from intracranial injury. Willy-nilly tossing of products into the patient is not the scientific approach. Send coag studies and a TEG. A study of these, in an ideal world, will tell you exactly what you can give. For example, if primary fibrinolysis is the cause of the bleeding, then epsilon aminocaproic acid may stop the bleeding better than cryo. In the real world, if the bleeding were really causing a disaster, I blush to disclose, you would probably treat empirically and give cryo. Messy, not terribly scientific, but the usual and customary treatment.

10. Look for a cause, rounding up the usual suspects first, hypoxemia, hypercarbia, electrolyte disorders (mannitol, for example, could have dragged a lot of potassium out with it in the urine). Treat the ectopy empirically with lidocaine while going through this rapid diagnostic process. Did your Swan slip back into the right ventricle? Cerebral injury on its own can cause cardiac weirdness, such as ST segment changes, but you must rule out treatable causes of ectopy before saying, "No big deal, that ectopy is just from the neural injury. Ho hum."

Examiners' Questions

Postoperative

1. In the OR, the patient is not responding; the surgeon wants to do a neuro exam. What next?
2. ICU or PACU?
3. Urine output falls 2 hours postop. The CVP is 2. The surgeon reminds you to "keep him dry." What now?
4. Urine output falls 2 hours postop. The CVP is 20. Your move.
5. A new nurse is having a hard time trouble-shooting the intracranial bolt. She pages you and says it reads 50. Tell me, tell me, give me the news, whatchoo gonna do now, Doc?
6. An internist places a Swan, unbeknownst to you, and you hear overhead a stat page. Patient's gone into complete heart block. What happened and what do you do to help the internist?
7. A med student asks you, "How long are you going to hyper-ventilate this guy?"
8. A concerned family member asks you if the operation "hurt" and what you're doing to make sure the patient isn't in pain on the breathing machine. What do you say?
9. Two days later the patient is extubated, but 4 hours later has labored breathing. What is the differential diagnosis and man-agement of this dyspnea?
10. What are the criteria for extubation?

Answers to Postop Questions

Time for a little honesty check. Who went right to the answers in that first "Answers to Intraop Questions?" Raise your hands! OK, I see a few hands here. There's one in Chicago. I see a few hands in LA, a hand or two in Seattle, Detroit. There's a couple in New York, Chattanooga, Denver…. Bad! You should not do that. If you were really clever, you wouldn't even look at these answers at all, you'd answer them for yourself and ignore what we say. OK, I hope you feel duly admonished. On to the postop answers. I wonder where Waldo is?

1. First, remember ABC. Don't rush to extubate, lose the airway, and undo a *lot of good surgery* with a *little bad anesthesia*. Keep the airway until the patient's neuro status allows extubation. To facilitate the surgeons request, do what you can to assure no "anesthesia" causes are keeping the patient unresponsive—muscle relaxant, inhaled agent, IV agent, hypothermia, hypoglycemia. Once all that is taken care of, if the patient is still not responsive, the most likely cause is cerebral edema from the injury and the traction of surgery. Support the patient until he is responsive, but keep asking the question, "Is there anything I've overlooked that could be keeping this patient from responding?"

2. Humongo neuro operation? ICU. Ideally a neuro ICU where the staff are familiar with intracranial pressure monitors. Try to avoid sending the patient to a "generic" ICU, particularly on a weekend when hospitals flesh themselves out with travelers and agency people who might not be familiar with the vagaries of neurosurgery.

3. The tug of war between a "dried out brain" and a "pruned out kidney" can be problematic. Discuss with the surgeon your concern and use a modest fluid bolus to get the urine output up. (Assuming you have done your prerenal, post-renal, and renal checklist. Make sure the Foley is in the right place.) Start renal dopamine to make yourself feel better. Check a hematocrit. If the patient needs blood (recall, he has a cardiac history and you don't want to exacerbate ischemia with inadequate oxygen carrying capacity), transfuse blood.

4. Back to the oliguria algorithm. Once you've ruled out the usual stuff, and it looks like the patient really is full, give Lasix. As a cardiac patient, he may be used to Lasix, and will need it to maintain an adequate urine output.

5. If the pressure is indeed 50, (check stopcocks, monitor cables, and transducer heights to make sure that is an accurate reading), you're in deep Kimchee. The patient may well need a reexploration. Tell the surgeon. To acutely drop the ICP, try the same medical maneuvers you use in the OR—hyperventilation, head positioning, diuresis. To this, add barbiturates in the form of pentathol.

6. Golly Moses, those internists. Pull the Swan back in case that is causing complete heart block. If the patient is in complete arrest, start

CPR, and follow standard ACLS protocol. Pacing would be just the thing, so use a Zoll external pacer (easiest and fastest to place) at the same time you are getting a pacing wire to put through the Swan introducer (there may be a panic as people try to find the right stuff).

7. Golly Moses, those medical students. Darn good question. Hyperventilation is just the ticket for causing a temporary decrease in cerebral blood flow and, hence, a decrease in intracranial pressure. That helps cerebral perfusion pressure and is just grand. But the kidneys, in their ceaseless quest to maintain homeostasis, start adjusting their excretion of bicarb and "undo" the effects of hyperventilation. Then, when you go back to normal ventilation, you will get a "rebound" effect; the kidneys will take a while to readjust, and you will have the exact opposite of what you want! So, enough dancing around the answer. When the cause of the increased intracranial pressure has been treated and the patient no longer needs medical therapy to "shrink the brain," then I would stop hyperventilation, look for any signs of a rebound increase in intracranial pressure, look for any signs of neurologic deterioration, and move toward extubation.

8. It's axiomatic in neurosurgery that the brain has no pain receptors, so you only have to anesthetize for the skin, periosteum, and dura. Those fine points are dandy for doctors, but don't help the family members to any meaningful degree. I'd tell the family members, "Anesthesia was given during the operation, just like it was for any operation like a hernia or a broken leg operation. While on the breathing machine, your family member receives regular, small doses of tranquilizing medicine so the breathing tube is not so bothersome."

9. First, do a bedside evaluation, and intubate if circumstances dictate. Better to have the patient's airway secured then have all the time in the world to tease out the cause of the respiratory failure. The dyspnea could be from fluid overload—he is a cardiac patient and just underwent a big stress, the myocardium may have further infracted somewhere along the hospital course. A rebleed could have caused a worsening of his neuro status. Any of the invasive lines could have caused a pneumothorax. His long hospital stay and immobility could have caused pneumonia, aspiration, or a pulmonary embolus. Two days of intubation could have left his upper airway swollen and his respiratory failure stemmed from upper airway obstruction. A chest x-ray, head CT, and blood gases should help make the diagnosis.

10. No need for positive pressure ventilation or PEEP. (Mask CPAP once extubated is an option here, but not usually a good one.) Neuro and upper airway status consistent with the patient holding his own as far as respiration and clearing secretions. In short, look at the patient and ask yourself, "Can he get by without that tube?" If anything says he can't, then keep it in. If everything says he can, then take it out.

Grab Bag Questions

1. During an appendectomy, an 8-year-old's temperature rises from 37.4 to 38.7 over 20 minutes. What is your differential diagnosis and how do you evaluate?
2. A preeclamptic patient is on magnesium and the newborn appears floppy, what do you do?
3. Two weeks after a cholecystectomy a patient develops jaundice. The internist says it is clearly a case of Sevoflurane hepatitis. You say?
4. A hospital pharmacist says, "That damn propofol is breaking the bank! Can't you use anything else?"

Answers to Grab Bag Questions

OK, no more guilt trips if you look. It's your life, do what you want.

1. Check the end-tidal CO_2. If that is rising and tachycardia is blazing, go with a diagnosis of MH, call for help, and start dantrolene. If the patient really has MH and you've waited until the temperature has risen, you're up a well-known creek without a paddle. A much more likely cause for this temperature rise is blankets, Bair-Huggers®, and a warmed room just causing the patient to get warm. Uncover the patient as best you can and cool the room.

2. Magnesium crosses the placenta and causes muscle weakness. Although calcium may reverse this weakness, the practical aspects of getting a line in the child and the need to support ventilation right away demand that you support the child's ventilation.

3. Before rolling over and saying, "We did it again," look for other causes of jaundice. The operation was on the biliary tree, make sure some surgical clip isn't in the wrong place. Then look for medical causes—Epstein-Barr virus, alcohol related liver injury.

4. Propofol is seductively easy to use for sedation in the ICU. But infusions of old standbys such as morphine, fentanyl, and midazolam can accomplish the same degree of sedation. And, if stopped for a few hours, these sedation regimens can provide for timely emergences and extubations.

First session done. A knock at the door, you look at your watch, and the examiners stop asking questions as if a light switch were thrown. You stagger out of the room, wondering how the hell you did, then you sit down at another desk with another stem question. This time you'll be facing the shorter version. You will be doing the preop and intraop drill this time. "Can I already be halfway done?" The few minutes fly, you try to forget about all the dumb things you said in the first room, then you jump into the next room and sit down with two more examiners. Your mouth tastes like cotton, your palms drip sweat, and your brain is amped out all the way to the red zone.

Don't you love this?

Session 2

An 18-year-old, 62 kg immigrant from Laos is admitted in labor. She is 6-cm dilated and screaming, "Baby! Baby!" Her BP is 170/100, HR 100, R 24, and temp 37.5°C.

Examiners' Questions

Preoperative

1. Which labs will you want and why?
2. What is the utility of a bleeding time?
3. How will you get "informed consent" from this patient?
4. Her husband is the "translator." When you ask him her name, he says, "Yes." When you ask him if she has any other medical problems, he says, "Yes." When you ask him which ones, he says, "Yes." No one else is available and it's 2 A.M. What do you do?
5. Is it "assault" to proceed without any better communication?
6. What special considerations do you have in the airway exam?
7. Between contractions, her blood pressure falls to 110/65. Does this patient have preeclampsia?
8. What is the difference between preeclampsia and eclampsia?
9. A tox screen shows cannabis in the blood. Any further workup needed given these findings?
10. Physical exam reveals a 2/6 systolic murmur but no other findings. Do you need an echo?

Answers to Preoperative Questions

1. Hematocrit—Want to know where we're starting in case blood loss gets problematic. As the patient is from a developing country, she could have malnutrition, parasitic diseases leading to malabsorption, and hence, even more anemia than the anemia of pregnancy. Her blood pressure may be that high due to the pain of contractions, but that pressure does qualify for preeclampsia, so I'd want a PT, PTT, and platelet count. No one of those will change my plan, but they will be good to know if, indeed, she has some form of coagulopathy.

2. Bleeding time supposedly ties it all together, but the hassle of doing it, plus the variability of the technician's interpretation, render the test of little use. I wouldn't get one.

3. Informed consent is a joke in this setting. The patient is half out of her mind with pain and the unfamiliar setting. For legal purposes, I'd let the nurse get the patient to sign whatever papers people usually sign, but you and I know that for the consent to be meaningful, all this stuff has to be spelled out well ahead of time in a calm setting. No go here. I would document everything in the chart with a fine tooth pen.

4. Textbooks in days of yore said that a language barrier is a contraindication to regional technique. Yeah, right. Try that on a busy floor with a high immigrant population. As best you can, try to convey the notion of how to hold still for the "shot" in the back. Keep hubby around to help. Watch for signs of toxicity, as you won't be able to ask about "ringing in the ears or a metallic taste in your mouth." Watch for tachycardia (hard to tell from the tachycardia of pain) and signs of dissociation or impending unconsciousness. Finally, the language barrier can be overcome by observing for signs of pain relief.

5. Cutting through the legal babble, the best care for the patient is the best care. Do the best to get some interpretation across, then do what will help the patient and baby. You're a doctor, not a Supreme Court judge. Time is of the essence here. Getting a well-functioning epidural in may save a life or two. Hesitating until next shift's Laotian translator comes in will not help anybody.

6. The pregnant patient has a swollen, friable airway. If she has preeclampsia on top of that, then the airway will be even worse. Large breasts may interfere with the laryngoscope handle. The gravid uterus reduces FRC and will lead to rapid desaturation. Finally, the stomach is full, posing an aspiration risk.

7. Preeclampsia encompasses the triad of hypertension, edema, and proteinuria. Edema may be hard to tell from the generalized swelling of pregnancy, but a urine dipstick will show if there is proteinuria. As this patient's blood pressure is not sustained, then she most likely does not have preeclampsia. Her blood pressure was most likely up from the pain of contractions.

8. Eclampsia means preeclampsia plus seizures. Should that occur, treatment focuses on, first, supporting oxygenation. The seizure itself is not as bad as its accompanying hypoxemia.

9. Just look for other, more sinister findings in the tox screen. If, for example, cocaine shows up, then the mother may suffer from hypertension or cardiac problems from long-term cocaine abuse. Nosebleeds, infectious hepatitis, and HIV could accompany IV abuse. The baby may be born addicted to cocaine and require intensive nursing care.

10. The high flow state of pregnancy often produces a "flow murmur." I would order an echo only if she had other symptoms, such as shortness of breath, orthopnea, or drop in exercise tolerance. Admittedly, each of these are hard to tell from the baseline state of advancing pregnancy.

Intraop Questions

1. To place the epidural, do you have her on her side or sitting up? Why?

2. What is the advantage of an epidural in this case? A disadvantage?

3. First pass elicits a clear, gushing liquid not entirely unrelated to some CSF you read about in history books. Do you place a catheter and do a continuous spinal? Why or why not?

4. You place the epidural elsewhere and aspirate blood. Do you now run a continuous toxic intravenous and just hope no one notices?

5. At 8 cm, the fetal heart rate drops to 60. While they're preparing for a C-section, you try to buy some time. The patient is on Pitocin. What measures can you take?

6. Heart rate stays down, now it's time to fix bayonets and perform a "normal spontaneous Caesarean delivery." What steps do you take in preparation? Do you give antacids? If so, which and why?

7. In the OR, the FHR returns to normal, you've already done a "section dose" and the patient is completely numb. What do you say in your discussion with the surgeon?

8. Incision is made and the patient screams in Laotian. What do you do?

9. You induce and can't intubate but can ventilate. What do you do?

10. Mom's now fine, but under general anesthesia. The pediatrician can't intubate the baby and asks for your help.

Answers to Intraop Questions

How did the preop questions go? Pregnancy questions can be killers. I wonder if any of those answers were the Waldo? Or if all of them were. Do you really have the definition of preeclampsia down cold?

1. Sitting up. The advantage is the ease of finding the midline. On the side, the midline can sag away from you and you can get lost. A disadvantage is the struggle to get the patient sitting up. Also, in the sitting position, the BP can drop or the fetal heart rate can drop. "The baby doesn't like it when she sits up," is not an unheard of response. Also, if something goes toxic when the patient is sitting up, the patient will topple, which is no fun. On their sides, there is no place to topple. But as I'm going for ease of insertion, I'd go with the sitting position.

2. An epidural provides an ongoing source of pain relief and avenue for C-section. A disadvantage is a less dense block if the case goes to C-section. Another disadvantage is the large dose of local anesthetic you need to use. If this large dose goes intravascular, you will have prolonged cardiac collapse. If the needle goes in too far…

3. Oops! Seems we have a gusher here. I would not place a continuous spinal, as this has been associated with nerve root irritation. Better to pull out, go to another level, and give it another go. Also, if you have a continuous spinal in and hand the case off, some well-meaning anesthesiologist may forget the catheter is intrathecal and give a whopping spinal. Note this patient's name, as you will be back to treat spinal headache later on. Explain, as best you can, what happened so she will know what to expect.

4. Aspirating blood means pull the catheter out. Flushing a little and pulling back a little may just land you in the epidermis, so better to pull out and try again.

5. Fix the basic stuff first; left uterine displacement. If that fails, she may be in the 10% that need right uterine displacement. Stop the Pitocin, this may be making the uterus contract too vigorously and cause uteroplacental insufficiency. Give supplemental oxygen. Treat hypotension with fluids and ephedrine. If still no go, try the all fours position to establish better placental perfusion.

6. In this quick, quick, quick to the OR, there is no time for antacids. Get the epidural dosed up if you can. Two percent lidocaine injected as you go down the hall can and does get you a level. The goal is to avoid a general if you can, especially since you have a working epidural in.

7. There you are, all dosed up and nowhere to go. The "section dose" can be allowed to wear off and you can go back to "laboring dose," though a few hours may pass. Of more interest is this discussion with the OB. "She has shown she has borderline uteroplacental insufficiency, shall we decide the issue now before she throws another scare in us, or should we risk sending her back to the labor room, and next time we're not so lucky." I would vote to do the section then and there. Better to do the section under controlled circumstances.

8. You have inadequate surgical anesthesia and surgery has begun. Perform a general anesthetic. Limping through on ketamine (the "Keta-dural" is a halfway attempt at salvaging a regional) is not a good idea.

9. At this point, there is no fetal distress, but in effect there is maternal distress (the surgical incision is there), so I would proceed with a general anesthetic with maintained cricoid pressure. If you attempt to wake her up and do an awake intubation, she will be in agony from the incision and cooperation will be hard to come by. I'd call for extra anesthesia hands, place an LMA, and sweat bullets the whole case. I'd tell the OB docs of my troubles and ask for their help, specifically, avoid externalizing the uterus. Try to close the incision without all that yanking. It's a stretch, but the extreme circumstances require extreme measures.

10. If my hands were still full with my mask ventilation, I would tell the pediatrician to mask ventilate the child, call for help himself (specifically, respiratory therapy should be able to provide a hand). If I had been able to intubate Mom, I'd have the pediatrician roll the high-tech bassinette over to me so I could intubate the baby while making frequent glances back at Mom.

OB, what a minefield. Doesn't take much to get painted in a corner there.

Grab Bag Questions

1. During a rocky labor, a 20-year-old multip suddenly becomes cyanotic and loses consciousness. What, pray tell, is most likely going on and what do you do?

2. A 4-year-old develops stridor in the recovery room after an uneventful node biopsy. How do you evaluate and treat?

3. A PACU nurse wants a sign out for a patient who had a radical retropubic prostatectomy. "Oh yeah, he hasn't put out any urine the last hour. It's shift change and I'm a nurse short, can you get off your lazy butt and sign this guy out?"

4. One year after a carpenter cut off his thumb with a band saw, he comes to you with complaints of unremitting pain in his whole forearm. How will you evaluate?

Answers to Grab Bag Questions

1. Tumultuous labor and sudden cardiovascular collapse could be an amniotic fluid embolus. Other less likely causes are a more generic pulmonary embolus or else aspiration (say the patient was a drug addict and had sneaked some heroin in her IV). Going with the most likely course, the treatment is none other than supportive, and if the amniotic fluid embolus is big enough, you could be sunk as mortality is high. If a code should occur, deliver the baby STAT as CPR is much more effective post delivery.

2. Provide bedside evaluation and supplemental oxygen right away. Look for something obvious in the upper airway, a tooth or a forgotten gauze pack. Mask ventilate, if necessary, with the caveat that you don't want to blow anything further into the airway. Suction for blood and emesis. If airway swelling occurs, use humidified oxygen and epi to reduce the swelling. Keep and observe the patient at least 4 hours. Keep the child overnight if you're spooked about recurrence of stridor.

3. No, I will not sign him out, I will look for the three causes of oliguria and will strike like the wrath of God at each of these causes. First I'll check the Foley and make sure it's functioning properly. The next most likely cause after a big operation like a radical retropubic prostatectomy is hypovolemia. Even if you kept up with blood loss, there could still be a lot of third spacing or ongoing oozing. If fluid challenges didn't produce some urine output, and if the patient didn't have a CVP in, I'd place one.

4. Your biggest concern is reflex sympathetic dystrophy. If unchecked, it could lead to severe pain, tissue loss, and eventually a useless limb. First perform a physical exam, looking for hyperesthesia, mottling, hair loss. If the exam is consistent with RSD, then plan a series of stellate ganglion blocks to interrupt the sympathetic discharge to the limb and, with luck, improve the arm pain and check the development of RSD. No guarantees in this department, though.

That's it! First test done. You did it! How was it? Surprising how straightforward it is, isn't it? Basically it's the same question over and over again. "*This* happens, what do you do and why?" "*That* happens, what do you do and why?"

And nothing comes from left field. You've done neuro cases. You've done OB cases. You've faced all these questions at one time or another. And yes, there are lots and lots of gray areas. You *could* do the first patient with a Swan, or you could with a CVP. And as far as the OB question goes, you could have gone a different route with the "can't intubate, can ventilate" scenario. It's all how you explain your reasoning.

Did you do the test out loud? Tape yourself? Do the test with a friend? Run the tougher questions past an attending and see what they would do? Did you do the test then look up the areas you stumbled in? All to the good.

Did you just punt and look up our answers? Shame on you. Those are the answers that *we* made up. *WE'RE NOT TAKING THE TEST, YOU ARE!* Get to work, you lazy slime mold!

One thing you will notice as the practice tests progress—you will see the same stuff recur (lost airway, treatment of various vital signs). Are these worth going over and over and over again? You bet your board certification they're worth going over again. Now, on to the second test.

Keep an eye out for Waldo.

SAMPLE TEST #2

Session 1

A 28-year-old, 75 kg, 5'9" tall male is brought for ORIF of a femur fracture.

HPI: Apparently a Three Stooges fan, this unfortunate fellow declares he is a "victim of circumstance." He just happened to be in a total stranger's house in the middle of the night and just happened to be carrying that person's stereo out the window. Alas, his footing not being what it used to, he slipped and snapped his femur while making his exit from said window. He suffered no other injuries and the stereo is also doing quite fine, thank you.

PMH: The stress of living under disability for a heroin addiction has led this man to drink. He blames a broken home and an unhappy childhood for this sad collection of substance-related maladies.

Physical exam: Airway normal. Lungs and heart normal. His femur reveals, not just a discoloration, but (gasp!) a bullet hole. Apparently the stereo owner took considerable umbrage at the loss of his property and "helped" expedite the man's jumping out the window with a little high caliber push.

Labs: Tox screen positive for cocaine.

He ate nachos bell grande 2 hours ago, but the surgeon states there may be ongoing blood loss in the thigh so surgery is emergent.

Intraop Questions

1. What will a normal hematocrit tell you about the man's volume status?
2. How will you induce? Is a spinal an option? An epidural?
3. How will you do a lighting volume assessment just before you induce?
4. Patient won't move to his side or sit up for a spinal, so you go with a general. Will you premedicate for aspiration prophylaxis?
5. You induce and the patient vomits through cricoid pressure. What do you do?
6. You are able to intubate, but suction out Mexican food. Some idiot in the room says, "Yo quiero Taco Bell." While you're killing the idiot, how do you treat the aspiration? Are prophylactic antibiotics indicated? Prophylactic salsa?
7. After suctioning, the SaO_2 is only 88%. How do you treat this?
8. What is the concept of "best PEEP"?
9. An hour into the case the HR is 130 and the BP is 80/45. Your move?
10. An OR tech sticks himself with a needle. What do you advise him to do?

Answers to Intraop Questions

1. If the man lost a lot of blood but he hasn't received a lot of IV fluids, the hematocrit may well be normal. So a normal hematocrit may mislead. His CVP might be 1, and by the time you volume replete him, the hematocrit could be much lower.

2. I'll go on the assumption of heap big blood loss in the leg and induce with etomidate. Yes, if the patient is on his absolute last gasp of sympathetic tone, nothing is completely safe, but etomidate should keep his blood pressure normal. Ketamine is another option, but the patient's tox screen is positive for cocaine. Ketamine's sympathomimetic effect plus cocaine's sympathetic stimulation could add up to tachycardia and arrhythmias, so etomidate is the choice. Moving the patient around for a spinal or epidural with a broken leg would hurt a lot, so I wouldn't do it. Also, performing a sympathectomy on a patient with uncertain blood loss status could result in serious blood pressure drop.

3. Examine the patient for signs of shock—pale, cool, clammy skin. No urine in his Foley or else dark, concentrated urine. Mentation—if in shock, he won't be able to communicate well. See if he has a narrow pulse pressure and if his pulse feels rapid and thready. Basically, you'll induce assuming some blood loss, you just want to make sure he is not so far gone that you'll kill him with induction and starting positive pressure ventilation. If that is the case, then you'll need to start blood and volume resuscitation prior to induction.

4. No. The man is in severe pain and probably got narcotics in the ER, so he won't empty his stomach, even if you give him some Reglan. Pouring a cup full of antacid into that stomach full of tacos will not help much either.

5. Bed into Trendelenburg, head to the side, suction. Once the emesis has stopped and the muscle relaxant has taken effect, then perform laryngoscopy, suction out emesis, place the endotracheal tube, and perform check for breath sounds and end tidal carbon dioxide.

6. Suction the endotracheal tube. If necessary, squirt saline down the tube to help suction out more stuff (this is controversial, as this maneuver may push food further down the bronchial tree). If there still seems to be a lot of stuff down there, perform fiberoptic bronchoscopy to direct your suctioning. If complete occlusion occurs and super grande size chunks are in the way, you may have to go all the way to extubating and performing rigid bronchoscopy to pull out the big tostada that's blocking the mainstem. Prophylactic antibiotics are as useless as a screen door on a submarine.

7. Yipes! Make sure the patient is actually getting oxygen, check the oxygen analyzer, make sure you have 100% oxygen going in. Check the endotracheal tube position. You don't want to go all the way to

ECMO and then find out you only had to pull the ETT back. Suction again, treat with bronchodilators (a beta agent down the ETT) to clear up any bronchospasm that resulted from the aspiration. Then apply PEEP. Place an arterial line, as you may be supporting his ventilation postop and you'll need to send gases. Get a chest x-ray right away (the surgeons are working on the leg so you won't bug them). In some cases, aspiration may show up predominantly in one lung (usually the right one since it's a straighter shot). For true refractory, refractory, refractory hypoxemia, you can sometimes turn the patient on their side, get more blood flow through the nonaspirated-into lung, and raise the oxygen level that way. (This is rare, but it happened to Chris once and is a great "real world" trick to keep in your back pocket.)

8. PEEP helps aerate the lungs but works against the thoracic pump. So PEEP can drop cardiac output and blood pressure. In an argument in the "reductio ad absurdum," you could oxygenate almost anybody with a PEEP of 100 cm H_2O, but you'd knock their blood pressure to zero and blow out their lungs. That is obviously not the "best PEEP." But, as in this case, if zero PEEP cannot oxygenate the patient, that is obviously not the "best PEEP" either. So, by trial and blood gas and blood pressure measurement, you try to get the PEEP high enough to oxygenate, but not so high as to hurt the circulation. A worthy goal is enough PEEP to keep the saturation above 90%, while keeping the FIO_2 50% or lower. (Greater than 50% O_2 is in itself harmful to the lungs if maintained for prolonged times.)

9. Sounds like hypovolemia. Replace volume and reduce the anesthetic inhaled agents. Check for more sinister things, such as a pneumothorax in case you placed a central line.

10. Clean the wound as best he can and go immediately (get another tech to replace him) to employee health. Prophylaxis for HIV may need to be instituted. Draw labs from the patient (rules may be sticky about this) to see if they are hepatitis or HIV positive. This is the best medical treatment. The legalities of drawing lab tests from the source patient would have to be tackled in an institution-by-institution basis. The main idea is to act on, not ignore, the needle stick.

Before you go on to the postop questions, do yourself a favor. Go back to the stem question. Make up another 10 intraop questions. Act like an examiner on that stem and go through every complication in the universe that could ever happen during that case.

Postop Questions

1. At the end of the case the patient won't arouse from slumber. What is the Dx?

2. You've given four units of blood and the orthopod says, "Better give him some fresh frozen." What do you say to that?

3. While writing his orders, the intern on the ortho service says, "This guy might go into DTs. What should I write for so he doesn't?"

4. In the PACU, the man's sat is 88% on room air, but 92% on 3 L nasal cannula. The nurse asks, "I heard he aspirated, OK for him to go to the floor or do you want ICU on him?"

5. The man's pain is hard to control but you're not sure this isn't just "drug-seeking behavior." What do you do?

6. The man smiles and says, "Hope you got a good dentist doc!" He shows you a broken off stump of a tooth, then coughs and the tooth flies out of his lungs and lands in your front pocket. How do you respond to this citizen?

7. Nausea and vomiting do not come under control with the usual droperidol. What steps do you go through to control his nausea?

8. The surgeon requests a femoral block to help with pain control. How do you do one and would you do one?

9. The next day the man has fluffy infiltrates in his right lower lobe. What is the treatment now?

10. Under what circumstances would you reintubate this patient?

Answers to Postop Questions

1. Simple things first. Make sure the vapors are off. Then check the end-tidal gas analyzer to make sure the vapors have been exhaled down to a low enough level to allow emergence. Then check off the other anesthetic agents—neuromuscular, hypnotics, narcotics. If all these are at a reasonable level (i.e., you didn't give 100 cc of fentanyl for this 2 hour case), then check for hypothermia or any metabolic cause of delayed emergence—hypoglycemia, hyponatremia (unlikely), low CO_2 from your hyperventilating him the whole case.

2. "What are you, nuts?" is what you say to the examiners. "Then if the orthopod gives me any grief, I rough him up a little, slap him silly." If that does not produce the desired response from your oral board examiners, then tell them—giving factors after an arbitrary number of units of packed cells is not necessary. You treat only if there is a clinical problem—bleeding—then you guide your therapy by what is most likely the missing factor. If a lot of blood is given, then the most likely cause of diffuse bleeding is a dilutional thrombocytopenia. A platelet count will tell you that and a TEG will confirm that you need to give platelets.

3. DTs result from acute withdrawal from alcohol. You can, and some places do, write for patients to get some booze while in the hospital. That is a perfectly fine way to prevent DTs, though many cringe at us "feeding the habit." An alternative is to write for Librium tid. As full blown DTs can be fatal, remind the intern to watch for signs of sympathetic hyperactivity. When the orthopod gives you a blank stare, just tell him to make sure an internist is on the case.

4. If aspiration occurred and is really going to progress to bad news, it tends to happen early. If after a few hours the lung damage appears "mild" (nasal cannula can maintain satisfactory oxygenation), then I would not send the patient to the ICU. An exception would be on weekends or holidays, when floor staffing suffers. Keep him on a pulse oximeter overnight.

5. This is no time to cure a patient of substance abuse. He has pain from a fractured leg so treat the pain. Pain is pain, no matter what you shot up before the injury. His requirements may be high due to tolerance, but you may just need to go high to treat the pain.

6. In the best of all possible worlds, you did a good airway exam ahead of time and noted any rotten teeth that were about to fall out. "Patient warned of risks to teeth," helps in this case. Take an x-ray to make sure there is not more dentition lurking in the lungs, then get a dental consult as soon as possible. (That's hard as hell in a real hospital, but if you can get the dentist to smooth down the tooth, it won't hurt as much.)

7. First make sure nothing is amiss, such as undiagnosed intracranial bleed leading to nausea (trauma means associated injuries!) If this is just plain old nausea, treat with a different anti-emetic such as Reglan or ondansetron. The newer antiemetic agents are more expensive, and the pharmacy may squawk, but a prolonged stay in PACU is also costly.

8. Sure. A femoral block is a good idea. Using a nerve stimulator for guidance, and looking for a good contraction of the quads, place local such as bupivicaine near the femoral nerve near the inguinal ligament. Placing the block *after* the case is a good idea. There's no delay *starting* the case. And if it's less than perfect, so what?

9. The aspiration is now "showing." Treatment is still supportive. No steroids. And no antibiotics unless he has a culture proven pneumonia or if he grows bugs out of a blood culture. Supplemental oxygen and ventilatory support are used if the patient cannot maintain his own oxygenation. Follow-up chest x-rays and clinical assessment are also appropriate.

10. If he needed PEEP, I'd intubate. I would not bother with mask CPAP. If he could not clear secretions or if his breathing became so labored that he looked like he would "wear out," then I'd also intubate. Better to intubate when he looks like he's going to wear out than wait until he actually does wear out.

Now you're getting the picture. Questions just like the stuff you do every day. Just explain what you do, be clear, and stick to the question asked.

Grab Bag Questions

1. You perform a stellate ganglion block and the patient becomes dyspneic. What happened and what will you do?
2. Before a fem-pop the K is found to be 2.9. The surgeon isn't sure if he should proceed or if you should attempt to normalize the K intraop. Your response?
3. A man is scheduled for an excision of a ganglion cyst in the wrist. He is on MAO inhibitors for depression. Do you proceed?
4. A surgeon asks you how to preoperatively "optimize" a patient with a pheochromocytoma. What do you say?

Answers to Grab Bag Questions

1. When you plunk a needle in and inject something, then either the needle is in the wrong place (pneumothorax; torn vessel leading to bleeding and a hematoma) or the injected material is in the wrong place (intravascular injection leading to CNS excitation, then progressing all the way to seizures and cardiovascular collapse; intrathecal tracking leading to a high spinal and respiratory arrest). This sounds like a pneumothorax. Check breath sounds, give supplemental oxygen, order a chest x-ray. If progressing to a tension pneumo, then place a 14 g angiocath in the 2 d intercostal space, midclavicular line to relieve the pneumothorax. (We read about that all the time, I did it just once and was there an "ooh, aah" in the room after that. Scared the living hell out of me, though.)

2. I wouldn't worry about the K. The patient is in all likelihood chronically potassium depleted. Attempting to replace the tons of potassium that would bring him back to "normal" would take forever. If done with sufficient dispatch, this potassium-o-rama could kill the poor guy. The guy needs the operation (ischemia threatens his limb), so just proceed with the case.

3. The big terror of MAO inhibitors is gone. Just avoid Demerol and avoid ephedrine. Other than that, the routine anesthetic regimen is fine. Taking a patient off his MAO inhibitor may deny them the only effective treatment for depression. In the two weeks they are off the MAO inhibitor (to facilitate a "safer" anesthetic) the patient may get so depressed he commits suicide.

4. A pheo is worth optimizing. Block both alpha and beta receptors with po meds, aiming to neutralize that giant sympathetic neuron. Once the patient comes to the OR, you should have less trouble if they are truly optimized, but you still have to be ready to handle big pressure swings as well as dealing with the removal of the sympathetic supertanker. In effect, when you cut out the pheo, you just did the same as cutting off a big epinephrine drip.

Halfway through your second test. Go have a smoke.
Unfiltered Camel. That's the stuff.

Session 2

A 5-year-old had a tonsillectomy at 2 P.M. It is
now 10 P.M. and he just pulled into the ER, bleeding from the mouth
and the mother is frantic. Vital signs are BP 80/50; P 150; R 30. The
child appears listless.

Preop Questions

1. How do you assess the volume status in a child? In *this* child?
2. How do you assess blood loss in a bleeding tonsil?
3. Do you premedicate for aspiration prophylaxis?
4. Should you insist the ER type and cross for blood?
5. The mother is a Jehovah's Witness and refuses blood. What do you tell her?
6. Do you transfuse in the ER or go straight to the OR?
7. Is there any "medical" way to slow the bleeding (Drug infusion, radiologic thrombosing?) while the surgeon is on his way in?
8. How do you establish IV access if the child rouses himself enough to fight the IV?
9. Any labs necessary before going to the OR?
10. Do you place a NG or an OG preop to empty the stomach?

Answers to Preop Questions

1. There are guides to tell you if a child is slightly volume depleted, very volume depleted, and a whole bunch volume depleted. Physical exam signs include sunken fontanelles (not in this 5-year-old, of course), mental status, and color. The divisions are arbitrary and the reality of a volume assessment boils down to this, "Has this kid lost enough blood that a standard induction will kill him?" You will have to perform an anesthetic on the child to let the surgeon stop the bleeding, so frittering away over "Is this 10% volume loss or 30% volume loss?" is a moot point. Look for signs of shock, that is, inadequate tissue perfusion. Ask the mother, has the child urinated? If not, that may mean the kidneys are inadequately perfused. If, in all the excitement, the child wet his pants on the way into the hospital, that tells you at least there is enough volume to maintain renal perfusion. Is the skin cool and clammy? That means inadequate skin perfusion. Is the child coherent? That indicates cerebral perfusion. Here, the child is listless and that means inadequate cerebral perfusion. Add it all up and say,

- volume status bad enough to require blood before we start,
- volume status bad enough to induce with ketamine (no guarantee with ketamine, but at least it is an attempt to induce and maintain your vital signs), and
- volume status not so bad, can induce the normal way.

This kid's most scary sign is listlessness. That means inadequate cerebral perfusion. That means you'll need blood ready and you'll have to do an induction aimed at maintaining blood pressure.

2. Blood loss, like volume status, is hard to peg. Blood loss could have been going on all day, with the child swallowing blood. Then a bleeder could have opened up and sped up blood loss. There could be hundreds of ccs "hiding" in the stomach. With placement of an IV, try to get a hematocrit, realizing that a hematocrit doesn't tell you the whole story. But seeing a preop hematocrit of 30 will put you in a better frame of mind than seeing a hematocrit of 20!

3. No. No time. Anything PO may cause emesis and worsen blood loss. Any IV medication won't have time to change anything.

4. Yes. You need blood. The tonsillar bed, recall, is just in front of the carotid artery. The bleeding can be furious and fatal. Of course you are reluctant to transfuse a child in these infectious days, but if you must to save their lives, then you must.

5. A Jehovah's Witness can refuse blood for themselves, but can't deny a minor a lifesaving transfusion. You assure her that you will do what you can to avoid a transfusion, but if necessary (say the child develops ectopy, a sign that the hematocrit is so low that the heart is not receiving enough oxygen), then you will transfuse.

6. I would get the blood ready and go straight to the OR. Better to be up there, getting monitors on, getting ready to go, than hanging out in the ER. Before I induced, I'd get one more set of vital signs, take another good look at the skin, and see how much blood is coming out of the mouth. At this point you have to weigh this dilemma—if I transfuse now, I'm replacing much needed volume, but I'm still *losing* volume. If I induce now, I'll get the evils of anesthetic induction and positive pressure ventilation, but at least the surgeon will now be able to *stop* the volume loss.

7. No. And any funky attempt at radiologic catheter weirdness will waste time and put you in the dark, creepy confines of the radiologic wasteland. Concentrate on IV, blood, and OR.

8. You will need an IV, so do what you can with people holding the patient. If you can't get anything peripheral, then go central. A femoral line may be easier to place that a neck line, for a struggling child will wiggle the head back and forth. Enlist help from pediatric people (ICU nurses, pediatricians from the ER, your own anesthesia people). This is a case where you pull out all the stops in terms of getting help.

9. A hematocrit. More important than that lab is a type and cross.

10. No. Poking around in a bleeding mess may just knock off a clot and worsen the whole situation. Plus, the child will cry and fuss with placement of the tube, and that will also worsen blood loss.

Note that the oral boards emphasize reasoning. The examiners want to know what you are thinking. A bleeding tonsil is tough, no doubt. Pat answers just aren't there. But you can explain your concerns, so the examiner *knows that you know.*

Intraop Questions

1. Which agent will you use to induce and why?
2. If the IV from the ER blows, what will you do?
3. Will you use an IM sedative if the IV placement is impossible?
4. Explain the rationale for intraosseous placement of an IV. Would you use it?
5. You induce but can't see anything for the bleeding. What do you do?
6. After induction the pressure is unobtainable, but the EKG is still going. How do you resuscitate?
7. Patient develops multifocal PVCs and the blood isn't yet crossed, what do you tell the blood bank?
8. What is your endpoint for transfusion and why?
9. What special considerations do you take to prevent recall in this difficult case?
10. Near the end of the case, the child starts wheezing and inspiratory pressures go up each time you try to "lighten" the patient. What do you do?

Answers to Intraop Questions

1. Ketamine. This drug tends to maintain sympathetic tone in the case of hypovolemia. No drug is completely safe, of course, but in this case, ketamine is the option. Could you get by with tiny doses of pentathol? Yes. Any drug, used with the patient's physiology in mind (patient has lost blood, therefore use smaller doses of all anesthetic agents), will work. Just as any drug, ignoring the patient's physiology, will fail.

2. Place another one. This kid needs an IV. Even if you don't have a big one at induction, place a bigger one postinduction.

3. If absolutely nailed to the wall, yes, I'd use an IM ketamine dart to get the kid to hold still enough to place the IV. That is an extreme measure, but this is an extreme case.

4. In cases of no IV access, a large bore needle jammed into the tibia gives access to the circulatory system via the bone marrow. I would not do it because I've only read about it but never done it. I'd have the surgeon do a cutdown first.

5. Suction like mad. I'd have two suction machines ready, in case one got clogged. If the bleeding were huge, I'd ask for pressure on the carotids to try to slow the flow enough to see. If, after changing blades, head position, and practitioners, I still couldn't intubate, I'd mask ventilate while the surgeon did a trach. Yes, the child will aspirate some blood, but that is better than going without any ventilation at all.

6. The child is in EMD. Volume, volume, volume. If blood is not yet ready, tread water with crystalloid but ask for trauma blood (uncrossmatched O negative blood) STAT if the child's own blood is not ready. If the child's blood is at the type and screen level, get that. Along with blood, remember to give calcium to counteract the citrate from the banked blood.

7. PVCs tell you that the child's myocardium is starving for oxygen. The incidence of adverse reactions from type and screened blood is no higher than the incidence of adverse reactions from type and crossed blood, so use the type and screen blood right away.

8. Follow hematocrits. Although any one number is arbitrary, I'd aim for a hematocrit of at least 25 and evidence that adequate perfusion has returned to all organ systems—urine output, normal vital signs, good color, no ectopy. If, at 25, there were evidence of inadequate perfusion, then I'd transfuse up to 30. The goal is to restore organ function but minimize exposure to blood products. "Settling" for a hematocrit of 25 versus the more often quoted 30 is a testament to my faith in youth. An otherwise healthy kid who has no other organ system disease should be able to get by on a lower hematocrit.

9. Watch what is said in the OR. Speak to the child, saying you're doing everything you can to help him get better. All this is to make sure that if he does hear something, it is comforting. Once the vital signs can support some medication, give midazolam in an attempt to block memories, realizing midazolam has no retrograde amnesia properties. Then later, once resuscitation has gone far enough, start anesthetic vapors.

10. This problem can set up a revolving cycle of problems. Lighten—wheeze, deepen—wheezing clears. Try to lighten again—more wheezing. Until you get to the point you can't ever wake the patient up! First, go through your "all that wheezes is not asthma" checklist. Once tube position, pneumothorax, and carinal stimulation are taken care of, you are left with the most likely diagnosis, aspiration of blood stimulating the bronchial tree. Once you've suctioned as best you can, including fiberoptic poking around, then make this decision—if the aspiration is severe enough, then support the patient's ventilation until the aspiration clears up. In this case, I would sedate the patient, keep him intubated overnight, and see if the pulmonary picture improves by the next day. Better that than extubate deep (the stomach is full), or extubating in a panic as the child wheezes and then try to reintubate through a bloody awful mess.

Back to the notion of explaining your reasoning. If you just say, "I'd induce with ketamine, because ketamine is perfect and never drops the blood pressure on anybody," then the examiners would peg you for a ninny. But if you say, "I have to induce with something, and one decent option is ketamine," then the examiners know that you know what's going on. And you can go on to mention that another option is an awake intubation, but that would be hard in a bleeding, moving patient. If the patient were moribund, then an awake intubation with no induction agent at all is an option.

I wonder if any of those answers were Waldo? When you take your exam, I advise against using the "Waldo gambit" with your examiners. They, in all likelihood, will not see the riotous humor.

Grab Bag Questions

1. You're filling the vaporizer and spill some. A housekeeper walks in, sniffs, and says, "Doc, I just found out I'm pregnant. That gas stuff going to hurt my baby?" What do you say?
2. You are asked to provide anesthesia for ECT for a man with severe, inoperable CAD. How will you conduct this anesthetic?
3. The head nurse of a preop clinic wants to save money on preop labs. "Just what do we need and on who?"
4. A series of lumbar sympathetic blocks is done on a man with RSD of the foot. There is some improvement but the man isn't sure if it's worth doing it again. What do you tell him?

Answers to Grab Bag Questions

1. As you conduct her out of the room, you say, "No one really knows, but it's advisable to minimize your exposure to any medications, inhaled anesthetic agents included. No one has ever shown harm to a baby, though some evidence shows that exposure to one of our gases, nitrous oxide, may cause some abortions. But no one is sure if it was the gas, or whether it was just the stress of working in the operating room."

2. Intense, brief sympathetic discharge from the ECT could worsen the myocardial oxygen supply/demand picture. But if ECT will prevent severe depression or suicide, then the benefit outweighs the risk. Use esmolol, labetalol, and nitroglycerin to counteract the brief blast from the ECT. This wealth of short acting drugs helps in the short period of hyperstimulation from the seizure.

3. Pregnancy tests in women of childbearing age. Every other test, without being flippant, is something indicated by the patient and the procedure. A carpal tunnel release? Doesn't need any labs if the patient has no symptoms or organ systems that need investigating. Diabetes and advanced age? There could be a heap of trouble hiding out, so you'll need to check glucose, creatinine (diabetics can have renal insufficiency), and EKG (silent ischemia). Work with the preop clinic nurse to work on a set of guidelines like these.

4. It's worth continuing at least a series of blocks. Improvement is not guaranteed, but if improvement is to occur, then it often takes patience, concomitant physical therapy, antidepressant medication, and return visits and reassessments. Chronic pain therapy is a process, not just an individual procedure.

Round two over.

For each and every case, you could ask, "Now you can't intubate and can't ventilate, what do you do?" Or you could say, "Intraop the patient develops MH, what now?" That's where your hard work comes in to play. Change the patient a little, make the coexisting diseases even more involved. Work it, work it.

PRACTICE EXAM #3

Session 1

A 73-year-old, 5'4" tall, 100 kg executive for Philip Morris is scheduled for bronchoscopy and right upper lobe resection of a squamous cell CA.

HPI: No stranger to tobacco, this poster child for the American Lung Association has smoked three PPD since he was 16. "It ain't the tobacco, you know. It's all those filters and chemicals the government makes us put in!" His exercise tolerance is unknown, for he only changes the channel on his TV. He has a chronic cough. He is allergic to PCN ("I don't know, my Mom told me."). No history of MI. He has "borderline diabetes" that he controls with diet. Yeah, sure.

PMH: TURP 3 years ago.

Physical Exam: Short, thick neck, large tongue, barrel chest, ample abdomen. Coughs like a fiend.

Chest x-ray: Mass in RUL. Atelectasis.

Lab studies: Hct 54; ABG shows pO_2 of 67 with a pCO_2 of 50; normal pH

Medical consult: The patient's regular pulmonologist says, "Look, don't hate me for sending you this guy. He's a wreck, but that's about as good as he gets. He hardly ever takes his meds, but he never will so better just do the deed. If you want, I'll do some PFTs, but the CA has to come out. It will start blocking his bronchus soon and will kill him with a postobstructive pneumonia. Sorry. Are we still on for tennis this weekend?"

Your resident has lined him up with an A-line and a 16-g IV in the forearm. The patient refuses a central line placement until "I'm asleep, damnit!" He also insists any spinal or epidural be placed once he's asleep.

Intraop Questions

1. Do you insist on placing the central lines or neuraxial drugs while the patient is awake?
2. You do an awake look and determine the airway is difficult, how do you secure a double lumen tube or at least lung isolation in this difficult airway?
3. Which size and side double-lumen tube will you use and why?
4. You intubate but cannot isolate the right lung, go through a logical progression of steps to isolate the lung.
5. What are the absolute indications for lung isolation?
6. What do you tell the surgeon if you can only get a single-lumen ETT in?
7. Intraoperatively, the ST segments rise 3 mm in both lateral and frontal leads. What is your Dx and Rx?
8. The surgeon enters the pulmonary artery and massive bleeding occurs. What do you do?
9. Urine output drops to 15 cc/hr, but the CVP is 16. What next?
10. With chest closure, the inspiratory pressure alarm goes off and blood pressure drops. What is your Dx and Rx?

Answers to Intraop Questions

1. The neuraxial work should be done with the patient awake. If you spear a nerve while fishing around for his epidural space and the patient is under anesthesia, he won't be able to tell you and you could cause permanent damage and permanent pain. That's a hell of a price to pay for a few days of postop pain relief. The central line post induction is fine. As long as you have enough peripheral access to induce and take care of induction problems.

2. One conservative approach is to do an awake intubation with a single lumen tube, then, once you have the airway safely secured and the patient relaxed, take a look with a laryngoscope and see if a double lumen is possible. Pass an endotracheal tube stylet down the single lumen tube as a safety net, then pull the single lumen out and try to place the double lumen. Another approach is to use a special endotracheal tube, designed by George Arndt, which has a built-in endobronchial tube blocker. If you don't have one, then jury-rig a Fogarty catheter to use as an endobronchial tube blocker.

3. Left sided, because they are operating on the right side. Going down the left side also obviates the problem of the high takeoff of the right upper lobe bronchus, that is, a right-sided tube, unless placed just right, can block off the right upper lobe and you end up with two lobe ventilation rather than one entire lung ventilation. Of note, Benumof questions that. For size, I want a tube that is not so huge that I'll have trouble placing the tube, yet not so small that I'll have difficulty, with the cuffs inflated, in isolating the lung. My choice, 39 French, with bigger and smaller tubes in the room.

4. Make sure you clamped off the correct side. Then make sure the lung is really being ventilated, the lung may be stuck to the pleura by infection, neoplasm, or old adhesions. If you truly are ventilating the right lung by mistake, then the endotracheal tube is probably too far up, and ventilation into the left lung is slipping over to the right. Look with the fiberoptic and advance the tube until you see the blue endobronchial cuff just past the carina.

5. Keeping wet stuff in one lung from getting over to the other, dry lung. That wetness can be purulence, blood, or, a real rare bird, irrigating fluid used to wash out the lung in patients with alveolar proteinosis.

6. Bow your head and say, "I am not worthy." Then suggest that, when he needs lung isolation, you will advance the single lumen tube into the left side under fiberoptic guidance. If that doesn't work, do pseudo high frequency ventilation (say, 20 breaths per minute at a smaller tidal volume) so the lung doesn't move terribly much. Then ask him to use lung retractors.

7. Intraoperative ischemia has reared its ugly head. Inform the surgeon, then do all in your power to fix the myocardial oxygen/supply demand situation. Make sure there is enough oxygen and hemoglobin in the blood. Make sure the blood pressure provides enough perfusion pressure to feed the myocardium. Treat tachycardia. Use nitroglycerin to unload the heart and diltiazem to treat coronary spasm. If all that fails to fix the problem, consider canceling the case, for you have just performed a "thoracotomy stress test" and have uncovered coronary disease. The patient may have left main disease and need revascularization before his lung operation.

8. If blood is not in the room, get it now. Uncrossmatched O blood will do in a pinch. Don't worry about O negative, O positive is fine if they don't have enough O negative. Get help. No one around? Pull a nurse from the ICU or PACU, they are a great resource in time of need. If access is inadequate, try to get in a femoral line, it will be too hard to get at the subclavian or the neck as the surgeon flails with the severed PA.

9. Do the prerenal, postrenal, renal dance. If all else checks out OK and the CVP reading is accurate, start dopamine and give Lasix. This is one patient you don't want to risk overloading. The reduced lung volume after the lobe resection means he'll tolerate excess fluids poorly.

10. Reopen. The chest tube they placed has somehow malfunctioned and your positive pressure ventilation has created a tension pneumothorax.

Note, as you wind through these questions, that most answers are pretty short. The examiners want to hear your answer to a specific question. Once they hear that, they want to move on. They have a lot of ground to cover. So don't jump up on a soapbox and pontificate for eons, you just don't have the time.

Postop Questions

1. You placed an epidural, but 2 hours later the pain relief is inadequate. How will you evaluate this?

2. The surgeon wants the double-lumen tube changed to a single-lumen but the airway looks edematous after the 4-hour procedure. What do you do?

3. ST segment elevation persists in spite of NTG. Do you call a cardiologist? What do you tell the cardiologist?

4. The patient describes intraop recall. What do you tell him?

5. The patient coughs and coughs. The surgeon is afraid this heavy coughing will disrupt his bronchial suture line and asks if you could help. What do you say?

6. In the PACU, the patient suddenly drops his pressure and arrests. What condition specific to a pulmonary procedure could cause this?

7. The patient tells you his "little thing in the back of the throat is all swollen." How do you evaluate?

8. During a line change in the ICU, you place a Swan introducer in the carotid. What do you do?

9. Three days later, the internist says, "This guy gained 5 kg since preop. You idiots drown my patients in the OR. What are you thinking?"

10. A nurse calls you to say the epidural you placed is leaking at the site. What do you do?

Answers to Postop Questions

1. Dose it once, inspect the site to make sure it hasn't come out, then yank it and replace it if there's still no pain relief. It's easier to place the thing again and make sure it's working than to agonize over where it might be.

2. For safety's sake, keep the double lumen in until the edema is down. To reduce carinal stimulation, deflate the bronchial cuff and pull the ETT back into the trachea. Once the edema is down then change the tube, but only after you have looked with a laryngoscope and make sure you'll be able to pass a single lumen.

3. Yes, call a cardiologist. This patient may be having an infarct and will benefit from some intervention. Which one, in the light of fresh surgical work? Heparin? Cath? Tough call. You need a cardiologist to make that call.

4. First discuss with the patient just what he heard. Sometimes a patient will recall something in the ICU and think it was in the OR. If it was indeed in the OR, then tell the patient that he did have recall, that is, validate his concern rather than dismiss it. Explain that safety concerns (the PA got cut and the blood pressure plummeted, so all anesthetics were turned off) sometimes mean the anesthetic drugs have to be turned off to maintain vital functions.

5. The best antitussives in the anesthetic realm are narcotics. Start with codeine containing PO meds if the patient can take PO. Lidocaine is another option. You could try a Lidocaine drip and see if that helps. No luck? A low level intravenous fentanyl infusion (in the ICU only) may work.

6. Cardiac herniation, seen most often in right pneumonectomy, can cause instant cardiac collapse. The heart slips through the disrupted pericardium, twists on itself, and cuts off all circulation. Treatment is opening the chest and untwisting the heart. As this patient had a tear in the pulmonary artery, another possibility is a stitch coming off the PA and the patient bleeding out.

7. Inspect his throat. If the uvula is swollen, explain to the patient what happened and assure him this should improve with time. Warm saltwater gargles may help, though I suspect this is an old wives' tale. If pain persists, get an ENT consult.

8. Look around to see if anyone is looking. Yank it out, then run away and don't write anything in the chart. AHA! You thought you just found Waldo, didn't you! Not so easy, my friend. If you plunk an introducer in the carotid, call your friendly neighborhood vascular surgeon, go to the OR, and under direct vision, with all the goods available for a vascular repair. The surgeon may repair the carotic under local, or under general. The main idea here is do not be cavalier. If you yank the sheath out, the subsequent bleeding could squish off the airway. Better luck finding Waldo!

9. Anesthesia depresses the circulation, as does positive pressure ventilation. To maintain vital signs, we always have to give more fluids than the internists like. Also, one response to the stress of surgery is ADH release. The patients "hang on to fluid." So, no surprise that the patients gain weight during the perioperative period. Check whether this internist regularly refers patients to you, if so, then say, "You're absolutely right, what was I thinking? I'll be more careful next time." If this internist doesn't regularly refer you patients, then tell him to take a hike.

10. Inspect the site. If it is leaking, pull the catheter out. Replace the catheter if the patient still needs it, but if he is a few days out and po meds can take care of his pain, don't replace it.

Grab Bag Questions

1. You are about to place an arterial line when a med student says, "You didn't perform an Allen test!" What words of wisdom do you lay on the well-meaning, snot-nosed brat?
2. What do you do to prevent an airway fire in a case with lasers?
3. What do you do to treat an airway fire when you forgot to prevent an airway fire in a case with lasers?
4. A 75-year-old, otherwise healthy man is scheduled for a TURBT. He has a loud systolic murmur. So you proceed with the case?

Answers to Grab Bag Questions

1. The Allen's test is of limited utility. Tell the med student to go get you a cappuccino and danish, or you will consider giving him a grade reflecting his limited utility.

2. Keep the FIO_2 as low as possible, preferably no higher than 25%. Don't use nitrous oxide, as that supports combustion. Use a laser tube that resists fire and inflate the cuffs with blue water. Pack the area with wet gauze. Know where the fire extinguisher is located. Wear safety goggles and make sure the door is posted so people don't come in and get zapped. (The goggle thing is not, strictly speaking, a fire safety measure.) Just for grins, if you do such a case around Halloween, get one of those big silver fireman outfits and put it on after the patient is induced. It'll crack up the whole OR.

3. Glad you're wearing that silver suit, aren't you? Turn off the oxygen, pull out the endotracheal tube, pull down the drapes, and use the fire extinguisher or else use water bottles (irrigation bottles) to douse the flames. Once the initial panic is over, now you have to rese-cure the airway. Recall that you now have the equivalent of a burn victim with a known airway injury, so you will need to reintubate before airway edema causes respiratory compromise.

4. Closely question him regarding, specifically, any episodes of dizziness or syncope. That could indicate aortic stenosis versus the more common "aortic sclerosis" murmur (whatever that is). Then look at his old record. If he has had a half dozen TURBTs in the last few years without any adverse OR events, then go ahead and conduct the anesthetic. If this is a first time, and anything seems fishy in the story, get the echo.

Halfway through number three. Getting the hang of it?

Session 2

A 60-year-old, normal sized male is scheduled for a right carotid endarterectomy. Except for the usual litany of hypertension and cigarette use, he is in good health. Vital signs are remarkable for a BP of 180/106.

Preop Questions

1. Any further workup necessary for the possibility of heart disease?
2. Does the hypertension mandate delay of surgery?
3. What if you found out the patient *normally* takes "some blood pressure pill" but didn't take it this morning?
4. If, in addition to his TIAs, the patient had a stroke 3 weeks ago, should surgery be delayed?
5. What preop labs are necessary?
6. Do you need any medical consultation preop?
7. Given the need for a "rapid wakeup," how do you premedicate the patient?
8. Do you insist an EEG be present?
9. What do you tell the patient regarding options for anesthesia?
10. What do you do if the patient insists he be asleep when the surgeon does almost all of these under a block?

Answers to Preop Questions

1. Anyone with vascular disease in one area (here, the carotids) is likely to have vascular disease in other areas (the coronaries). So the world's most conservative approach is to insist on a heart cath on anyone undergoing carotid disease. But if the patient has no symptoms, it's not worth it to go on a fishing trip. A carotid is a low volume shift operation that exposes the patient to a few minutes of hypertensive stress (as you raise the blood pressure during cross clamp). That degree of stress does not merit a heart cath. How about a noninvasive test, such as a dobutamine stress test? Again, with no symptoms, I wouldn't insist on it. Be aware of the possibility of coronary disease, but don't go ape trying to uncover it.

2. No. For baseline pressures, look to clinic charts or the vital signs mentioned at outpatient check-in. Use that to guide your blood pressure management. In the immediate preop area, the patient may well be nervous and have an elevated blood pressure. Canceling the case and sending the patient off to be further optimized will in all likelihood not end up optimizing him. And in the meantime, he may have another TIA or stroke. Lot of good canceling did him in that case.

3. Same answer. With labetalol, esmolol, and your anesthetics, you should be able to handle the hemodynamics. Getting all prissy about, "He forgot his thiazide diuretic this morning, case cancelled!" is ridiculous.

4. A recent stroke places the patient at risk for another stroke perioperatively. The farther out the stroke (say, years ago), the less the risk. The more recent the stroke (as in this case, a few weeks), the higher the risk. The percentages escape me. Whether to proceed or not hinges on your discussion with the surgeon. If the carotid lesion's anatomy presents grave risk for an embolus (a ragged edge or a plaque hanging in the wind), then the risk of waiting is greater than the risk of proceeding. If the carotid lesion's anatomy is more "stable," then you should wait. Voice your concern to the surgeon, explain the situation to the patient and family, then proceed.

5. Since other vascular areas could be affected, get a creatinine to check renal function. EKG as a baseline—if at the end of the case, someone notices the T waves are flipped, you'd be happy to have a preop EKG that showed the same thing. If he's on diuretics, get a potassium. Hematocrit. Why? In case ischemia occurs or uncontrollable hemorrhage occurs, it's good to know where you started.

6. No.

7. Midazolam 2 mg IV will help relax the patient preop, and shouldn't interfere with emergence. I would not want to go into a vascular procedure wide awake, and neither, I suspect, would you. Longer lasting agents, such as Valium, could interfere with the quick emergence and neuro evaluation that you want to do at the end of the case.

8. Yes. Although imperfect, the EEG will alert you to global changes that could indicate cerebral ischemia. Doing the case and "just hoping" he wakes up OK is not cool.

9. General versus local plus sedation. "A general anesthetic means you are completely asleep but we'll use a machine to watch your brain function closely. Local plus sedation means we'll put numbing medicine in your neck and you will keep talking to us, letting us know you're OK. No one has proven that one way is safer than another way."

10. The patient's preferences trump the surgeon's preferences. We can explain the surgeon's point of view, the surgeon's view of the advantages of doing the operation "his way," but ultimately, the patient has the call. (In certain cases, a patient may make a request that just won't fly. "I want a spinal for my shoulder operation and I want the Mormon Tabernacle Choir in the operating room with me." That won't work.)

Did you notice in answer 4—"the numbers escape me." This is not the written exam, this is the oral exam. You can punt on some of the specifics, the examiners want to know what you're thinking, not what you memorized for the written test. Convey your idea and your reasoning, don't worry about producing a spread sheet of percentages.

Intraop Questions

1. Do you use general or a block? What are the advantages and disadvantages of each?
2. If you perform a block and the patient suddenly gets agitated with carotid cross-clamp, what do you do?
3. You pull back the drapes and discover the patient has vomited, what next?
4. You induce with a general anesthetic, what blood pressure parameters do you follow?
5. The EEG tech says the pattern looks ominous under cross-clamp, what do you do?
6. At the end of the procedure, you ask whether you should reverse with protamine. The surgeon says yes, you give 50 mg IV, and the pressure goes to 60/30. What do you do?
7. Just after you've extubated, a huge hematoma forms, distorting the airway. What to do?
8. You attempt intubation, but the tissue is all distorted in the pharynx. You can ventilate and the surgeon says, "Just let me tie off one bleeder! I see it!"
9. Now you can't ventilate anymore and the patient is all blue. The surgeon says, "Just one more minute!"
10. How would you diagnose damage to the recurrent laryngeal nerve in the operating room?

Answers to Intraop Questions

1. General. My primary concern with a block is twofold—I haven't done many blocks so I don't think I could do a good one, and second, if the patient gets in trouble, I want that airway already secured. The advantage of a block is that you can more closely monitor true cerebral function, rather than EEG waves that *imply* good cerebral function. Also, a block will have fewer hemodynamic swings and will have no coughing on the ETT at the end of the case.

2. The agitation implies inadequate cerebral perfusion leading to confusion. Induce general anesthesia and secure the airway. That will imply pushing back sheets and all kinds of headaches.

3. Suction, head down and to the side. Clear the airway as best you can, then proceed to induce, relax, and intubate the patient.

4. Keep the blood pressure about the same as the patient's baseline blood pressure. During cross-clamp, raise the blood pressure 10% to 20% above baseline and keep in touch with the EEG technician.

5. If your anesthetic is not interfering with the EEG waves (your vapors should be under 0.5 MAC), then raise the blood pressure and inform the surgeon that you have evidence of ischemia. He may choose to place a shunt to minimize (though it doesn't eliminate) ischemic time.

6. That little protamine shouldn't cause such a dip, unless the patient has been exposed to protamine before, or unless he has had a vasectomy and has antibodies to protamine (that's a little theoretical). Treat with fluids and phenylephrine. If the blood pressure doesn't respond and it looks like a dyed-in-the-wool allergic reaction, treat hypotension with epinephrine early and aggressively. Add Benadryl and steroids if you feel compelled, but stick with the mainstay of allergic reaction treatment, the big E.

7. Open the stitches to release the pressure. Reintubate as soon as possible as the airway will proceed to fantastic distortion in no time.

8. "Trach, now," is the response. That airway will only get worse.

9. Kick the surgeon in the keister and say, "Didn't you hear my answer to question number 8? When the airway is distorted and even opening the surgical stitches doesn't help, you have the world's worst airway nightmare. Even a good fiberoptic jockey would get lost in that swollen airway.

10. At extubation, as you pull out the endotracheal tube, look with a laryngoscope to see if the vocal cords work. That's what the surgeon will ask you to do, but if you think about it, it's very hard to do—your laryngoscope in the mouth just as the patient is waking up? Who are you kidding, the patient will be biting down on the scope and you'll be tempted to just say, "Yeah, sure, I saw them move!" when you didn't see a thing. If the surgeon really wants an evaluation, place the fiberoptic through the nose and look down on the cords as you extubate, that way you'll be able to see something without having to pull out the oral laryngoscope right away. Ask the patient to say "Eeee," and see if both the vocal cords move.

This line of questioning demonstrates one thing the examiners can and will do. I said I'd go with a general, then they said, "OK, now you did it under a block and these complications occurred." I didn't say, "But wait just a darned tootin' minute pardner, didn't you hear me? I said I'd do a general!" No, I adapted to the change in plans and talked my way through the complications. The examiners want you to explain an alternative anesthetic.

Grab Bag Questions

1. A woman presents to the OB suite with painless vaginal bleeding. What are the initial steps in her evaluation and preparation from an anesthetic standpoint?

2. A child with congenital diaphragmatic hernia suffers from low saturation after intubation. Peak inspiratory pressures are high. What must you do?

3. A diabetic scheduled for a hernia repair asks in preop clinic what he should do about his morning insulin. What do you tell him?

4. A 7-year-old will have eye surgery, but there are no more uncuffed tubes available at your surgi-center. Will you use a cuffed tube? Will you insist someone drive up to the main hospital and get an uncuffed one?

Answers to Grab Bag Questions

1. Get big IV access and get blood ready. This bleeding is a placenta previa until proven otherwise. After initial echo exam, the vaginal exam should be done in an OR ready for a stat C-section.

2. The good lung probably has a pneumothorax, so the child will need a chest tube. Of course check for all the normal stuff, endotracheal tube in the right place, oxygen being delivered. But a pneumothorax is the specific, high-likelihood problem in this case.

3. Hold the morning insulin. Although tight control may help a little in wound healing, tight glucose control (the "take half your normal insulin then we'll start a glucose infusion" technique) is not worth the risk of hypoglycemia in the perioperative period. Prevail upon the surgeon to do this case first.

4. Use a cuffed tube, just don't inflate the cuff. No big deal. Go with the usual guidelines—make sure there is still a leak at 20 cm H_2O. Don't force the tube and stir up edema in the airway.

Relax. Three down, seven to go. Have you spotted the deliberately wrong answer (or answers?) yet? Do you have a Waldo written down, or a list of Waldos? Enough to make you think. Maybe the answers are *all* Waldos and you should look up each and every answer yourself.

Hmmm.

PRACTICE EXAM #4

Session 1

The cath lab calls you to help sedate a patient for a PTCA. She is a 70-year-old, 55 kg woman with severe arthritis.

HPI: The patient complained of chest pain while watching a professional wrestling match. Apparently, lost in the excitement of the match, she stood up on her chair and was shouting, "Rip his throat out, Hulk! Rip his throat out!" She then grabbed her chest, fell back, and is now getting her coronaries examined.

PMH: Arthritis with neck and jaw involvement. Also, claustrophobia. Will not hold still for the PTCA.

Physical exam: Limited airway movement.

Labs: Remarkable for a hematocrit of 27.

She is on the cath lab table, wiggling to beat the band. She has groin lines in and a tiny peripheral IV. A propofol pump is ready and waiting.

Intraop Questions

1. How will you sedate this patient? Is propofol a good choice?
2. What if the patient continues to be agitated and you need to secure the airway. Is awake intubation the best option? Nasal approach or oral? Advantages and disadvantages? Special considerations given the heparin?
3. In spite of sedation she develops a heart rate of 140 with ST changes, what do you do? What do you tell the cardiologist?
4. The case goes to the OR and the patient has received TPA and all sorts of other *baddies*. How will this affect your anesthetic?
5. At induction you can't intubate but can get an LMA in. What next?
6. As the surgeon is taking down the IMA, the PA pressures rise, and blood pressure falls. Mixed venous sat goes to 45%. What do you do?
7. On bypass the patient starts to move. Your move. Is recall likely?
8. On bypass the urine output stops cold. What now?
9. Coming off bypass, design a logical mix of inotropes in case the heart does not separate from bypass.
10. At chest closure, the nurse notes that 250 cc of blood have drained in the last 15 minutes. How will you recognize tamponade?

Answers to Intraop Questions

1. This patient is beyond the "sedate" phase. She has cannulae in her groin, catheters floating around in her coronaries, she is laying on a rock hard table worthy of the Spanish Inquisition, and she is already wiggling out of control. In short, the cardiologists, the cognitive specialists, the wizards of the myocardial set, have painted the patient, and you, into a corner. Move to definitive control of the situation, which means securing the airway, getting access to the good lines in her groin, and getting in the best possible position to move definitively should she crash and need her chest opened in a hurry. Once you have her airway, then propofol may be OK. But not now, it will just make a bad situation worse.

2. Arthritis can present airway difficulties at the jaw, neck, and arytenoid cartilage level. The gobs of heparin make a nasal intubation problematic. Although the nasal approach "lines up" the endotracheal tube right above the cords, and avoids the sharp angle of the oral approach, the possibility of bleeding makes a nasal intubation a problem. And once the bleeding starts, she'll bleed like there's no tomorrow, like a stuck hog, like a runaway freight train, like too many clichés run together. Go orally. Although in her agitated state, you can, with an extra pair of hands, secure the tube awake. The key is to have the assistant hold the chin up, clenching the oral airway in place, so you can go in and stay midline with the scope. As she is still awake, you should be able to see the cords working, even if she is moving around. No easy task, but the safest option if the airway appears difficult.

3. Tachycardia with ST changes—tell the cardiologist that if she has an operable lesion, time's of the essence (time is myocardium). Of course address the usual causes of tachycardia (hypoxemia, open inotrope, pain). With the airway secured, you can give as much pain relief as the blood pressure can take, and as much nitroglycerin as the blood pressure can take, but the definitive move (yes, a stent may buy time, and yes, an intra-aortic balloon pump may improve perfusion and afterload reduction) is to get to the OR, open the chest, rest the heart on cardiopulmonary bypass, and get blood past the occluded vessels. With a maximum of tact, tell the cardiologist, "Quit fooling around, let's get to the OR!"

4. How do you spell "coagulopathy"? You'll need tons of blood products post-bypass. A scientific approach to this coming bleed-o-rama will be to send coags, get a TEG, and treat specifically. In the cold, cruel world of reality, you will pour platelets, cryo, and fresh frozen plasma at this patient until the blood bank screams bloody murder.

5. The LMA can be a bridge to intubation or a way to ventilate until you secure by trach (a bloody mess you'd just as soon avoid given all the antibleeding stuff from the cath lab). First, take stock of the whole scene as you ventilate through the LMA. Saturation OK? Good, then there's no screaming rush. Vital signs and STs any worse? Treat them and get the vital signs under control before you plunge into the airway. Then, once a modicum of calm has settled upon the land, load a long 6.0 endotracheal tube onto a fiberoptic, pass the fiberoptic through the spokes at the end of the LMA, and with any luck, you're there. Pass the 6.0 to secure the airway, then place an endotracheal tube changer in it just in case you dislodge the tube as you work the LMA out. Once the 6.0 is in place, if you can ventilate OK, leave it in. You can change to a 7.0 later using an endotracheal tube changer when under less emergent conditions.

6. You're in the death spiral. Treat with inotropes, but inform the surgeon that if your magic doesn't work, you'll need to heparinize, get cannulated, and get on bypass pronto. They may have to take down the IMA later. Buying time with inotropes will, in one way or another, flog the myocardium, and this, before the definitive revascularization. My choice of *the drug* when this situation arises is Primacor, 3 mg IV push, then have Levo ready to keep the BP up. If there is any drug in the world that can save your butt when you are up to your ass in alligators, it's Primacor. And I say that without even demanding that the Primacor (milrinone) salesperson bring donuts to our office next Monday.

7. Give more anesthetic. Either inhaled agent on the cardiopulmonary bypass machine, or injected anesthetic. Don't just paralyze, or you will risk recall. The most dangerous time for recall is as the patient rewarms. Some anesthetic should be on board then. Will BIS monitors or some new technology help us in this gray zone of "anesthetized or not?" Jury is still out on that one. For now we have to go with common sense.

8. This is a toughie. Of course make sure the Foley is OK (post renal oliguria) but then the dilemma is this. Some patients will not resume a good urine output until pulsatile flow is reestablished when you are off bypass. If you nail them with Lasix, then the urine output becomes a torrent later on, you'll lose a lot of potassium (read, ventricular irritability later on) and volume (read, chase your tail in the ICU). In this case, I would start renal dose dopamine, realizing I was just maybe making myself feel better, then wait it out until pulsatile flow restarted.

9. Give Primacor as the patient starts to rewarm, it will give you a few hours of phosphodiesterase inhibition. Have norepinephrine in line, as the SVR will sink like a stone from the Primacor. (Try not to think too much about the fact that you are *unloading* with the Primacor and making it *hard to unload* with the norepinephrine. For some reason, it works, even though it seems like you're driving with your foot on the brake and the gas at the same time.) Have epinephrine in line and going. Epi will give you blood pressure and kick. What more could you want? It is the mother's milk of inotropes. Have dobutamine in line, realizing that dobutamine is a *sissie* compared to the others. But with all those in line, you can honestly tell the surgeon, "Look captain, I've got all the guns blazing, if we can't come off with this, it's time for 'Balloons by the Bunch.'"

10. The earliest sign of tamponade is increasing inotropic support without another discernible cause. The PA pressures will equalize with the CVP, the mediastinum will widen (hard to tell in a fresh heart's portable chest x-ray), and all that is well and good. But the best way to pick up tamponade is early, before you're going ape in the unit, cutting open the wires with the unit secretary's nail clippers. Before you go screaming down the hall, CPR in progress, pouring undiluted epi into the patient with a firehose, then ducking as the blood pressure shoots to 6.02×10^{23} as soon as the surgeon opens the chest.

Even if you don't do cardiac all the time, (especially if you've been out of training for a few years and your hospital doesn't do hearts) at least brush up on the main points of doing a cardiac case. It's perfectly fair of the examiners to take you to the mat on inotropic questions.

Postop Questions

1. The surgeon wants the patient extubated as soon as possible. Will you give reversal agents for the neuromuscular blockers or for the narcotics?

2. In the ICU, the initial ABG shows a pO_2 of only 65. How will you adjust this?

3. The nurse cannot get the Swan to wedge. How will you help the nurse?

4. Cardiac output has dropped from 5.4 to 3.6. Should you give blood?

5. Renal dose dopamine will have what effect on the other hemodynamic parameters?

6. Patient has a run of V-tach that resolves spontaneously. What, if any, intervention do you institute?

7. The patient is waking up but doesn't appear to be moving the left side. What do you do?

8. The next day the patient is splinting and not taking deep breaths. How can you help this situation?

9. During the case the patient became, at times, pacer dependent. What settings do you put on the pacer box and what special instructions do you give the ICU staff?

10. The patient tells you, "I don't like your attitude one bit, buster, I don't want you to ever do my anesthesia again!" Then she gives you the finger. How do you defuse this irate wrestling fan?

Answers to Postop Questions

1. Fast tracking is all the rage now, getting patients off the ventilators as soon as possible. That is fine, but I'm not in that big of a rush. During the case, I would tailor the anesthetic to a reasonable extubation time, say 3 to 4 hours postop. That will give enough time for bleeding to "declare itself" in most cases. That will also give time for the patient to fully rewarm, get over shivering with its attendant high oxygen consumption, and let the labs come back. In short, I want the patient kosher and dandy for a few hours before I make a move. That length of time will allow the intraop narcotics and relaxants to wear off, no need to reverse them.

2. First, check the endotracheal tube position. Edentulous folk in particular are likely to have the ETT sink into the right mainstem. Then suction, administer breathing treatments, and give a few manual breaths to clear up any atelectasis. Increase the PEEP and the FIO_2. Often the pump run by itself can cause a "mini-ARDS" with high A-a gradient for a few hours postop. But that is a diagnosis of exclusion, so first fix anything else that can be fixed.

3. Don't bother with a wedge. Inflating that little balloon can cause a pulmonary artery rupture with fatal consequences. Getting a wedge isn't a priority, setting the patient right is a priority. Use the wealth of other information at hand, (PA pressures, rate and rhythm, blood pressure, acid-base status, urine output, cardiac output, lab values) to fix what needs fixing.

4. That depends on everything else. For example, if the hematocrit is low, say 24, and the PA pressures are low, say 12/6, and blood loss is continuing, and the mixed venous is falling, say to 55%, then that entire picture adds up to—give blood. It is the entire clinical picture, not just one value that determines the need to transfuse. But to just give blood because one value, the cardiac output, fell from one number to another number, is the decision of a feeble minded ninnie. At such a person and such a line of reasoning, I laugh.

5. The potpourri of effects from dopamine (renal at low levels, beta at middle levels, alpha at higher levels) is hard to predict, for each of those effects has its own bell-shaped curve. A low dose in one patient may cause a troublesome tachycardia, whereas a high dose may be necessary to really help the kidneys. Perhaps a diseased kidney needs a higher perfusion pressure (the alpha, high-dose effect) to make a real difference in, say, urine output. So the best you can say for dopamine is that you have to give it and see what happens. You can't just dial in a dose and be sure the dopamine will do what you want.

6. Scour the postoperative minefield for a cause of that V-tach. Yes, it may just be a "reperfusion irritability," whatever the hell that is, but you must look for a cause. Start simple—oxygen, hematocrit, potassium, pH. Magnesium levels are often low in these patients on chronic diuretics, so a magnesium level and subsequent replacement are in order. Finally, if all has checked out OK, start an antiarrythmic, such as lidocaine.

7. Spooky. Could be a stroke. Short of supportive care and making sure the blood pressure is adequate, there isn't too much to do. The aortic cannula or cross-clamp could have broken off flecks of calcium that embolized to the brain. A neuro consult is necessary to document the extent of the infarct. Good supportive care and time do resolve some of these CVAs. Make sure, if this patient is in the ICU, that while the big workup is under way, simple things are not forgotten. If there is going to be a meaningful recovery, then good nutrition, timely line changes to avoid sepsis, and good skin care will all play a major role.

8. If pain control is a real impediment to adequate respiration, you could place intrathecal or epidural narcotics and local anesthetic. There is no concern about "the big heparin bolus" now, for the operation is over. You could also localize the pain, often a chest tube, and perform an intercostal block so that the chest tube site will hurt less. Finally, a PCA may help the patient, particularly because she will have more ability to take care of herself rather than asking the nurses.

9. Keep the pacer connected and have an extra one in the ICU in case a battery fails. Set the pacer at the inhibited mode at a rate, say, of 50 with dual chamber pacing and inhibition. That way the pacer should not interfere with the native rhythm, but if the heart rate plummets, at least the pacer will kick in with a rhythm (A–V) that provides atrial kick.

10. After a run-in with a cardiopulmonary bypass machine, many patients have some cognitive difficulties. "Uncle Joe just never was the same after his heart bypass." Any number of explanations exist for this, microemboli, calcium thingies, air bubbles, demonic possession, CIA conspiracy, who knows what? If a patient is acting bizarre, make sure all is well with them before writing them off as a nut. Could this patient be septic, for example? If nothing appears amiss, and your mojo and the patient's just didn't get on track, try to keep your cool and accept her request that you not do her next anesthetic. Then offer to buy her the World Wrestling Federation's next pay-per-view extravaganza. That ought to make it all square between you two.

WATCH AS MAGILL "THE FORCEPS" GOES HEAD TO HEAD WITH THE TAG TEAM OF MAC "THE CURVED BLADE OF STEEL" AND HIS STRAIGHT MAN MILLER "THE KILLER"! $39.95. Kids, get your parents' permission.

Grab Bag Questions

1. A 45-year-old man with pancreatic CA and intractable abdominal pain is referred for a nerve block. What do you do?

2. You are setting up for a twins delivery. What special precautions do you take versus a singleton delivery?

3. You are doing an eye case and the patient won't hold still. What next, my friend?

4. For a Harrington rod procedure, a surgeon requests a wake up test. Why is this necessary if you already have evoked potentials?

Answers to Grab Bag Questions

1. After making sure with the oncologist that there is nothing treatable, say with radiation, then plan an approach of blocks and narcotics. Celiac plexus blocks using fluoroscopic guidance may help. Given the relatively rapid fatal outcome of pancreatic CA, high dose oral narcotics should be tried to alleviate the patient's pain. Concerns of addiction are, of course, invalid in this setting.

2. Twins are more likely to be premature, small, and therefore, have respiratory difficulties. Have twin bassinettes and two teams ready, and have an experienced nurse (not a student or a "new person") watching the monitor. Those two traces can get confusing. At delivery, be in an operating room, rather than a delivery room, because the possibility of cord tangling, breech presentation, or sudden decompensation is higher in twins. In short, your "pucker factor" should be higher for twins.

3. If regional isn't working, do a general anesthetic. Better to just stop, regroup, and make it right, than to limp along. Trying to sedate, sedate, sedate your way out of trouble, with the airway hidden under the drapes, will just lead you down the road to perdition and damnation, brothers and sisters.

4. Evoked potentials only test the sensory tracks, not the anterior, motor tracks. So the SSEP can look fine the whole case while the motor area is getting ischemic from the traction on the spinal column. The wake up test will tell if the motor track is functioning. If the test shows a problem, then the surgeons will "relax" the fixtures a little.

Halfway through number 4. Grab a frappuccino latte with cinnamon flakes and a biscotti. Put on some Birkenstock sandals, put your feet up, and pretend like you're trying to see Mount Rainier through the rain.

Alright, the break's over, back to work.

Session 2

A 5-year-old is scheduled for strabismus surgery. Normal growth and development. Mother says his brother died under anesthesia at the age of 18 when he had his appendix taken out.

Preop Questions

1. What is the differential diagnosis of "dying under anesthesia?"
2. What steps would you take to peg just how the brother's death occurred?
3. Would you insist on a CPK preop? A muscle biopsy? A test for pseudocholinesterase deficiency? A test for porphyria?
4. Is preop dantrolene indicated?
5. Would you do this case at a stand-alone surgi-center? Why or why not?
6. What other preop tests would you order?
7. How would you prepare the room, the OR, and the PACU staff for this case?
8. What is malignant hyperthermia?
9. What do you tell the mother about the risks of anesthesia?
10. Do you allow the mother to go into the OR?

Answers to Preop Questions

1. Anything from a lost airway to a Zeppelin crashing into the operating room while the surgeons were closing. Percentages lean toward the lost airway as Zeppelins rarely, if ever, land on an OR table. The best evaluation of this "mystery death" is the old record. In this day of faxes and e-mail, you should be able to find out, but in the rarified atmosphere of the boards, you will not have access to that information.

2. Question the mother as best you can to find out specific tip-offs—"The anesthesiologist said he couldn't put the tube in," "They said he had a high fever," "He vomited and the food went into his windpipe." In all likelihood, the mother will know nothing and you will be flying blind. Obviously, this should raise the hackles on your neck, looking specifically for the big MH.

3. If you suspect MH, you should do a trigger-free anesthetic. No muscle biopsy. Again, if you suspect MH, treat as if they have MH. The time, expense, and hassle of the biopsy are not worth it. A baseline CPK is also not necessary. If it's high, so what? Now your "suspicion" is raised a little, and you'll do a trigger-free anesthetic anyway. So the test made no difference so it wasn't worth doing. Voila! The other two "anesthetic diseases," porphyria and pseudocholinesterase deficiency, are possibilities. But taking tests to uncover them will also not merit the time, hassle, and cost. Those diseases are also unlikely to have caused a death.

4. Dantrolene is expensive, hard to draw up, and turns the patient orange and weak. Ay chihuahua, what a pain! Giving dantrolene prophylactically is not indicated. Have it around, know how to use it, but do not give it. Just do a trigger-free anesthetic.

5. Yes. The world's most cautious soul would say, "But what if MH happens and the whole world goes to hell in a handbasket and you're trying to do all this invasive stuff and resuscitate a patient at a little rinky-dink place!" A more realistic approach is if you do a non-triggering anesthetic, you'll be OK, and with all the short acting options we have now, specifically propofol, you should be able to conduct the anesthetic just fine without a prolonged wake up.

6. As the child is otherwise healthy, no other labs are necessary. Hematocrit? No need, this isn't a blood loss procedure. Electrolytes? Again, no need.

7. Warm the room (the ultimate irony when malignant hyperthermia is a consideration) because a 5-year-old child may become cool in the frigid confines of the normal polar icecap of an OR. Do a dry run of what you do in case of a MH emergency. You should do this a few times a year in whatever setting you work in anyway. Explain to the staff the concern in this case and what early signs to look for in case of

MH. Get a clean anesthesia machine—soda lime changed, fresh gas flows for 10 minutes, and tape over the vaporizers so some fool giving a break doesn't crank on the inhaled agents by mistake.

8. A disorder of muscle membrane. When triggered by succinylcholine or potent inhaled agents, the muscles go into overdrive, releasing calcium, and becoming hypermetabolic. Oxygen consumption, carbon dioxide production, and lactate production all go sky high. As a result, the muscles become rigid, the saturation drops, the heart rate rises, the end-tidal CO_2 rises, and last of all, the temperature rises. In the days before dantrolene treatment, mortality was high. Since dantrolene therapy, mortality has dropped but can still occur.

9. A direct but compassionate approach is best, in this as in all medical discussions with family members. "Anesthesia has risks, just as driving a car has risks or flying a plane has risks. We do everything we can to reduce the risks and conduct a safe anesthetic and a safe operation. Since your other son died under anesthesia, we will watch out for a disease specific to certain anesthesia drugs and we will avoid those drugs." 'Nuf said.

10. No. In the case of an inhalation induction, I would; but this child will need a trigger-free anesthetic, which means an IV preinduction. The placement of that IV will probably cause some crying and upset and I'd as soon avoid placing that on the mother.

Intraop Questions

1. Will you use a trigger-free anesthetic? What is a trigger-free anesthetic? What was the name of Roy Rogers' horse?
2. Does a nitrous narcotic technique run the risk of awareness versus an anesthetic with potent inhaled agents?
3. You decide on a trigger-free anesthetic, but the patient fights you off at IV time. What are your options?
4. At induction the child holds his breath and desaturates, do you give Sux?
5. Which muscle relaxants do you use and why? How will you reverse them?
6. The heart rate drops to 30 as the surgeon is tugging at a muscle, your Dx and Rx?
7. While you were out on break, your break person turned on sevoflurane because you, ninny that you are, forgot to tell them. Now the patient's heart rate begins to rise. What do you do?
8. The surgeon is not through with the case but full-blown MH is in progress. What do you tell the surgeon? How do you treat the MH?
9. Ventricular ectopy starts. Your treatment?
10. Cardiac arrest occurs. Go through the entire resuscitation you would give.

Answers to Intraop Questions

1. Yes. Using a clean machine and avoiding Sux and potent inhaled agents, I'll avoid the big bad boys of MH causation. Do I worry that "stress" alone will cause MH? (As in the porcine model?) No. And Roy Rogers' horse was named, uh, I forget, but I know for sure that I'd do a TRIGGER-free anesthetic.

2. Yes. Nitrous narcotic is more likely than potent inhaled agents to result in awareness. Propofol and midazolam to the rescue. I'd use these two agents in addition to a nitrous narcotic technique to protect against (there is no absolute guarantee against) recall.

3. One good option is, before IV time, give some PO midazolam, that could help calm the patient down. IM sedation may cause some upset by the shot itself, but after that upset is over, you may have an easier time with the IV. Options include IM midazolam, in case the child wouldn't take PO meds, or IM morphine. If the line becomes a real thrash-o-rama, then ketamine would be an option. The sympathomimetic effects of ketamine, specifically the tachycardia, could be seen as problematic, since an early sign of MH is tachycardia. But if you are doing a trigger-free anesthetic anyway, I would not hesitate to use the ketamine. And that may be the only way to sedate the child enough to get the IV in. Finally, mask administration of nitrous is an additional sedative you can use. Fifty percent nitrous alone cannot get a child to hold still enough for an IV, but that could supplement your other maneuvers. Topicalization options? Topical lidocaine cream is useful, but must be in place and sealed for 45 minutes ahead of time to work. And one kicker is, say the first site is a swing and a miss. Now you have to go elsewhere, and *that* site won't be numb!

4. No. Other relaxants, the nondepolarizers, will take a little longer to work, but keeping positive pressure on, the cords will loosen enough to admit some oxygen ere too long. And a child can only hold his breath so long. Of course, use 100% oxygen at this time as you will be doing an intravenous induction. If you break down and give Sux, you run the risk of triggering the very thing you are trying so hard to avoid.

5. Cisatracurium. This is short acting and easily reversible. Are any other agents possible? Certainly. Rocuronium, vecuronium—as with any neuromuscular agent, monitor train of four and make sure the patient is adequately reversed prior to extubation.

6. Oculocardiac reflex. Ask the surgeon to cease and desist for a moment, which should stop the vagal response. Give atropine if the heart rate doesn't respond.

7. Some breaks are more problematic than others. Tachycardia without another cause (hypoxemia, light anesthesia, hypovolemia) can be an early sign of MH. Cast a watchful eye on the end-tidal CO_2, for if that also starts to rise, you have more evidence of developing MH. If your suspicion is raised, then make the call and start treatment for MH. Better to raise a false alarm than wait until it's too late in the course.

8. This is not emergent surgery, so tell the surgeon to stop the operation. Call for help. (It will take one person alone to mix the dantrolene.) Turn off the Sevo, go to 100% oxygen, place an arterial line and send blood gases. Acidosis will be a real problem. Monitor potassium. Cool the patient. Keep giving dantrolene, that is the key to the treatment. Consult the little card on the anesthesia machine that tells what to do in case of MH (just to make sure you're not missing anything). Get a clean machine, a new ventilator from the ICU may be faster than rolling in a new anesthesia machine. Faster still is an ambubag. Make sure ICU care is arranged for. After the MH crisis has passed, observe the patient for signs of recrudescence.

9. Look for the cause of the ectopy; here, acidosis, hypoxemia, or hyperkalemia being most likely. Treat whatever appears abnormal. Use standard antiarrhythmics (none is implicated in causing MH). Give lidocaine and start a lidocaine drip, if ectopy persists. At the risk of sounding like a broken record, keep looking for metabolic abnormalities. For example, if you treat acidosis, remember that acidosis may recur. Just because you corrected a pH of 7.23, the acid-producing process is continuing. In spite of the bicarb you gave, the next pH may be 7.12.

10. ABC. Assure adequate oxygenation. Start compressions and perform CPR. Treat hyperkalemia with bicarb, insulin, and glucose. This is one time you would not give calcium, because calcium release is the problem. In giving resuscitative drugs, calculate that this 5-year-old is a little less than half an adult (the rule of thumb—a 7-year-old gets roughly half an adult dose in a code). Shock, shock, shock, epi, shock. Lidocaine, bretylium. If asystole, attempt pacing. Keep doing CPR and ACLS.

Once again, the examiners have the luxury of pulling you out of your normal plan. You did everything you could to avoid causing MH, you had high suspicions, and yet the examiner still dragged you kicking and struggling right into a full-blown MH crisis. So adapt. Go with the flow and explain your way out of the trouble.

During the exam, trouble will be your middle name.

Shagadelic.

Grab Bag Questions

1. A 15-year-old at term is flat on her back, watching a *Ricki Lake* show entitled, "My Brother Got Me Pregnant, Again." The fetal heart rate shows a late deceleration. What do you do?

2. An obese man undergoes hernia repair. The surgeon insists you extubate deep to avoid coughing and breaking the sutures. What do you say to that?

3. A T4 paraplegic woman is about to undergo cystoscopy. The surgeon says a little sedation will do because she "can't feel anything anyway." Your response?

4. In a code, someone hands you norepinephrine instead of epinephrine. You berate the person and they say, "Hey, take a chill pill. What's the dif?"

Answers to Grab Bag Questions

1. Left uterine displacement. The *Ricki Lake* show is probably riveting everyone in the room and people forgot that the gravid uterus compresses the vena cava, cutting down on venous return, dropping the blood pressure, and causing the pressure-dependent placental vascular bed to receive inadequate perfusion. That translates into fetal distress, and subsequent slowing of the fetal heart rate.

2. Deep extubation leaves this obese patient at risk for aspiration. You could debate the surgeon, "If your sutures pop when he bucks, what do you think will happen when he goes home and coughs, or vomits from his Percodan, or strains at stool." But most surgeons won't appreciate your rapier thrust of intelligence. So do your best to get a smooth, but still awake extubation. Narcotics, titrated until the patient's respiratory rate shows that he is comfortable (say a rate of 10 to 12) plus some IV lidocaine, may yield a patient opening his eyes to command but not fighting the endotracheal tube.

3. That level of spinal cord injury, coupled with cystoscopy, could trigger autonomic hyperreflexia. The patient should have either a general anesthetic or a spinal anesthetic. Myself, I would do a general anesthetic, avoiding Sux for concerns of potassium release.

4. Norepinephrine does have a little beta effect, but is primarily an alpha agent. Epinephrine has much more beta effect. In a code, epinephrine is what you want. You need that beta thunderbolt if you're going to restart the ailing heart.

Round four done. Getting the hang of the format? Use it as springboard to your own tests. Go farther out on each answer, too. Don't stop where we stop, pretend the examiner pauses after each of your answers, waiting for more.

I wonder if Waldo was somewhere in the last test. Maybe in the pediatric code? Have you leafed through an ACLS book lately? Think that might be a good idea?

SAMPLE EXAM #5

Session 1

A 55-year-old woman is scheduled for resection of a cecal carcinoma.

HPI: This woman toasted her good fortune at graduating from high school with a bottle of sloe gin and a pack of unfiltered Camels. And she never stopped toasting that good fortune. During one of her many admissions for alcohol-related problems she developed a lower GI bleed and was found to have a cecal CA.

PMH: Alcoholism with all the trimmings, to wit, ascites, cirrhosis, upper GI bleeds

Physical exam: Ascites. Normal airway. Lung exam consistent with COPD.

Chest x-ray: COPD. Nothing active.

Labs: PT slightly elevated. SGOT double normal. Hct 28.

She is in the OR with a 16-g IV in the antecubital fossa. She smiles at you and says, "You know the song, 'Night Night, Sweetheart'? Well, doc, night night."

Intraop Questions

1. What additional monitors will you place? Any neuraxial opiods?
2. At induction you notice a saturation of only 95% on 100% O_2. Why might this be?
3. The surgeon encounters enormous hemorrhaging, but the blood bank has only type and screened blood available. What to do?
4. What problems are associated with massive transfusions?
5. The end-tidal CO_2 rises from 35 to 45 in spite of no change in the vent settings. What gives, Jack?
6. A blood gas after the big transfusion shows a base deficit of 12. How will you treat this? Is THAM a good option?
7. What IV fluids will you use, given the patient's history of alcoholism and ascites?
8. Will this patient likely demonstrate tolerance to narcotics? How will you tell? How will that alter your anesthetic?
9. The patient bucks violently, tearing open a suture in the field. You notice the Forane vaporizer is dry. What do you do, and what do you tell the surgeon?
10. The patient's heart rate rises from 85 to 140 as she is emerging. What do you do?

Answers to Intraop Questions

1. After induction, I'd place an arterial line. The shunts around her cirrhotic liver could cause a big A-a gradient. So blood gases will be necessary intraop and postop. Also, once asleep, I'd place a central line. If my surgeon were good and fast, I'd place a CVP. The fluid shifts when the abdomen is opened and the ascitic fluid is drained off may make volume assessment tricky. If the surgeon were slow, then I'd place a Swan, because a cirrhotic may need high cardiac outputs to maintain organ perfusion. I would not place neuraxial opioids. The history and lab values all say, "Red alert, red alert! Danger Will Robinson!" I wouldn't want to risk a neuraxial bleed.

2. First, the usual stuff may be wrong—endobronchial intubation, wheezing, aspiration—but if these, more prosaic causes are eliminated, then the patient is revealing extensive shunting around her hepatic bed.

3. Call for the type and screen stuff. There is no higher likelihood of an adverse reaction with type and screen blood than there is with type and cross blood. Also, if you wait for the type and cross blood, the patient will already be on her way to the marble mattress downstairs in the pathologist's surgical suite. If you use up the type and screen stuff, get universal donor blood, that is O negative. If there is not enough of that (which can often be the case) don't fuss too much, use O positive. The chance that this patient will be pregnant again is somewhere between remote and no way.

4. Hypothermia if you don't warm the blood. Hypocalcemia from the citrate binding. Dilutional thrombocytopenia. If the blood is old and cell lysis has occurred, a pretty decent slug of potassium can be delivered, too. The most feared problem of blood transfusion is a transfusion reaction, most often from mislabeled (or in the heat of a disaster, inadequately checked) blood. The adverse effects from a transfuion reaction—hypotension, oozing, and hemolysis—can be hard to pick up if the patient is already hypotensive, oozing, and hemolyzing from an ongoing massive transfusion.

5. Either more CO_2 is being produced (malignant hyperthermia, intravenous bicarb was given, fever, shivering) or less is being eliminated (hypoventilation, but the question states the ventilation hadn't changed). My guess is bicarb administration resulting in more CO_2 production. In the course of a rapid transfusion, if hypotension and hypoperfusion resulted, then acidosis results. Giving bicarb to treat that without increasing the ventilation will result in a higher end-tidal CO_2.

6. The best treatment for acidosis is treating the cause of the acidosis. So treat hypovolemia, hypoperfusion, anemia, or whatever else could be causing the "evidence of cellular distress," that is, acid production. In a bow to reality, though, you still treat the metabolic acidosis with bicarb if the pH is low, for cellular enzyme systems do not function well in an acidotic environment. For example, as you start an inotrope to increase perfusion, that inotrope may not work well until the acidosis is at least improved. I would use THAM if a blood gas showed a high sodium, as THAM is a sodium-free base. Bicarb without the Na, as it were.

7. Free water is a no-no, so no D5W, as if I need to tell an examiner that. Other than that, there is no proof that one method of volume replacement (colloid versus crystalloid, the ancient debate) is better than another at "preventing" the ascites from returning. The main point in this patient's volume replacement is to give enough, as demonstrated by adequate urine output, good blood gases reflecting adequate perfusion, and adequate blood pressure. Given the multisystem disease she has, I'd be more generous on blood with her than I would with an otherwise healthy patient.

8. The tolerance question will depend on where her liver is in the natural history of liver failure. If her cytochrome p450 system (yes, technically the p450 system is a laboratory construct, but the descriptive term is useful) is jazzed up from her alcohol use, then she will demonstrate tolerance to narcotics. As you give, say fentanyl, you'll notice a short time of MAC reduction and you'll have to give "more than usual," vague though that may sound. If, however, her liver is quick fried to a crackly crunch and has no more functioning hepatocytic "oomph," then hepatically metabolized drugs will linger for a long time.

9. Give an intravenous bolus of sedative-hypnotic, refill the vaporizer, and tell the surgeon, "Thank God, the patient survived the intraoperative wake-up test. Thank you for being a part of it." Then try to change the subject and talk about whatever the surgeon does outside the operating room.

10. As the patient regains consciousness, she will also regain sensibility to the large incision in her abdomen. Therefore pain is the most likely cause of the tachycardia. Before you write off the tachycardia as exclusively from pain, make sure nothing else is amiss—hypoxemia, anemia—then proceed to treat the pain. Sufficient narcotics to reduce the spontaneous respiratory rate to 12 or so usually tells you that the patient has enough pain relief. (Respiratory rate is a great indicator of pain, and a useful measure for you to titrate narcotics.)

Remember the heady days of medical school? There, the best way to prepare for tests was to get ahold of old tests and study them. "They're bound to ask more or less the same thing. Right?" Same here. Even partway through this fifth exam, you're already starting to hear the same things asked—oliguria, vital sign aberrations, bleeding, monitors. As you drill and drill and drill the answers to these, you should start to gain confidence in your ability to answer just about anything.

Postop Questions

1. When will you know you've transfused enough? What endpoints or lab values do you look for?
2. The patient takes a hard inspiration against a closed glottis. Shortly afterwards pink, frothy material is seen coming from her mouth. Dx and Rx?
3. Urine output falls in spite of a normal CVP. What do you do?
4. What is delirium tremens?
5. She develops gram-negative sepsis and goes into ARDS. What is ARDS and how do you treat it?
6. What other metabolic abnormalities are seen in the alcoholic?
7. While in the ICU, her BP drops to 70/50 and heart rate stays at about 100. How will you Dx and Rx this?
8. High output failure is diagnosed with an SVR of 450. What is SVR and how will you treat this condition?
9. Your resident tells you he's sick of changing lines every three days on this patient. What do you tell your resident?
10. Do you need to change the arterial lines? Why or why not?

Answers to Postop Questions

1. No individual lab will tell, the overall clinical picture will tell. Blood pressure OK, urine output OK, heart rate near baseline? All these indicate a circulatory system not stressed to the max. Hematocrit of 30 is a good guideline, since you are likely to transfuse if below 30, but again, this is a guideline. Blood gases should reflect a normal acid-base status.

2. Negative pressure pulmonary edema. The respiratory effort sucks fluid out of the vascular tree into the alveoli. Treatment is supportive, that is, intubation if you are unable to maintain oxygenation and you require PEEP. Administer Lasix and let the damage repair itself. If the patient doesn't require intubation, then administer supplemental oxygen and Lasix and observe.

3. Do the prerenal, postrenal, renal shuffle. Place a Swan and evaluate the cardiac output. If the output is "normal for a normal person" it may be "subnormal for an ascitic person" and you will have to increase the cardiac output with inotropes. Renal dopamine may help (controversial) but I would start it.

4. Alcohol withdrawal can cause a state of sympathetic overstimulation resulting in tachycardia, arrhythmias, and go on to cardiac failure. Coupled with that is the likelihood of seizures, leading to high oxygen consumption plus running the risk of aspiration, hypoxemia, and death. DTs are no joking matter and can be fatal.

5. Adult respiratory distress syndrome stems from many causes (infection, aspiration, fat embolism among others), but ends up in a common condition—the lungs become an ineffective oxygen exchange organ. Air spaces fill with fluid and a large A-a gradient develops. Treatment of ARDS is, first, treat the cause of the initial insult, here, the infection. Then support the patient until the lungs can again become an efficient oxygen exchange organ. Intubation, PEEP, and close fluid management (too much fluid will worsen the lungs) are the mainstays of ARDS treatment. In a worst case scenario, extracorporeal membrane oxygenation can be used, but that's pretty heroic.

6. Low protein, either from poor nutrition or from the liver's inability to produce proteins, occurs in an alcoholic. This lack of proteins can lead to less protein binding of drugs, more availability of these drugs, and hence to a greater effect of drugs. Vitamins A, D, E, and K, the fat soluble vitamins, may be in short supply, leading to bleeding problems. In general, consider the alcoholic as malnourished, so wound healing is a problem, as is infection.

7. Most likely, if she is getting high amounts of PEEP, then her intrathoracic pump is severely impaired and the patient is thus hypovolemic. Treat with fluids and inotropes. Also, check breath sounds to make sure the PEEP hasn't caused a pneumothorax.

8. Systemic vascular resistance can be broken down into three functional categories, too low, just right, and too high. (Surgeons go nuts when they ask me what the SVR is and I say, "Just right.") Too low, as in this case, means the vascular tree is too dilated, you have plenty of cardiac output, but there is not enough blood pressure to provide a sufficient pressure head to perfuse the organs. In addition to volume monitoring, you will need to tighten the vascular tree with a predominantly alpha agent, norepinephrine. The other two categories of SVR are too high—plenty of blood pressure, not enough cardiac output, and just right—enough blood pressure, enough cardiac output.

9. Give the whining resident some cellulose therapy, which is a 2 × 4 board that you use to smack him upside the head. Central lines need regular changing because they are a source of infection. The slow flowing venous side of the circulation allows skin flora to track down the line and colonize the line site. Regular changing is the only way to keep these lines from becoming a problem. New gizmos have been used to breathe longer life into central lines, but the jury is still out on that.

10. The arterial side of the circulation is a high flow system, and skin flora have a tougher time colonizing A-line sites. A-lines should be inspected regularly, as should all lines, but you don't need to change them so often as venous lines.

Definitions of common things are not unheard of on the boards. Over the course of the week, you probably mention SVR and ARDS a few times. Make sure you have a definition, either semi-scientific (see answer 5) or at least functional (see answer 8) for the common things you mention every day.

Grab Bag Questions

1. A 7-week-old baby with communicating hydrocephalus is scheduled for a VP shunt. Which anesthetic agent will you use to minimize an increase in ICP?
2. You induce a 20-week-pregnant woman for appendectomy and the fetal monitor registers a loss in variability. What do you do?
3. You've just finished a stat C-section where you had to trach the mother to secure the airway. What do you say to the husband?
4. What are your discharge criteria from your PACU?

Answers to Grab Bag Questions

1. All potent inhaled agents increase ICP. If the child has no IV in, and you do an inhalation induction, I would use the agent that will cause the least coughing and struggling, and the agent that will provide the quickest induction, namely sevoflurane. Once the procedure has begun and an IV is in, I would keep the potent inhaled agent to 0.5 MAC and would supplement with intravenous agents. Narcotics in this young age group are tricky, since you don't want to overnarcotize and cause respiratory depression, so I would stick with short-acting narcotics (fentanyl, versus longer acting morphine).

2. Loss of variability is a normal response of the fetus to induction of general anesthesia. I would, of course, make sure Mom is OK in every way (oxygenation, blood pressure), since the best way to take care of the fetus is to take care of the mother.

3. Emphasize that mother and baby are doing well. Detail what happened and why, that the procedure was necessary to save both mother and child. Make sure the mother gets a Medic-Alert bracelet that tells she is a difficult intubation. Have an ENT see the patient in consultation to make sure the trach site heals as best as possible.

4. Stable, pain under control with oral meds, nausea under control. The patient should be able to ambulate, if they were ambulatory preop, and should be in the hands of a responsible adult with adequate instructions in case an emergency should arise.

Hands get clammy with any of those questions? Take a peek at the criteria for discharge in your own PACU. That's another example of a common thing you do every day, then if the examiner asks you, you'll go, "Uh, I...uh...I discharge people all the time...but...but..." There will be no "buts" come board time. Know those criteria. Get a handle on the new stuff too, the move toward doing away with the PACU entirely. It's the wave of the future, and sure to be coming to a board exam near you soon!

Session 2

A 74-year-old man is scheduled for a TURP for BPH. Five months ago he had an uncomplicated MI. He takes metoprolol and rarely needs sublingual nitro.

Preop Questions

1. What is this man's risk for another MI? What if he had angioplasty in the interim?
2. Is it worth delaying this case for a month so he's past the "magic" 6 months?
3. What further evaluation would you want from this man's cardiologist?
4. An EKG shows nonspecific ST-T wave changes. Does this alter your plans?
5. His preop Na is 131. Does this increase the risk of "TURP syndrome"?
6. Are any bleeding parameter studies necessary, given that a spinal is a likely anesthetic?
7. The patient asks, "Is a spinal safer than going to sleep?"
8. The surgeon asks, "Is a spinal safer than going to sleep?"
9. The patient had black coffee 3 hours ago, do you change your plans or cancel the case?
10. Do you request postop ICU arrangements, given his cardiac history?

Answers to Preop Questions

1. The short answer is, "I don't know what his risk is." The classic Rao article says the risk is 15% in the 3 to 6 month period after an MI. The latest *Audio Digest* says there is no increase risk in perioperative myocardial events in outpatients who are at least 3 months out from their MI. And if the patient had a successful PTCA, then his risk for an MI is smaller still. But to address the question head on, I would say the patient is at increased risk for a myocardial infarction over a patient who has had no myocardial event. That is all the more specific I can get.

2. No. The deciding events here are the uncomplicated MI and the rarity of his angina. At some point you have to make a common sense decision. If the man had an MI complicated by CHF, then he needed a multiplicity of medications and he had ongoing angina, going through a lot of nitro, then I would delay. The crowning glory would be the physical exam. If the patient looked hale and hearty, that would push me toward proceeding.

3. All I would want is the answer to these questions, "Does the patient need his coronaries studied by angiography?" "What is your estimate of the patient's ventricular function?" If the cardiologist can answer these questions without technology, then fine. If he needs an echo or a stress test to answer these questions, then fine. My goal is to steer the questions and let the cardiologist employ the necessary means to answer those questions. Just as I don't want him to tell me, "Patient OK for spinal only," I don't want to tell him, "Do an echo to tell me his LV." If he tells me, "Based on history and physical, his ventricle is good," that's all I need.

4. No. The history and the physical, plus the input from the cardiologist, answer my needs. An old EKG would be useful for comparison, but will in all likelihood not change anything.

5. Of more relevance than his baseline sodium is how much the sodium will change during the course of the operation. A long operation with extensive dissection, hence large absorption of free water, will increase his chances for symptomatic hyponatremia. It will be worth mentioning to the surgeon that the sodium is starting out low, and it will be worth drawing at least one sodium intraop.

6. Preop blood tests should be guided by the history and physical. If the patient has no bleeding problems, no liver disease, and is on no Coumadin, then bleeding tests are not needed.

7. "No study has shown that a spinal is safer than a general anesthetic. For this procedure, a spinal has a few advantages. You can talk to us during the operation and tell us how you're doing. That helps us make sure your blood chemistry is OK. Also, if at any point during the operation you should feel shoulder discomfort, that will also tell us something. So your being awake helps us take better care of you."

301

8. "No study has shown that a spinal is safer than a general anesthetic. Bladder rupture can be diagnosed under a general anesthetic, usually by bradycardia, but diagnosis of bladder rupture is better made by an awake patient informing you that he has shoulder pain. Also, a good hint that the sodium may be falling too low is the patient's consciousness. If he starts to get agitated, that will be an early warning sign of hyponatremia. For that reason, I steer the discussion towards acceptance of a spinal anesthetic for a TURP."

9. No changes. A clear liquid like black coffee will be cleared in a few minutes from the stomach. If he had taken a fatty drink, then I would wait at least 4 hours.

10. No. Once again, the history and physical argue against undue concern in this case. If trouble should arise, you can always get the bed later.

Question 9 brings up a point. The NPO guidelines at your hospital are different than mine. And the NPO guidelines have probably changed a few times in the last few years. When you give your answer, give an answer with a physiologic reason behind it, not a "that's the way we do it" reason.

Intraop Questions

1. You can't get the spinal with a 25-g needle. What do you do?
2. First pass gets a bloody tap, but the CSF clears, do you do anything different?
3. As you lay the patient down, he gets dyspneic and mouths the words, "I can't breathe, you incompetent schmuck." What do you do, Dr. Schmuck?
4. You attempt to induce the patient but the IV blows. He is getting blue. What now?
5. You attempt to intubate but the Sux hasn't hit yet and his vocal cords are slammed shut against your endotracheal tube. What do you do?
6. After an hour of dissection, you notice ventricular ectopy. Dx and Rx?
7. The lab sends you back the following, "Na 110. What are you guys doing to this patient?"
8. Blood pressure drops to unobtainable and the surgeon says he needs to make the channel "just a little wider." What do you tell the surgeon and how do you treat the patient?
9. Muscle relaxant has worn off and the patient is seizing. What do you do?
10. At the end of the case, the patient is obtunded. What is your management?

Answers to Intraop Questions

1. First reposition the patient to maximize your shot at cerebrospinal city. Curl the patient up better. Try a different position. Put more local in the area to keep the patient from tensing up. Give more sedation to see if that will help them relax and get in a better position. If it's still no go, go to the knitting needle, the 22 gauge. Turn the bevel sideways to minimize the risk of a spinal headache.

2. No, if the CSF clears, go ahead and place the local.

3. Either the spinal has gone too high or the patient is hypotensive. Place the mask on and prepare to assist ventilation as you press the blood pressure button. If the shortness of breath is from hypotension (medullary ischemia is invoked, but I don't really know how to separate medullary ischemia from cerebral ischemia) then treat the hypotension with fluids and phenylephrine. If the spinal is too high, then secure the airway. Keep in mind, a too-high spinal will also have hypotension from the complete sympathectomy you've just performed, Dr. Schmuck.

4. Mask ventilate, ask for help in starting an IV. If the patient is in laryngospasm and no IV is forthcoming, you can give succinylcholine IM.

5. Maintain positive pressure, if nothing else, once the patient gets hypoxemic enough, the vocal cords will relax, allowing ingress of oxygen. Going right to cricothyrotomy and jet ventilation is a bit extreme. The risk of causing vascular damage, bleeding into an airway, and causing subcutaneous emphysema is too high. Better to stick with the more bread-and-butter maneuver of positive pressure to "break" laryngospasm.

6. Free water absorption causing electrolyte abnormalities is most specific to this case. Sodium, potassium, or both could be low, so send off these labs. The more generic causes of ectopy could also be in play—hypoxemia, hypercarbia—so check your saturation and end-tidal CO_2. Send off a blood gas. Treat the cause of the arrhythmia, then if it still persists, give lidocaine. Inform the surgeon that the case has perhaps, just perhaps, gone about as far as it should go and he should wrap up the TURP pronto to prevent further absorption of free water.

7. The problem is excess free water, not too little sodium, so get rid of the free water by administering a diuretic—Lasix. Consider giving 3% sodium if the patient develops seizures or cardiovascular collapse from such a low sodium. But even if you do give the hypertonic saline, keep working on the real problem, getting rid of the water.

8. Case done! Give the surgeon something to do to get his mind off the vera montana. Tell him to start CPR because the patient has no blood pressure. Start hypertonic saline as his low sodium has indeed led to cardiovascular collapse. For inotropic support, go to the big E. Place an arterial line and a central line to guide and abet the resuscitation.

9. The other indication for hypertonic saline has reared its ugly head. If the blood pressure allows it, give thiopental to stop the seizure activity. Don't just give muscle relaxant to "hide" the seizures, for the seizure activity will continue in the brain even if you can't see it in the body. Assure adequate oxygenation throughout this time. The seizure will not kill the patient, the hypoxemia from the seizure will.

10. ABC. Keep the patient intubated. Redraw the sodium (he may still be hyponatremic; also, you want to make sure you didn't correct his hyponatremia too fast, leading to central pontine myelinolysis), the glucose (the seizure activity may have left him hypoglycemic), and blood gases (the seizures may have left him acidotic). Finally, make sure all your anesthetic gases are off. If all this results in continued obtundation, go to CT to see if the seizures led to an intracranial bleed.

Examiners can take any anesthetic and kill the patient. The lengths that they can take you are limited only by their imagination. So imagine all the wild disasters that could possibly happen in the course of your review. Talk through the disasters ahead of time; then when the test comes, you breeze right on through.

Grab Bag Questions

1. A myasthenic is scheduled for thymectomy. What special considerations will go into the anesthetic plan?
2. You're asked to consult on pain relief for a patient with sleep apnea. He is splinting after an open cholecystectomy and not saturating well. Your advice?
3. A 9-year-old status post extensive burns is scheduled for multiple debridements. The surgeon suggests ketamine. Your response?
4. A 2-year-old with neuroblastoma needs anesthesia to hold still for a round of radiation treatments during which she'll be prone. Design an anesthetic plan for her.

Answers to Grab Bag Questions

1. The hallmark of myasthenia gravis is muscle weakness, with morbidity stemming from respiratory insufficiency. Muscle relaxants for the myasthenic, therefore, must be titrated with more care than your usual case. The muscle relaxation from an inhaled agent alone may be sufficient for intubation, if not, then give a small dose of muscle relaxant and see what happens. Two milligrams of *cis*-atracurium, for example, might be enough for intubation. Watch the train-of-four like a hawk, and have a high index of suspicion for respiratory insufficiency or aspiration in the postop arena.

2. Supplemental oxygen, head up, and breathing treatments to try to get as much mileage out of the lungs as possible for starters. Intercostal nerve blocks are a way of providing pain relief without the concern of neuraxial opioids in a patient with sleep apnea. So I would do intercostal nerve blocks.

3. Ketamine alone may do the trick, but a better bet is to examine the patient first, see how much work needs doing, see how good the airway is, and make sure the patient has some good access, like a central line. A propofol drip with mask ventilation available may provide more pain relief and a smoother course than a single blast of ketamine and a moving, uncomfortable patient.

4. Sedating the prone patient who must stay still is fraught with hazard. The most conservative approach is to do a general anesthetic each time with intubation and IV access. For such a child, so many IVs will be difficult, so some permanent access (a Groshong) should be placed. Then, the child should be induced via mask while the mother is present, to keep the child calm. A continuous infusion of propofol should keep the child sedate. You can attempt to avoid multiple intubations, by placing the child prone with nasal cannula and seeing if ventilation is maintained by watching end-tidal CO_2 and watching the chest rise and fall. A little styrofoam cup with a little flag on top will allow you to see the chest movement from a distance.

Halfway there. As an exercise, if you have the energy, go back to each test, pick out one answer you disagree with, and explain an alternative strategy. Then once you've done that, give yourself a break, go to Baskin Robbins and get a hot fudge sundae.

PRACTICE EXAM #6

Session 1

A 68-year-old, 85 kg, 5'10" man is scheduled for an AAA repair.

HPI: Ah, the wicked tobacco companies, they've struck again. This man *did* inhale, tobacco smoke, that is, for many a year and his blood vessels are paying the price. Workup of abdominal pain revealed a 7-cm aneurysm, above the renal artery takeoff.

PMH: CABG 2 years ago with no angina since. No pulmonary meds, though he's been told to stop smoking by several doctors. He was also told to take a white heart pill, or was it blue? In any case he doesn't take his meds.

Physical exam: Normal

Labs: Hct 49, ABG shows a pO_2 of 73

He is on the OR table with a Swan, A-line, and epidural catheter in place.

Intraop Questions

1. Will you dose up the epidural with local anesthetic, narcotics, or both? Will you use it intraop or just at the end of the case?
2. How will you induce? What are the goals of induction?
3. After intubation, the patient wheezes and feels "tight." Dx and Rx.
4. At aortic cross-clamp, what changes do you expect to see?
5. How does mannitol work? Would you give mannitol pre-clamp? What other measures would you take to "protect" the kidneys?
6. At cross-clamp the blood pressure, PA pressure, and ST segments rose at the same time. What would you do?
7. Is NTG or SNP better for dropping the blood pressure in the above case? Why?
8. At unclamping the blood pressure dropped to 60/30. What do you do?
9. During cross-clamp, the urine output dropped, but after cross-clamp removal, the urine is bloody. What do you tell the surgeon and what do you do?
10. Just as you are getting ready to move the patient, you aspirate blood through the epidural. What would you do? What if you aspirated CSF?

Answers to Intraop Questions

1. Local anesthetic (bupivacaine) plus narcotic (fentanyl, to be given as an infusion). Dose the local anesthetic while the patient is still conscious, first, to tell you whether the dumb thing is working, and second, to tell you a level. I'd continue to run the narcotic/local anesthetic as in infusion throughout the case and in the postoperative period.

2. The goals are to keep the heart rate low and the blood pressure high enough to provide good coronary perfusion. And keep the blood pressure from shooting to the moon, which would make the aneurysm pop, and oh wouldn't life be grand then.

3. His smoking history argues for reactive airways as the cause of the tightness. First, go through the "all that wheezes is not asthma" checklist (endobronchial intubation, carinal stimulation, aspiration, pneumothorax from one of your lines), then treat bronchospasm. Deepen the anesthetic with inhaled agent and give beta inhalers down the endotracheal tube.

4. If the aorta is already clamped (aorto-occlusive disease versus a bona fide aneurysm) then you'll see no change. If the aorta still has a little life in it, then you'll see the effects of sympathetic stimulation and afterload increase, namely, increased blood pressure, increased PA pressures, and often a decrease in urine output as the renal blood flow gets impaired. Even if the clamp is below the renal takeoff, the kidneys still suffer decreased blood flow.

5. Mannitol enters the kidney tubules and is not reabsorbed; therefore it works as an osmotic diuretic. Mannitol also alters blood flow distribution in the kidneys and may provide some renal protection in that way. I would use mannitol preclamp and would use renal dopamine, both maneuvers so I could chart that I was doing all I could to protect the kidneys, but realizing that adequate volume replacement is the most important and the only proven method of protecting the kidneys.

6. Afterload is killing you, so off-load. Isoflurane will help as will nitroglycerin. IV agents, such as fentanyl, will also help reduce the blood pressure. As you are already planning for postop pain relief with the epidural, I would lean more on the inhaled agent and the nitroglycerin.

7. SNP will work more quickly to reduce the blood pressure and is certainly a fine option. NTG allegedly has coronary dilation up its sleeve, but whether that actually happens or the off-loading effect occurs is hard to tease out. The important point is not to get married to one or the other. Use what works and change as necessary.

8. Turn up the volume. Get a blood gas to see if acidosis is contributing to your hypotension. Tighten the patient's vascular tree with norepinephrine. And keep pouring in the volume. If all your clever ruses come to naught, then inform the surgeon that he'll need to place the clamp back on while you get your volume act together.

9. Tell the surgeon that you are thrilled that urine output has returned, but that the urine is blood-tinged. Get a blood gas and if there is any acidosis, treat with bicarb; this may alkalinize the urine and make the surgeon feel that you are doing something useful. You know in your heart of hearts that volume replacement is a hell of a lot more meaningful to preserving kidney function than bicarb.

10. Administer no more goodies through the catheter. But before you take it out, make sure the patient's coags are all in order. That catheter may be acting as a stopper, and if you pull it out in the face of a coagulopathy, you could get an epidural hematoma.

You don't need to memorize Goodman and Gilman before your test, but make sure you can at least give a thumbnail sketch of drugs you use commonly. An examiner can ask you how mannitol works (see question 5), how the inotropes work, how *anything we give* works. Can you say in a sentence or two how Pentothal works? Atropine? Epinephrine?

Postop Questions

1. An hour after surgery, the ICU nurse tells you the patient is ready to extubate. How will you evaluate this?

2. Postop chest x-ray shows the Swan is in the RV. How else might you pick it up? What are the risks associated with a Swan?

3. Urine output again falls. What would you do? At what point would you make a diagnosis of ATN and start restricting fluids rather than pushing them?

4. A chest x-ray shows an infiltrate in the RLL. In spite of a normal intubation, it appears the patient has aspirated. What do you do?

5. The patient complains of numbness and tingling in his left arm. How will you evaluate this?

6. The first time the patient tries to get up, he gets short of breath. How will you determine if a transfusion is necessary?

7. Pain relief from the epidural is good, but the nurse is concerned about the extent of somnolence in the patient. How will you assure a safe course of epidural narcotics?

8. Three days postop the patient has an MI. A concerned family member asks why you didn't prevent this. What do you tell that person?

9. The patient develops weakness in both extremities and back pain. Evaluate this.

10. You are asked to place a "more comfortable" central line. Discuss the pros and cons of an internal jugular versus a subclavian line.

Answers to Postop Questions

1. Act like you are a pilot checking off a plane for takeoff. ABGs indicate that the patient will maintain his O_2 and CO_2 once he is off the ventilator? Check! Neuro status indicates he can maintain his airway and clear secretions? Check! Hemodynamics and bleeding indicate he won't go screaming back to the OR anytime soon? Check! Weaning parameters indicate a dandy lung function? Check! Patient wasn't so hard to intubate that you'll be hard pressed to reintubate? Check! All righty then, take off!

2. The wave form would look different, specifically the diastolic pressure would be all the way down to 0. Ectopy would also tip you off to irritation in the ventricle. Swan problems include rhythm disturbances, including complete heart block if the patient has a baseline LBBB. While placing the Swan, you can get a carotid puncture, jugular thrombosis, pneumothorax. As with any line, you can get bleeding and infection. If placed in the left side, you can hit the thoracic duct and get a chylothorax. If the balloon is inflated at an inopportune time, a PA rupture can occur, and oh, what a bummer that is.

3. (By now you should have this oliguria thing down.) Check the Foley and make sure there is not a postrenal cause of the oliguria. Manage volume and inotropes to optimize everything that needs optimizing. Transfuse to at least a hematocrit of 30. If urine output does not respond to all these measures, then ATN has probably occurred and you must go to fluid restriction. This is a difficult 180° turn to make, because you tend to pour in volume, pour in volume nonstop in an attempt to breathe life into the kidneys. Then *SCREEEEEEEECH!* Now you restrict fluids.

4. First, supportive care, maintaining intubation to assure adequate oxygenation, adding PEEP if necessary to keep an adequate pO_2. Don't give steroids, and don't give prophylactic antibiotics. Suction as best you can, include via bronchoscopy, to get as much aspirate out as possible. Treat accompanying bronchospasm and have the respiratory folk do deep breathing exercises with the patient to minimize atelectasis. In short, support the patient while he cures himself of the aspiration.

5. See the patient and do a neuro evaluation. Look specifically for the most likely neuro injury, an ulnar nerve stretch. The patient may have difficulty opening up his finger and may have numbness in the pinkie and half of the ring finger. Explain to the patient what happened and assure him that most of these injuries resolve themselves, though the time frame may be weeks or months. If the pain persists or chronic pain develops, then the patient should be referred for chronic pain management treatment.

6. Check a hematocrit. If it is below 30, you will have to transfuse if he is symptomatic. The dizziness from sitting up the first time may just be from his autonomic system not kicking in quickly enough after prolonged bed rest. If you still have a Swan in and you can measure mixed venous saturation, that may tip you one way or another. For example, if his hematocrit is 29 and his mixed venous is low (say, low 50s) then that would incline you toward transfusing. As with any transfusion, the whole picture, rather than any one lab, determines the decision.

7. If the nurse is concerned, you are concerned. Examine the patient, see how arousable he is. Look at his respiratory rate over the last shift. If he looks oversedated, then reduce the rate of the epidural infusion. Reexamine him and see how he's doing on the reduced rate.

8. "For reasons we do not entirely understand, the third day out from an operation seems to be the time of highest risk for an MI. People suggest that the inflammatory response from surgery makes the platelets 'extra sticky' and that may lead to blood clots in the coronaries. In spite of everything we do—watching the hemodynamics intraoperatively, watching all the blood tests around the time of surgery—people will still have MIs."

9. Back pain accompanied by neurologic findings means epidural hematoma until proven otherwise. Examine the patient yourself and make damned sure a neurosurgeon is all over this like white on rice, for time is of the essence. Get the CT *now*, take the patient there yourself if you have to. If there is to be any hope of a meaningful recovery, you have to drain that hematoma within a short time of the diagnosis.

10. A subclavian is less hassle for the patient. They can move their heads around and not have a tugging at their neck and they can sleep better. The drawbacks are in the placement. A subclavian is more likely to cause a pneumothorax. Also, if you hit the subclavian artery, it is hard to put pressure on it to stop bleeding, as the artery is covered by the clavicle.

Grab Bag Questions

1. A patient for carpal tunnel release has a pacemaker. He asks what could go wrong with it during the operation on his hand.
2. A 500-pound man is scheduled for gastric bypass surgery. He is MH susceptible. One of your partners says, "Hell with this noise, cancel it." Your response?
3. A patient with chronic back pain is frustrated because "Everyone tells me to lose weight. I just can't!" What do you advise?
4. A bright 14-year-old sees a bubble in the IV tubing and says, "Hey, that bubble could kill me!" What do you tell this bright student of physiology?

Answers to Grab Bag Questions

1. First, evaluate the patient by history, physical, and looking at the EKG. If the pacer has worked well until now, then it is unlikely to fail during the case. If the pacer has been sputtering and the patient has been symptomatic (say, he faints in the preop holding area) that would indicate that this pacer might need a tuneup. Once in the OR, the main problem that could occur with a pacer is interference from the electrocautery. By placing the grounding pad away from the pacer, that problem usually does not occur, but the savvy anesthesiologist always gives the EKG a good once over the first time the Bovie fires.

2. Coward! The man needs the surgery, as untreated morbid obesity carries with it a host of medical problems. Simply do a trigger-free anesthetic with a clean machine with the special considerations of morbid obesity in mind. The most central problem will be the airway. Since you can't use Sux, and a long-acting relaxant could get you in trouble (if you can't intubate) then do an awake intubation and do the case with IV agents. Nitrous might be problematic as it will decrease your FIO_2 and could interfere with oxygenating these hard-to-oxygenate patients.

3. Treatment by a chronic pain specialist. With a series of pain blocks, physical therapy, medications, the patient's back pain may get under control, allowing the patient to get more exercise, and thus lose weight. Just chastising a chronic pain patient to lose weight, period, is not effective treatment.

4. An air bubble needs to be pretty substantial to cause an air lock and kill the patient. If the patient has a probe-patent foramen ovale, a small bubble could sneak across to the left side and cause a problem. To allay the fears of this junior scientist, stop the infusion, suck out the air bubble, and win a few brownie points.

Having done a lot of these now, you can see how no individual question is so bad. IJ versus subclavian, how to handle an epidural hematoma, these are the daily bread of anesthesiology. But (here goes the broken record again) *you have to explain it clearly and reasonably.* Now you're over half way. If you haven't practiced aloud yet, you had better press the reset button on your head and rethink your studying. It's *aloud* that you'll prepare.

Session 2

A 47-year-old man with severe ankylosing spondylitis is scheduled for arthroplasty of the MP joint in his left hand. The surgeon says the case will take about 2 hours.

Preop Questions

1. What are the anesthetic implications of ankylosing spondylitis?
2. Is further lab work necessary, for example, PFTs, given his restrictive lung pattern?
3. What do you tell the patient are the special risks associated with this procedure?
4. Should you obtain a neuro consult before proceeding?
5. What, if anything, would lead you to cancel the case?
6. How soon before the operation should antibiotics be given for maximal prophylactic benefit?
7. If the patient had nausea in the preop holding area, how would you treat it?
8. If peripheral access were unobtainable, where would you get a line?
9. If you are planning a regional, how would you premedicate?
10. The director of the outpatient center you're at tells you, "If you're spooked, don't proceed, we can't afford any transfers to the hospital. It'll hurt our numbers." What do you say?

Answers to Preop Questions

1. The primary difficulty is airway, airway, airway. From the cervical spine fusing to the downward curve of their overall spine. This severe curvature leads to restrictive lung disease that in turn can lead to right heart failure. Aortic regurgitation can also occur, along with cardiomegaly and cardiac conduction problems.

2. Yes, get PFTs plus an ABG, an echo, and EKG. The PFTs are to document the degree of restrictive defect. The ABG is to have a baseline; in particular, you want to see if the patient retains CO_2. This workup is necessary, even though a regional technique may be used. If you have to convert to a general, you'll be happy to have this workup of the patient's pulmonary and cardiac status.

3. The procedure planned is a block of the arm. The risks associated with that are nerve injury from a needle stick, intravascular injection of the local anesthetic, infection, vascular injury, and failure of the technique, which would mean induction of a general anesthetic.

4. No. Do your own neuro exam. Document well any neuro problems that exist before you plunge your dagger into the patient's axilla, but a neuro consult is an unnecessary expense.

5. No insurance. Negative wallet biopsy. What is this, a soup kitchen? But seriously folks. I would cancel this if the patient were pregnant (low likelihood in this man), questionable NPO status, or if the patient were febrile and sick with a URI. I would cancel if he were not medically optimized, specifically, if he had evidence of CHF (recall ankylosing spondylitis can have cardiomegaly) or if he had a malignant arrhythmia (AS patients can have conduction problems).

6. Within one hour of the incision; that is, *before* the incision.

7. Make the diagnosis first. Is the patient suffering from nausea from influenza (then you would postpone the case)? Or is the patient just nervous? After all, you just told him you would be his anesthesiologist, and it's only natural that he should be nervous. If the diagnosis were nausea from nervousness, give an anxiolytic such as midazolam. I would also give metaclopramide to treat the nausea. Droperidol? Hmm. Would you really give this as a preop medication? Might cause the patient to freak out and bolt.

8. Central line. This may be difficult as the patient's AS may make neck movement difficult (hard to get at the IJ). Also, the degree of curvature may make it hard to get at the subclavian area. If these were not options, place a femoral line.

9. First I'd take care of that nausea. Then I'd premedicate with midazolam, keeping a pulse oximeter on the patient. Recall he has a restrictive lung pattern. Also, place oxygen on the patient as you pre-medicate him.

10. The overall transfer rate from outpatient centers is about 1%. Outpatient centers are doing sicker and sicker people. The old adage that you only do ASA 1s and 2s for removal of lumps and bumps is history. Now they do AICDs, 600-pound patients, and 106-year-old people (I kid thee not). An ASA 3 or 4 who is medically compensated is OK for an outpatient surgery center. That is the reality of today.

Intraop Questions

1. Do you perform a regional anesthetic, and if so, which type? Compare axillary versus interscalene versus Bier block.
2. The surgeon says, "Even if your block fails, I can do this with local." Your response?
3. How will you sedate this patient?
4. So do you give antisialagogue or any other preparations for an awake intubation?
5. The regional starts to wear off. Now what?
6. What is the mechanism of tourniquet pain?
7. You have to induce a general anesthetic. What agents will you use?
8. How will you secure the airway? Will an LMA suffice?
9. You place an LMA and the patient vomits. What will you do?
10. With the LMA in place, you suddenly can't ventilate. Evaluate this.

Answers to Intraop Questions

1. Axillary block. Axillary is safer in this patient because the anatomy of the neck is abnormal, and the interscalene block could be difficult. Problems with an interscalene block include pneumothorax, a high spinal if the local tracks up to the CSF, and vascular injury in the neck. A Bier block is dandy, but after an hour or so, tourniquet pain could be a problem. Since the surgeon said the case will last 2 hours, a Bier block is not a good idea. Both axillary and interscalene share the danger of intravascular injection with subsequent cardiovascular collapse. The axillary block, in general, is good for procedures "lower down" in the arm, but the axillary can miss the musculocutaneous nerve.

2. Given the peripheral location of this operation and the ease of blocking the involved area, I would say this is a good way to go. The hyperparanoid response is, "The block will fail and we'll have to intubate and we won't be able to and the patient will die. Oh me, oh my!" But a reality check says this is unlikely given the operative area. If the surgeon were doing a larger procedure, then the paranoia would be merited.

3. Propofol drip, starting low and titrating to effect. The advantage here is a rapid disappearance of effect if the patient becomes oversedated and respiratory compromise occurs. Any number of other sedative plans is acceptable, as long as you stick by the old sedation dictum, "Give a little and see what happens." And also remember that, "If the patient is talking, he must by definition be breathing."

4. Yes. Call it overreaction, but in the back of my mind is the outside, outside chance that weirdness might happen. And if you do have to go with a fiberoptic, you will want the mouth dry. At least you will want no secretions in your way. The downside, a dry mouth, shouldn't bother the patient too much, especially with the propofol infusion running.

5. Take the surgeon up on his offer and have him put more supplemental local anesthesia in. Better to place this earlier than later. Don't fall into the trap of sedating the whazoo out of the patient and performing a pseudo-general anesthetic, also known as a room air general.

6. Ischemia leads to sympathetic stimulation. Treatment of the sympathetic stimulation can be done with labetalol. The pain part of tourniquet pain is more problematic. You can increase the inhaled agent if a general anesthetic is under way. In this case you can give narcotic. If the pain becomes unbearable, ask the surgeon if you can let down the tourniquet. Once again, the overriding concern is the patient's bad airway; if you narcotize to the nth degree, you'll end up in trouble. This is a case that requires a lot of communication with the surgeons.

7. Damn! Just what you didn't want to do. This patient needs an awake intubation. As he is already sedated with propofol, you don't need any more of that. Topicalize with lidocaine, place an oral airway, and place the endotracheal tube under direct vision. Once intubated, you can let the patient breathe spontaneously an inhaled agent.

8. No. An LMA will not suffice. This airway needs definitive securing. If you place an LMA in this difficult airway and the patient vomits, you'll be stuck.

9. Damn! How do I get in these jams? Pull out the LMA, turn the patient's head to the side (as much as you can with AS), put the bed into Trendelenburg, then once the airway is cleared, provide mask ventilation.

10. That damned LMA! Let the cuff down and reposition it. If that doesn't work, get an intubating LMA, place that, and move toward a definitive airway, that is, endotracheal intubation.

That case reemphasizes a point—the examiners can make you do what you wouldn't normally do. Then you have to explain yourself out of an uncomfortable position. Don't panic. As the Nike commercial says, "Just do it."

Grab Bag Questions

1. What is a "Tet spell" and explain the best treatment if this occurs under anesthesia.

2. A healthy patient drops his pressure a little, so you give a little Neo. The heart rate drops like a stone. What happened and what will you do?

3. An orthopedic surgeon asks whether his total hips, until now done under general anesthesia, will do better with some regional techniques. What do you say?

4. What is the best anesthetic technique for a patient with porphyria?

Answers to Grab Bag Questions

1. In a child with a cardiac shunt, the relative vascular resistances can determine which way the blood flows. In a hypercyanotic attack, the pulmonary vascular resistance is too high, relative to the systemic vascular resistance, and the child becomes cyanotic. Insufficient blood is flowing to the lungs. Children learn to treat this themselves by squatting, increasing their systemic vascular resistance, and, in effect, "pushing" more blood into the lungs to relieve the cyanosis. Under anesthesia, the treatment of increasing systemic vascular resistance can be accomplished by giving phenylephrine. The other treatment is a beta-blocker such as propranolol.

2. The vascular system is reacting with an appropriate reflex. Blood pressure goes up so the body responds by dropping the heart rate. For this reason (it's scary when it happens), treatment of a minor drop in blood pressure may better be done with a mixed alpha and beta agent like ephedrine.

3. Hips done under regional techniques have been shown to have fewer pulmonary emboli and DVTs. It may indeed be safer to do these with regional techniques. Combined regional and general? That may be just as advantageous and has the added benefit of securing the airway in a patient on their side. That is, if the spinal or epidural malfunction halfway into a hip, you hate to have to intubate with the patient in such an awkward position.

4. Avoid those agents that will induce the cytochrome p-450 system, namely barbiturates, sedative hypnotics, and benzodiazepines. The classic induction of a porphyria patient is an inhalation induction. If airway or full stomach concerns are a consideration, then sedate with narcotics, secure the airway awake, then use the inhaled agents.

Six down, four to go. Starting to sound the same, aren't they? That's why it's good to get exams from a lot of different sources. No matter what, one examiner, or in this case, two examiners, will tend to go back to the things they know. But go to another examiner—then you get a fresh perspective, a new take on things. So spread the joy a little, get exams from lots of different people. Get one from an OB specialist, one from a peds specialist, one from someone that does hearts or vascular. Be sure to get an exam from someone who knows pain inside and out; a lot of examinees are seeing pain questions.

PRACTICE EXAM #7

Session 1

An unfortunate young woman with metastatic breast CA is scheduled for prophylactic pinning of her femur.

HPI: Breast CA has metastasized all over this 45-year-old woman and now a large tumor mass goes right across and nearly replaces her femur at mid shaft. A pathologic fracture is imminent, so, in an attempt to keep her as comfortable as possible, a pinning is planned.

PMH: Good health until the cancer struck.

Physical exam: Cachexia. Obvious malnourishment.

Labs: Mets in the ribs, back, all over. Her Hct is 28 and her albumin is low.

She comes to the OR with an 18-g IV in her hand.

Intraop Questions

1. What anesthetic will you choose, regional or general?
2. What special concerns are there in placing a regional block in a patient with mets in the back?
3. How will you induce?
4. What effect will malnourishment and low albumin have on the bioavailability of drugs?
5. You induce and the pressure goes down. How do you react?
6. Now you lighten the anesthetic ever so much and the patient moves. How will you do this anesthetic?
7. What precautions do you take to prevent recall with such a "light" anesthetic?
8. As they are reaming out the femur, the $ETCO_2$ disappears. Dx and Rx?
9. Later, the ETT fills with straw colored fluid. What has happened?
10. Explain the pathophysiology of a fat embolus.

Answers to Intraop Questions

1. General anesthetic.

2. With metastases all over her body, she could have metastases in her spinal column as well. You could palpate a soft area, think it's a space, and put a spinal needle right through a metastasis, thereby seeding her CSF with cancer cells. Although this is just a proposed method of spreading mets, I would avoid that procedure. Also, the patient must be in great pain from all these bony involvements, so rolling her over or sitting her up to place the spinal would cause further pain.

3. After preoxygenation, and with placement of cricoid pressure, I would perform a modified rapid sequence induction. All the pain meds she is on means she may have altered gastric emptying, so I'd maintain the cricoid, mask, and intubate.

4. Less protein means less protein binding and more pharmacodynamic effect. In short, you will get more "bang for your buck," so reduced doses are the order of the day.

5. Volume and ephedrine. Routine drops in blood pressure with induction are nothing but "anesthetica imperfectica." Also, keep the agents off until the blood pressure has returned to baseline.

6. Clearly this patient is touchy. The least anesthetic and her pressure drops. Just paralyzing her to make it "look good" is not an option because she may have recall. Give fluids and start an inotrope to give her enough blood pressure to "support" an anesthetic.

7. Preoperative midazolam will help, but there is no guarantee against recall in this or any case. Keep that in mind as you do this case, make sure all the conversation in the OR is professional, keeping in mind that anything said in the OR may be recalled by the patient.

8. Grinding up the marrow, particularly with a tumor mass in it, could give you a fat embolus. Other causes of the end-tidal disappearing are monitor disconnect or malfunction, ventilator disconnect or malfunction, and complete cardiovascular collapse.

9. The pulmonary vascular tree has filled with debris from the marrow.

10. Vascular integrity of the lungs now gets all shot to hell, and the air spaces fill with fluid. The heart must now work against high pulmonary arterial pressures, and right heart failure can result. Oxygenation is impaired and ARDS can result. Fat emboli have probably also traveled to other vascular beds, including the brain, kidneys, liver, and eyes.

Postop Questions

1. Should you suction out the fluid from the ETT at the end of the case? Explain the Starling forces at work.
2. The patient's muscle relaxants do not reverse at the end of the case. What's the differential diagnosis?
3. What are your initial ventilator settings and which mode will you use?
4. Design a rational protocol for weaning this patient from the ventilator.
5. In the hours postop, the hemodynamics worsen. How will you intervene?
6. One of the housestaff points out that the patient is a "no code." Does this affect your management?
7. Her left hand, site of a radial art line, starts to look dusky. What do you do?
8. Blood gases reveal a large shunt. What is shunt and how will you attempt to manage it?
9. On high PEEP, the urine output drops. What will you do?
10. A family member asks what happened and why no one told him this might have happened with the operation. What do you say?

Answers to Postop Questions

1. No. The Starling forces describe the balance of forces that keep fluid inside the vascular tree and out of the air spaces. The fluid filtration rate across the alveolar-capillary membrane is described by fluid filtration = Kf {(Pmv-Ppmv) – Rho (pi mv-pipmv)} Yipes! That means the pulmonary capillary hydrostatic pressure, the pulmonary interstitial hydrostatic pressure, the pulmonary capillary colloid osmotic pressure, and the interstitial colloid osmotic pressure, are all functioning to maintain a balance. Suctioning will move the equation towards the accumulation of more fluid in the air spaces. In cases of pulmonary edema, suction only when the endotracheal tube is completely obstructed and no air movement is possible.

2. Recheck your doses to make sure you didn't overdo it. She may be hypothermic. The patient may have such a small muscle mass that even small doses of relaxants may keep her weak. And finally, she may have an Eaton-Lambert syndrome, a myasthenic-like syndrome that accompanies some cancers and results in prolonged effects of muscle relaxants.

3. Tidal volume of 10 ml/kg, rate of 10 per minute, 5 cm of H_2O PEEP. 100% oxygen. Look at the oxygen saturation immediately and increase the PEEP if the saturation isn't at least 90%. Get a blood gas in 15 minutes and adjust from there.

4. As she is weak, cachectic, and just had a fat embolus, wean slowly. Start weaning when she is hemodynamically stable and no further fluid is issuing from her lungs. Wean first the FIO_2, getting her to 50% as soon as possible. Then wean the PEEP to no greater than 5 cm H_2O. Once she's square with that. Start weaning the IMV, two at a time, checking blood gases and saturation as you go.

5. Go invasive, with a Swan, arterial line, and a transesophageal echo. She will need inotropic support until she has overcome the fat embolus.

6. No. In the OR and under your care, no one is a no code. If, after the patient has been in the ICU for a while, you may reevaluate with family, surgeon, and all interested parties. But for now, she came down for an operation and that means you will take care of her full bore.

7. Inject a small amount of nitroglycerin through the arterial line to see if you can dilate the vessel. If it works, great, if not, you don't lose much. Then take out the arterial line and get a vascular surgery consult. If she still needs an arterial line, place one in a larger vessel, such as the femoral artery.

8. Shunt means blood is going to areas without oxygen exchange. Areas of pure shunt are not as common as areas of ventilation-perfusion mismatch. Treatment consists of fixing what you can fix (treating pneumonia if that has occurred) and supporting oxygenation with PEEP and ventilation until the patient overcomes her injury.

9. Check the Foley to rule out postrenal causes of oliguria. The high PEEP is hurting the patient's intrathoracic pump, so she is effectively hypovolemic. She will need volume replacement and possibly inotropic support to make up for the effect of PEEP.

10. Just explain the physiology and tell the family member that this is a rare complication of surgery. Assure them that everything is being done to better the condition.

Things happen, complications happen. Think through everything you do, the complications that can happen from what we do, and explain them to your rearview mirror on the way to work. Explain them to your pet ferret at home. Explain them to your tree in the backyard.

Grab Bag Questions

1. At what point is it safe to give Sux to a patient with a spinal cord injury?
2. What purpose does a magnet serve in case of pacemaker dysfunction?
3. If a patient develops A fib with a rapid response, what is the medical treatment of choice? At what point would you shock?
4. How does a pulse oximeter work? How can ambient light give a false reading?

Answers to Grab Bag Questions

1. For the first 24 hours after a spinal cord injury, it is safe to give Sux. After that, Sux may cause a massive potassium release so it is best to be avoided. Is there a safe time later on to give it? After a few months or years? I don't want to be the one to find out.

2. A magnet should (emphasis on should) make the pacer fire at a fixed rate of 70 in the VOO mode. This will be of use if the electrocautery goofs up the pacer function. Today's hypersuper ultra cool pacers that do everything but walk the dog may not respond so passively to a magnet, however, so caution is the byword.

3. Adenosine is a thundershock treatment (in the parlance of Pikachu the Pokemon) but can be a bit much, read asystole. Verapamil is the drug of choice. Use cardioversion if conventional medical methods don't work. If blood pressure drops with the rapid response, then cardiovert emergently.

4. Pulse oximetry measures the absorbance of the pulsatile component of blood flow. Two wavelengths of light are shone through a vascular bed (fingertip, earlobe, or lip) and through some miracle of technological wizardry, the amount of light absorbed is proportional to the oxygen saturation.

You don't have to build a Wheatstone Bridge for the examiners, and you won't need to bring your soldering gun, but it does pay to know at least the rudiments of our electronic gadgets.

Session 2

A 26-year-old woman at 24 weeks' gestation requires clipping of an AV malformation at the base of her skull. Labs and vital signs are normal and the gestation is also proceeding normally.

Preop Questions

1. Is it best to delay this operation until after the delivery?
2. What lab work is necessary here? What labs may appear "abnormal" with a normal pregnacy?
3. What do you tell the patient and her husband about the risk to the baby?
4. Does the location of the aneurysm affect your anesthetic plan?
5. What "understanding" will you have with the obstetrician in this case?
6. How will you plan to monitor the fetus and how long postop will you continue that monitoring?
7. What is subarachnoid hemorrhage and how is it managed medically?
8. Will you have plans in store for a C-section should it become necessary?
9. What drugs will you avoid given the pregnancy?
10. How will you premedicate this patient?

Answers to Preop Questions

1. That is a question only the neurosurgeon can answer. You must consider the risks of delaying a burst AV malformation against waiting for the child to be more mature. Complicating things is the coming delivery. Sympathetic tone may be high with the pain of contractions, there will be Valsalva maneuvers with pushing. All this could put a lot of strain on that AV malformation and lead to an intracranial wipeout mid-delivery.

2. This is a big Kahuna operation. Get electrolytes and a creatinine. With intracranial work it will be worth knowing the baseline renal function as well as starting electrolytes. Get a hematocrit, which may be low with the "anemia of pregnancy."

3. No one does elective operations during pregnancy since you "don't expose the baby to any drugs unless you have to." But this operation is not elective, the AV malformation must be fixed. Many operations are done on pregnant patients with no ill effects whatsoever. The gravest risk is precipitating premature birth, but that is seen most often with operations near or on the uterus. Nothing is guaranteed in this world, but the best way to take care of baby is to take care of Mom.

4. The aneurysm at the base of the skull means access to the operative site will be a bear. The surgeons may need to open her whole face to get adequate exposure. The airway may be problematic and you should plan on postop ventilation (have an ICU bed ready).

5. Have an OB nurse who knows her stuff in the room and watching the fetal monitor throughout the case. The obstetrician should know about the case, should talk with the patient and her husband ahead of time, and all should be clear about what will happen if an emergent delivery is necessary. The OB should also talk with the neurosurgeon. He may suggest waiting at least a couple weeks to allow the baby's lungs to mature. The goal is to avoid surprises and avoid last minute calls to docs who know nothing about the case.

6. Place the fetal monitor before induction, and plan on monitoring throughout the case. Keep the fetal monitor on until the patient is at least 4 hours postop. That is no magic number, just an attempt at a practical number. By 4 hours postop, most of the excitement should be done, most hemodynamic wildness should be over. From a practical standpoint, you can't keep the fetal monitor on forever.

7. Bleeding under the arachnoid causes vasospasm of cerebral blood vessels and subsequent cerebral ischemia. A leaking AV malformation can cause subarachnoid hemorrhage. Treatment is difficult and involves sedation, surgical repair of the cause of the bleed, and maintenance of adequate perfusion pressure. Some argue for placement of a Swan and managing the patient with high filling pressures and a low hematocrit. But arguments bounce all over the place, reflecting how hard it is to draw a clear conclusion as to the optimal treatment. Nimodipine, a calcium channel antagonist, has shown some promise.

8. At 24 weeks, the baby would be right at the edge of viability. If the neurosurgeon could wait just another week or two, the child might produce enough surfactant to manage better if a C-section were necessary. If push came to shove and the mother is in trouble, the attention will be focused on saving the mother (say the aneurysm bursts) and not toward some wild attempt at doing a C-section while they are still operating on her cranium.

9. Tetracycline. Duh! As if you were going to give that anyway. No anesthetic drugs have been implicated as problematic except for possibly the benzodiazepines and a weak link to cleft palate. This late in gestation the cleft palate issue is moot. I would avoid nitrous, as that may be linked to spontaneous abortions. In general, I'd stick with old standbys like fentanyl, vecuronium, and isoflurane. The idea is, the longer the track record, the fewer surprises.

10. Morphine. You want the patient calm, especially as you will be placing invasive lines. And you will want some pain relief on board for the same reason. Arterial lines and central lines in a wide awake patient could result in increased blood pressure and strain on that AV malformation.

Neuro stuff can be pretty dicey. Barash's *Clinical Anesthesia* sums up all the high points. That book also has the distinct advantage of being all in one text, so you don't have to go looking stuff up in the index of one volume and then finding the spot you want in another volume. Barash is one-stop shopping.

Intraop Questions

1. What lines will you have in this case?
2. How will you monitor the fetus and what position will the mother be "allowed" to be in?
3. What drugs will you use to induce? How will you make sure the "shear pressure" doesn't change across the aneurysm?
4. At induction, mother desaturates for 30 seconds and the fetus develops bradycardia. What do you do?
5. Surgeon requests deliberate hypotension. What agent is safe to use?
6. Describe the perfusion of the placenta and how deliberate hypotension will affect it.
7. The aneurysm bursts and massive bleeding occurs. The surgeon demands maximal hypotension until he can clip the aneurysm. The fetal heart tracing looks awful. What do you do?
8. At the end of the case, the patient can't move one side. What has likely happened and what do you need to do?
9. The patient develops DIC. What is DIC, why did it develop, and how do you treat it?
10. At the end of the case the fetal heart tracing is unobtainable. What do you tell the father?

Answers to Intraop Questions

1. Arterial line. Swan (in anticipation of large volume shifts in case of a big bleed, and to monitor fluid status postoperatively, when a subarachnoid bleed may occur with its attendant vasospasm). Big lines. At least two peripheral lines and one extra cordis. If the AV aneurysm pops, there will be no time to go fishing around for more IV access.

2. Place a fetal heart rate monitor on the patient's abdomen, letting the OB nurse find the optimal spot. Left uterine displacement should be used. Even if the mother doesn't show supine hypotensive syndrome, there can be compression of the lower aorta if she is flat on her back during the second and third trimesters, so keep her tilted to the left.

3. The goal is to avoid wide swings in blood pressure and intracranial pressure. If the ICP drops (you induce and mask ventilate too fast, dropping the CO_2, and hence the ICP), and you intubate a poorly anesthetized patient (inadequate narcotics, lidocaine, or inhaled agent on board) then the blood pressure will increase. Net result, more pressure inside the aneurysm wall, less pressure pushing against the outside of the aneurysm wall. Pop goes the aneurysm. To avoid that, I'd induce with fentanyl, thiopental until the patient's eyes close, a nondepolarizing relaxant (if the airway looked OK) then easy mask ventilation with inhalation agent on board. A minute prior to intubation I'd give IV lidocaine. All the time I'd watch the blood pressure, reacting if the pressure dropped too much (bad for cerebral perfusion) or rose too much (bad for the aneurysm). As the patient is at risk for aspiration in the second and third trimesters, I'd apply cricoid pressure throughout the induction, but would do a modified rapid sequence rather than a generic rapid sequence. This ties in with the goal of a smooth induction without wide swings in the blood pressure.

4. Don't panic and focus attention on the baby. Take care of the source of the bradycardia—hypoxemia in the mother. Keep the FIO_2 at 100%, assure the endotracheal tube is in the right place by auscultation and observing the end-tidal CO_2 trace. If you fix the problem in the mother, that will fix the problem in the baby.

5. Two concerns arise in using deliberate hypotension in the pregnant patient, will the blood pressure drop hurt the pressure-dependent uteroplacental blood flow, and will the actual agent (nipride and its potential for cyanide toxicity) cause a problem? Drop the blood pressure to a mean of 50 (the usual goal in a deliberate hypotension neurological case), but keep in touch with the OB nurse. If the fetal heart rate shows distress, then inform the neurosurgeon and raise the blood pressure. Use narcotics, one half MAC of inhaled agent, and labetalol to drop the blood pressure. Finally, add nipride to get the last drop in blood pressure you need. Will cyanide toxicity occur? Unknown. (Nipride *is* used in treating severe preeclamptics.) The best guess is a short run of nipride (a few hours) at a low dose (most of the hypotension coming from the other agents) should not harm the baby.

6. The placenta is a large, low resistance, pressure dependent system. If the deliberate hypotension drops the pressure so low that the baby gets in distress, the fetal heart rate monitor may show bradycardia. A loss of variability won't help you, because a loss of variability is a normal response to anesthesia.

7. This is a bind. If you raise the blood pressure and the surgeon can't clip the aneurysm, both baby and mother will die. So bite the bullet, give maximal hypotension in an attempt to save them both. If it is so bad that the child is lost, that is a tragedy, but your first patient is the mother. A mother can have more children. But if she dies, there won't be this child or any others. As soon as the aneurysm is clipped, do what you can to raise the blood pressure, restore blood volume, correct acidosis, and normalize the mother. That is the best bet for saving the child.

8. The clip may be on the wrong branch of a vessel. The patient needs immediate reexploration (the surgeon may insist on an angiogram first) for removal of the erroneous clip and placement of the correct one. Time is crucial.

9. Disseminated intravascular coagulation is a meltdown of the coagulation system, with crucial clotting factors getting used up in little mini clots all over the place. That results in an exhaustion of platelets and elements of the coagulation cascade. Diffuse hemorrhage results. DIC can result from a multitude of causes, including intracranial pathology such as a subarachnoid bleed. (Just how a subarachnoid bleed triggers DIC is unknown.) Treatment is, first, eliminating the triggering cause. As you treat that cause, you must also attempt to correct the clotting deficiencies, no mean feat. Using PT/PTT, platelet count, fibrinogen split products, and TEG guidance, correct what you can correct. That will usually involve some judicious mix and match of platelet transfusions, fresh frozen plasma, cryoprecipitate, and aminocaproic acid. Scientific as we may discuss this in the board setting, in real life, you pour in the products, recheck labs, and hope the bleeding stops.

10. First confirm that the trace is really flat and not just hard to find. The baby may have turned and made it hard to find the trace. If the baby is indeed lost, tell the father that all was done to save the mother. Refer to the OB as to the next move, as the fetus may need to be delivered to prevent development of yet more DIC.

Rough question. Forgotten about Waldo yet? Maybe my explanation about nipride (question 5) was made up. How *would* you do this case? Don't take my word on any of this. *Make sure you answer these questions yourself!*

Grab Bag Questions

1. What are the adverse effects of hypothermia on the cardiac patient shivering away in the PACU?
2. What is a trigger point and how is it treated?
3. How would you induce an actively wheezing asthmatic requiring a rapid sequence induction for emergency abdominal surgery?
4. An EMT asks you why they can't use a little nitrous in the field for pain relief for their trauma victims.

Answers to Grab Bag Questions

1. Hypothermia can cause shivering, resulting in an increase in oxygen consumption of up to 500%. That can shift the myocardial oxygen supply/oxygen demand curve into the danger zone. Control hypothermia, first, by preventing it with good temperature maneuvers in the operating room. If shivering occurs in the PACU, treat it with meperidine and with warming blankets.

2. A trigger point is a distinct tender point in the muscle. It feels ropy and often reproduces a distinct painful sensation (shooting pain for example). Treatment is an injection with local anesthetic and steroid to reduce the inflammation.

3. Preoxygenate, cricoid pressure, lidocaine, narcotic, and intravenous ketamine. The goal is to get deep fast and to avoid eliciting more bronchospasm.

4. Nitrous reduces the available FIO_2 and that can be a problem in the field. Also, nitrous could obtund an already obtunded patient. And a final kicker is, nitrous could further expand a pneumothorax.

DING! Round 7 is over. How's it going? The more you do, the easier it gets. Like practicing a musical instrument or speaking a foreign language. Think of it as muscle memory for your brain.

SAMPLE EXAM #8

Session 1

A 25-year-old man with normal body habitus is brought to the ER after a diving accident. Posterior cervical fusion is planned. BP is 72/40, P 60, T 37.5°C.

HPI: A dive into a shallow body of water visited tragedy on this previously healthy young man, now quadriplegic and in a neck brace.

PMH: Occasional EtOH. Occasional tobacco.

Physical exam: C5 quadriplegic. Adequate but shallow respirations. No other injuries visible.

Labs: C5 fracture

He is brought to the OR with two large bore IVs in place.

Intraop Questions

1. What is "spinal shock" and how will it affect your anesthetic induction?
2. What is the concept of "secondary injury" and how will you try to prevent it in this spinal cord injured patient?
3. What is the innervation of the larynx and how can you topicalize this airway with minimal coughing?
4. After induction, the pressure becomes unobtainable. How will you treat it?
5. The pressure is normal, now the surgeon wants the patient to be sitting upright for the case. What special precautions must you take?
6. How do you secure the endotracheal tube to guard against accidental extubation? What do you do if accidental extubation occurs?
7. In the middle of the case, the patient goes into complete heart block. What are your treatment options with the patient in the awkward, sitting position?
8. What is a venous air embolism? How will you detect and treat it?
9. Saturation drops to 80% near the end of the case. What steps do you take?
10. The patient goes into V fib in the sitting position. How do you resuscitate?

Answers to Intraop Question

1. The sympathetic nervous system is sectioned, thus a complete sympathectomy results, with attendant hypotension. The normal reflexes are disrupted, so in spite of the low blood pressure, heart rate is slow. Induction, with the attendant hypotension, should be careful (as if you need to be reminded of that) and you may need phenylephrine to keep the BP up. Ephedrine and epinephrine are equally useful. Volume resuscitation will need to be generous, as the patients can't vasoconstrict, hence they are functionally hypovolemic.

2. Hypotension, defined as a systolic less than 90, can exacerbate central nervous system injury. Hypoxemia, too, can worsen neural damage. Avoiding both of these (like the cardiologist's stern admonition to "avoid hypoxia, avoid hypotension") is crucial to protecting what function you can. Steroids, specifically methylprednisolone, is a standard of care and should be given soon after the injury, within a few hours.

3. The internal branch of the superior laryngeal nerve provides sensation down to the vocal cords. The recurrent laryngeal nerves provide sensation below the vocal cords. Topicalizing the airway and magically avoiding coughing is, alas, not usually possible. I would topicalize orally by first giving a drying agent so my local would work. Then spray with lidocaine, asking the patient to pant like a dog so he would breathe way in and topicalize down in the trachea. Sooner or later, some local will get below the cords and cause some coughing. Better a little coughing as you topicalize than a huge amount of bucking when you place the endotracheal tube.

4. Volume, raise the legs, turn the anesthetic agents off, go to 100% oxygen, phenylephrine in geometrically higher doses. If no response, then epinephrine in geometrically higher doses (8 mcg, 16, 32, then stop fooling around and go to 100 mcg at a time.)

5. With no sympathetic tone around, the upright position will pool a lot of blood and plummet the blood pressure. Raise the patient gradually, checking the blood pressure at each incremental tilt. Tighten the patient with vasoconstrictors as you go.

6. Since the surgeons will be operating at the back of the neck, you can't wrap the tape around the neck, which is a real bummer. Tape the tube as best you can, using sticky stuff to keep the tape in place. (Tegaderms on the tape helps.) God forbid the tube comes out when the patient's in a weird position, have the surgeons place a bandage on the neck wound, tape the bandage in place, put the patient supine, and reintubate. Oh, the horror, the horror.

7. Floating a pacing wire through one of your cordises. If that technology is not available, put a Zoll external pacer on. There is also a system of esophageal pacing, which has the distinct advantage of ease in placing the probe (it's like an esophageal temp probe) and ease of use. Of course, your hospital may not have this. Medically, you can give atropine while you are arranging the pacing systems. The patient may not respond but it's worth a try. Another medical option is an isoproterenol drip.

8. When the surgical site is above the heart, air can entrain into the circulation and occlude the blood flow. The best monitor is a precordial Doppler, which will make a whooshing sound. Treatment is a family affair. The surgeon must flood the field to stop further entrainment of air. You as anesthesiologist must support the circulation and evacuate the air if possible. Place the patient on his back. Jugular pressure may raise the pressure enough to cause back bleeding, and PEEP may help (PEEP is controversial, that may push air through a probe patent foramen ovale). If CPR is necessary, that may have one additional benefit, the compressions sometimes break up the air embolus and restore circulation.

9. Make sure the patient is on 100% oxygen. Hand ventilate and auscultate to make sure the endotracheal tube is in the correct place. Listen for signs of pnuemothorax. Check the oxygen analyzer to make sure you are actually delivering oxygen. After all that, then check the saturation monitor to make sure it hasn't come off.

10. Start compressions and place on 100% oxygen with all anesthetic agents off. Attempt defibrillation (it is possible in the sitting position) while you call for help and try to find out why the fibrillation occurred (hypoxemia, venous air embolism, the effects of the patient's sympathectomy from the spinal cord injury, electrolyte imbalance?). Have the surgeons pack the wound so you can move the patient to the supine position and do CPR in a more normal modality. In abbreviated form, the ACLS will be shock, shock, shock, epi, shock, lido, shock, bretylium, shock. Keep that up and don't be shy with the epi.

You could spend the entire 35 minutes of your exam discussing question 8 and venous air embolism. But in the exam there is a "get a move on" atmosphere. The examiners aren't really interested in getting a Ph.D. dissertation on any one of the questions. They just want to know that you know, then they want to get along to the next issue. In my exam, I definitely sensed when the examiners felt, "OK, he got it," then they zoomed right into the next question. It will seem abrupt and you might feel like saying, "But wait, I haven't finished!" but that is actually a good sign.

Postop Questions

1. What are your criteria for extubation?
2. Continued intubation is decided on. What will you sedate the patient with to keep him from fighting the ETT? Is propofol a good idea?
3. A few hours postop, the urine output falls to 10 cc/hr. What do you do?
4. Blood pressure swings are wild, sometimes 200/100, sometimes 60/40. What accounts for these swings and can you do anything to prevent them?
5. An ICU nurse notes what looks like a corneal abrasion. How will you evaluate this?
6. During placement of a subclavian line, the inspiratory pressure alarm on the ventilator goes off and the patient's pressure drops. What is your immediate move?
7. After extubation, the patient is hoarse and the surgeon says, "Your damned tube knocked off his superior laryngeal nerve!" How do you respond to this and what do you do for the patient?
8. The surgeon is undecided whether a trach is necessary or not. Help him decide.
9. The patient complains of severe neck pain and needs some maintenance plan for long-term pain relief. Design such a plan.
10. The patient comes back for debridement procedures years later. Is Sux an OK drug to use?

Answers to Postop Questions

1. Special attention to the neuro status. Make sure the patient is alert enough to keep his airway patent and that he has enough respiratory strength to clear secretions. With this high of a spinal cord lesion, he may very well require long-term ventilatory support. If, however, the swelling goes down and he didn't have a complete transection, and if secondary injury was limited, then he may be able to get off the ventilator if he shows good weaning parameters (adequate FVC, good ABGs, normal respiratory rate).

2. A propofol drip provides good sedation, but can get a bit pricey, and the pharmacy people will be all over you. Also, since most propofol can support bacterial growth, the tubing needs frequent changing. I would sedate with a fentanyl infusion plus prn orders for midazolam if the patient requires supplemental sedation.

3. Check the Foley to make sure there are no kinks, clogs, or wheels sitting on it. Administer a fluid challenge. If that doesn't work, place central monitoring (remembering that the sympathectomy from the spinal cord lesion creates a hypovolemic state) and start dopamine.

4. The entire feedback loop of the nervous system is interrupted. I know of no magic bullet to prevent these swings, the best you can do is keep the fluid status optimized. For procedures that could cause pain, hence autonomic hyperreflexia (bladder manipulations), topicalize and just be aware of the potential for blood pressure swings. For operative procedures, the patient, even if he has no sensation, will need anesthesia to prevent autonomic hyperreflexia.

5. Examine the patient. If he feels like he has "something in his eye," that is a corneal abrasion until proven otherwise. If you're burning with ambition, place some fluorescein in the eye and take a look yourself with your handy dandy pocket slit lamp. If you're like the rest of us, call your friendly neighborhood ophthalmologist to examine the eye and recommend whatever eyedrops or patches are necessary. As with any complication, document, explain, get appropriate consultation, and follow-up.

6. Presume you have caused a tension pneumothorax. Place a 14-gauge angiocath in the midclavicular line at about the 2d interspace to relieve the tension, then get help to put in a chest tube. Oh, and do remember to put the angiocath on the side that caused the pneumothorax. It is rumored that dropping the *other* lung has little or no therapeutic effect. As this is going on, make sure the patient is on 100% oxygen.

7. First make sure the patient is maintaining an adequate airway. A sore throat is a common occurrence after intubation, most often just irritation of the trachea and pharynx. Time, saline gargles, and lidocaine swish and swallows usually suffice. If hoarseness persists, call in an ENT to see if there is any vocal cord paralysis.

8. If intubation has gone over a week (there is no magic number of days, a week is just a guideline) and the neurologic lesion is "set," and the patient does not have the ability to generate a good cough, then the patient will need a trach. All the intercostals muscles, so necessary to generate airway clearing coughing, are out. So this patient will most likely need a trach.

9. Chronic pain will require long-term follow-up with a pain specialist. Starting out, the plan should include antidepressant medication, trigger point injections, physical therapy, and most importantly, seeing the same doctor and pain team on a regular basis. This patient may need multiple modalities (cervical facet blocks, TENS unit), and the only way to create an effective plan is to try a mode, assess, try a different mode, assess, and keep working at returning the patient to as functional a role as he can achieve.

10. No. When exactly the patient no longer is at risk for massive potassium release is an open question. Don't be the one to find out.

Grab Bag Questions

1. What are the anesthetic implications for a patient in DKA who requires emergent surgery?
2. How fast can you replace K? Say a post CABG patient pouring out urine has a K of 2.1 and ongoing ectopy.
3. What is reflex sympathetic dystrophy?
4. What heart rate considerations apply for a patient with tight aortic stenosis? Why?

Answers to Grab Bag Questions

1. Volume loss can be tremendous in diabetic ketoacidosis. As the glucose functions as an osmotic diuretic, the urine output may be misleading. You may feel that your fluid replacement is adequate—"See, the urine output is great!"—when you are just fooling yourself. You'll need central monitoring. The metabolic acidosis, if severe enough, can lead to hypotension unresponsive to your usual medications (inotropes don't work as well when the pH is 7.04). Plus, the stress of surgery and whatever is the cause of the surgery (open fracture, intra-abdominal woe) will exacerbate the difficulty in controlling the glucose.

2. With symptomatic ectopy from low potassium, you can actually push potassium (Ah! More heresy!). In a fast running central IV, push 1 cc, 2 meq of potassium, then look at the EKG. It's handy to remember that "the potassium lives under the T wave" at times like these. Wait a minute, then push another cc. In this way, you can get 20 meq into the patient in, say 10 minutes, which is not much different that doing a somewhat brisk "potassium run." Another thing to remember at a trying time like this is that the magnesium may also be low and require replacement too.

3. Pain, autonomic disturbances, and eventually muscle and bone wasting that usually results from an injury. The injury itself may be trivial, but in subsequent weeks, the patient notices skin changes, first erythematous, then as the disease progresses, the skin becomes cool. Intense pain occurs, even the slightest touch can be excruciating (the weight of a sheet on an affected leg, for example). If unchecked, muscle and bone loss occurs. The mainstay of treatment is sympathetic blocks.

4. The exit ramp from the heart is a pinhole, so you have to avoid tachycardia. There will not be enough time to squeeze blood out of that pinhole. It's also worth remembering that if the patient should code (say you drop the SVR too fast) you'll now be attempting to squeeze blood through a pinhole by the decidedly inefficient chest compression technique. A code in *any* patient is an unhappy affair. In a patient with aortic stenosis, a code is most unpleasant indeed.

Think, think, think. Just like Pooh bear. Think, think, think.

Session 2

All right, you've gone at it for 300 pages plus. Put your feet up. Pop a cold one. Or, if you're like me, break out some ice cold milk and whip up a batch of Toll House Chocolate Chip Cookies. Break time.

Forget for a minute the exam, the lost airways, the uncertain C-spine, the oliguria.

One of the benefits of doctorhood is listening to some great stories from the patients. At a VA hospital I heard this from an old vet and it still gives me shivers when I think about it. If you're hard core studying, skip this part and go right to Sample Test #9. But if you want to cool your jets for a while, read on.

The Salute

HPI: Warren Hackner is a 71-year-old male with BPH scheduled for TURP.

PMH: MI 6 years ago with subsequent CABG. Now symptom free.

Physical Exam: Remarkable for a blurry tattoo on his left upper arm.

Anesthetic course:

"Lean forward a little, partner," I say, encouraging the patient to incline forward ever so gently. "There'll be a little prick here."

"Ouch!" the patient jumps. "What you puttin' in there, Doc, a railroad spike?"

"Yes," I admit, "but a small one."

"Aw hell, Doc, do what ya gotta do, long's my you-know-what works afterwards. It *will* work afterwards, won't it?"

CSF starts dripping out of the needle.

"Don't you worry about your you-know-what, partner. After this operation you'll be a stallion like no other. People will pay ten dollars at the county fair just to see you in action."

I tap the tattoo on Mr. Hackner's shoulder.

"Where'd you get that?"

We're laying him down and the spinal is kicking in. I fire up the blood pressure cuff.

"Iceland," Warren says.

"Iceland?" I ask, "What were you doing up in Iceland getting a tattoo?"

Blood pressure 85/50. In goes a little ephedrine and I open the IV up. I don't want this case to turn into an oral board scenario.

Warren cranks his head back and looks at me.

"You really wanna know, Doc?"

"Contact, bearing oh-one-fiver!" the navigator shouted.

Warren Hackner, pilot of the Catalina flying boat, on anti-submarine patrol over the North Atlantic, September 15, 1943, adjusted his headset.

"Any good?" Hackner asked. The radar equipment, when it had all the right replacement parts, when it hadn't frozen in the bitter air of Iceland, and when it wasn't feeling cranky, could occasionally pick up a surface contact. And when the radar made a surface contact, it might be an enemy submarine. Then Hackner would dive the plane, arm his 500-pound bomb, swoop in on the target, and find…nothing. Most often the radar contact would be a fog bank, a whale, a freighter, or just nothing at all.

"Yeah," the navigator said, "It's a good one. I mean it's real good."

"OK," Hackner reached to arm the bomb. His left arm still stung a little from his fresh tattoo. Hackner had never dropped a bomb in anger, though he'd done the best in his squadron at hitting both the land targets (boxes marked with an X) and later the floating targets (big rafts marked with an X). Hackner wondered if the German submarines had big Xs painted on them.

Not that Hackner had ever seen one. Nor, for that matter, did he expect to see one now. It was daytime, and no U-boat skipper would be on the surface in the daytime.

The Catalina flew into a fog bank; everything went milky white.

Maybe the U-boat skipper was down there, hiding in the fog. Hackner's stomach rose into his throat as the plane continued to dive on the contact. The altimeter spun as the plane dropped, dropped, dropped.

"It's good, it's good skipper," the navigator said, the excitement making his voice rise and crack. He sounded like a junior high kid with his voice changing. "No kidding, skip, this is a good one."

Hackner thought, "I don't think so. He had been crisscrossing the North Atlantic now for six months, and was coming to believe that you could never find a submarine in mid-ocean. Hour after hour (the average patrol lasted 18 hours), day after day, month after month. A big fat nothing.

Six months of patrolling and nothing to show for it. Six months on freezing, treeless Iceland, eating food that always, always got cold before you got it in your mouth. Wind, cold, bad food, patrol, wind, cold, bad food, patrol. Patrolling over the empty, empty ocean with a crackly radar box that showed a snowy, blurry bunch of specks. Maybe we should fly around with a divining rod and wait for it to point to a sub, Hackner thought.

"Almost done, Mr. Hackner," the surgeon said in the soft shout used by all doctors to all patients in all ORs. "Few more minutes. You doing OK?" the surgeon asked/shouted.

"Just fine Doc," Hackner said, "make sure I ain't singin' soprano at the end of this."

"No problem."

I tapped Hackner on the shoulder.

"What did you see when you came out of that fog bank, Mr. Hacker?"

"God Almighty!" Hackner yelled, his arm going automatically to the bomb release.

Dead ahead of Hackner's Catalina was a surfaced German submarine, its aft doors open and some smoke drifting out. In the split second Hackner had before the bomb release, he could tell the sub had surfaced with some kind of engine trouble, possibly a fire.

Hackner's plane was at right angles to the sub, the perfect attack position. The conning tower was straight ahead.

No "X" painted on the target, but there were some numbers.

Hackner's hand pulled the lever, the plane lightened, floated up a bit as the bomb fell away. He couldn't miss. This sub was as big as ten of the practice targets.

The explosion pushed the aircraft forward, but the sound was different than in the practice runs. This time there was a crack, audible even over the engine's roar. A crack like a redwood tree snapping in two. A redwood tree made of metal.

Hackner banked steeply to port to look. The conning tower was gone, the two ends of the sub now pointed crazily upwards. Black oil spread on the grayish ocean water. Then the milky white fog enveloped the plane again and Hackner saw no more.

"All done, Mr. Hackner," the surgeon chirped, standing and thwacking his gloves into the garbage can. "You'll have a urine stream that can put out a fire on the seventh floor now."

"Thanks Doc."

In the PACU, as I dropped him off, Hackner grabbed my arm.

"Wanna know something, Doc?"

"What's that, Mr. Hackner?"

The PACU nurse put on monitors. I wrapped a BP cuff around his arm.

"He saluted me."

I looked puzzled, "Who saluted you?"

"The captain," Hackner said, "The captain of that sub I sank. I could see him there, standing in the conning tower. I can see him like I see you now. He had on a black rubber slicker, and one of those captain's hats. And he had a beard, a dark beard. He looked right at me and saluted. Saluted as I dropped a bomb down his throat."

Hackner looked at me. "What do you make of that, Doc? Why did he do that?"

"I don't know. I don't know why he saluted you."

SAMPLE EXAM #9

Session 1

A 58-year-old diabetic with inoperable CAD is scheduled for outpatient knee arthroscopy.

HPI: Long-standing diabetes has left this man with a host of problems, panvasculopathy, if you will. His coronaries have been worked up but the vessels are so involved and the lesions so numerous that no surgeon will touch him. His kidneys are borderline, and he has neuropathy in both legs. The orthopedic surgeon knows of all these risks, but the patient has what looks like a bad meniscal tear. "Look," the surgeon says, "I don't want to do this any more than you do. But if he can't walk, he can't do his rehab. Then that will be it."

PMH: The angina pattern is spooky, but stable. He takes a nitro at least one time per day, but at least it's not changing. The cardiologist's concoction of calcium channel blockers, beta-blockers, and nitrates seem to be holding their own.

Physical exam: Slight obesity.

Labs: D-stick this morning shows 212. "That's about what I normally run if I skip my AM insulin," the patient reports.

He is on the OR table with an 18-g IV in.

Intraop Questions

1. Will you place any invasive lines? In an outpatient setting does it make a difference?
2. Will you run prophylactic NTG by infusion or as a patch? Why or why not?
3. What are the anesthetic options? Regional versus block versus spinal or epidural? What are the advantages and disadvantages of each?
4. You place a 3:1 block and an intraarticular block. As the surgeon twists the leg around the patient moans. What will you do?
5. You place an LMA. Describe how you could convert an LMA to an endotracheal tube if necessary.
6. During the procedure the ST segments start to climb. What do you do? At what point would you cancel the case?
7. Heart rate goes to 120 and blood pressure goes to 200/100. How do you treat?
8. Monofocal PVCs begin to appear. As you draw up your lidocaine, you see multifocal PVCs. How do you treat?
9. A D-stick comes back 5. You stare in disbelief and repeat it. It is still 5. What do you do? Just after you give some D-50, the nurse who got the D-stick admits she did it wrong and repeats the D-stick. Now it's 500. What do you do?
10. At emergence the patient violently twists off the table and falls to the ground. What do you do?

Answers to Intraop Questions

1. No invasive lines. Routine monitors will do. The outpatient setting doesn't make a difference. An ASA class 3 or 4 who is medically stable is OK for the outpatient setting.

2. Yes. Since he takes nitro every day, you want to get as much coronary vasodilation as you can.

3. The best option here is a knee block. The knee block can provide adequate pain relief (there are just two or three surgical sites to anesthetize) and provides minimal sympathetic disturbance. Of course, with any regional you have to be ready for a general anesthetic. Another option is a spinal, but that might provide too much of a sympathectomy too fast, dropping coronary perfusion pressure. So a better option is an epidural, that way you can titrate in the sympathectomy more gradually. And the last option is a general anesthetic. That has the advantage of "always working" (it's rare to hear of a "failed general"). Knowing his coronary history, if the regional technique failed, I'd put in an arterial line.

4. With any luck, you've tested your block beforehand. The patient's moaning may not represent complete failure, you may further sedate. Also, this case is amenable to the surgeon putting more local in the field. If the patient continues to have pain, that pain may cause too much sympathetic stimulation and you're better off converting to a general rather than milking the regional technique.

5. There are two ways of doing it. First, take the LMA out and do regular laryngoscopy to place the ETT. The second way is to place a fiberoptic down the LMA and slide a long 6.0 ETT. (If you have the good fortune to have an intubating LMA, then you can advance a larger ETT.)

6. Optimize the patient's oxygenation, blood pressure, and heart rate. Start nitroglycerin IV. If the patient became unstable (blood pressure down, continued ST elevation) then I'd tell the surgeon to get a move on. Still unstable? Cancel then and there. Tell the surgeon he'll have to make his BMW payment off another patient. Then I'd send the patient to the CCU and send off isoenzymes and get a cardiology consult. Place invasive monitors if instability continues.

7. If there are no contraindications, give beta-blockers to help the myocardial perfusion (slower heart rate gives longer diastolic time, hence more perfusion time). Increase nitroglycerin to decrease the blood pressure.

8. First, look for the cause of the arrhythmia—hypoxia, hypertension, hypotension, electrolyte disturbance, high CO_2 leading to acidosis. Once you've fixed the fixable, then go to antiarrythmics. Give the lidocaine. If you see improvement, start him on a lidocaine drip. If that doesn't help, go to bretylium. Don't forget the algorithm of arrythmia treatment. People now are quicker to go to bretylium.

9. Ay chihuahua! A high glucose is better than a low glucose. People survive high sugars, but that glucose of 5, *aaaaaaaaaaaaaaggg!* Once you've pegged that the glucose is indeed 500, then give IV insulin (remembering that some will rain out in the tubing) and follow glucoses with a sliding scale.

10. Woe is me. Go through the ABCs first, and if need be, secure the airway. Check vital signs. Get him on a stretcher, keeping the C-spine protected. Examine the patient, document the living hell out of everything, then send him for indicated x-rays. What you have become is an ER doctor evaluating a trauma patient.

What do you say we skip all the rest of the questions and just do cool stories from the VA for the rest of the book? But NO! Back to the task at hand. You have a test to take.

Postop Questions

1. In the PACU the glucose from the lab comes back 500. What are the dangers of hyperglycemia and how do you treat it?
2. From the fall off the OR table, the patient has a bruise on the back of his head and he has slurred speech. It is just 5 minutes postop. What do you do?
3. ST segments are still elevated and the man now wakes up enough to complain of chest pain. Your Rx?
4. In spite of 3 L nasal cannula, the man's saturation is only 92%. What do you do?
5. All seems well and then the man has a seizure. How do you treat?
6. His seizure ends, he remains confused. What is your next move?
7. As you are putting him into the ambulance to go to the real hospital, his wife comes screaming through the door of the PACU saying, "What the hell happened here? He was just having his knee scoped! What bozo did his anesthesia?" Your move, Dr. Bozo?
8. The orthopedic surgeon asks if this man is a candidate for lumbar sympathetic blocks if his knee pain continues. Your answer?
9. In the ambulance now for transfer, the EMT asks, "Has he always been flat line?" You answer?
10. You resuscitate the patient. As you are driving up to the hospital, a Fuji blimp, flying over a nearby stadium, loses power, crashes into your ambulance and kills everyone but you. What will you write on the incident report?

Answers to Postop Questions

1. No one dies right away from a high glucose. But if left unchecked, that high glucose could lead to diabetic ketoacidosis, and that could be fatal from a combination of fluid loss, acidosis, and electrolyte imbalances. A high glucose in the perioperative period leads to wound healing. In the case of neurologic injury, high glucose can worsen secondary injury to the central nervous system. And of course, in the very long-term, diabetes itself, through an unknown mechanism, leads to vasculopathy in all vascular beds.

2. A head injury implies a neck injury, so stablilize the C-spine in a collar. Slurred speech could be residual anesthetic, but if you just did a knee block, you've got a heap of trouble on your hands. The patient will need a CT to see if there is an intracranial bleed. Rule out metabolic causes first, of course.

3. Inoperable disease with ongoing chest pain, good time to sign this patient over to the on-call guy. Since medical therapy is your only option, maximize your vasodilation with nitroglycerin, treat tachycardia to keep myocardial oxygen demand down, and give supplemental oxygen. If none of this works, consider whether a cardiologist would want to put in an intraaortic balloon pump.

4. Before going whole hog to intubation, there are some increased FIO_2 options. A mask, then a rebreather mask, and finally mask CPAP are the options for giving more oxygen outside of artificial ventilation. See if there is some other cause of hypoxemia, such as a pneumothorax, bronchospasm, or congestive heart failure.

5. Seizures in themselves don't kill, but the resulting hypoxemia, high oxygen demand, and risk of aspiration may kill. Stop the seizure with thiopental, mask ventilate, then secure the airway. Figure out what caused the seizure (low glucose, that pesky intracranial bleed from pitching off the table).

6. Back to the broken record—try to find out the cause of the confusion, whether it is metabolic or from intracranial pathology. Address the ABCs to make sure the confusion isn't from a correctable vital sign problem, such as hypotension or hypoxemia. Protect the airway, for a confused patient may not have the neurologic wherewithal to avoid aspiration.

7. Explaining unexpected complications to family members is a daunting task. The best approach is a direct recitation of the facts without assigning blame anywhere. Then assure the family member that everything is being done to diagnose and treat the problems that arose. Avoid sneakiness or whitewashing; remember what happened to Nixon.

8. If the man shows evidence of sympathetically mediated pain, then a series of lumbar sympathetic blocks could be helpful. If, however, his pain is from a meniscal tear or other surgically correctable cause, then the lumbar sympathetic block would be less helpful.

9. First look at the patient to see if the clinical picture correlates with the monitor. If the patient is sitting up, pulling his nasal cannula off, then he is most assuredly not in asystole. If the monitor correlates with a pulseless, blue patient, then initiate CPR and ACLS. And you would be well advised to tell the driver to step on it.

10. Just when you thought you'd made it—it's always something, isn't it?

As you can see, making up your own tests can be a blast! The weirdness of your complications is limited only by your imagination.

Grab Bag Questions

1. A firefighter, fresh from rescuing people from a mobile home fire, has singed nasal hair, and is coughing up carbonaceous material. He sees what you are thinking and says, "Oh no, you don't need to stick that tube in me! I'm breathing just fine, thank you." What do you say to him and what do you do?

2. A man with tight aortic stenosis is scheduled for AVR the next day. The surgeon asks, "Should we stick him in the unit with a Swan tonight and tank him up?" What do you say?

3. On a preop EKG in your preop clinic, a patient has new onset atrial fibrillation. Do you cancel her planned ulnar nerve transposition?

4. A patient calls you and complains of a terribly sore throat. Your record shows he had an uneventful LMA anesthetic for an ankle arthroscopy. What do you do?

Answers to Grab Bag Questions

1. The firefighter has all the earmarks of an upper airway burn. Though he may be fine now, the swelling from the burn may convert him to an airway nightmare in no time. Intubate the firefighter now, before it's too late.

2. No. That is expensive and will have no benefit. You can place the Swan in the morning, look at and treat the numbers then, and then induce carefully with the physiologic concerns of aortic stenosis (slow heart rate, maintain SVR) in mind.

3. Yes. Atrial fibrillation is a sign of some kind of cardiac distress. The causes are manifold and include myocardial infarction, pericarditis, thyroid dysfunction, and electrolyte abnormalities. The fibrillating atrium can harbor clots that can progress to strokes. No matter how *minor* the planned surgery, this patient needs a thorough workup to find out what caused her heart rhythm to change.

4. See the patient personally. Examine the mouth yourself and explain to the patient what happened and why you chose an LMA for the anesthetic. If the exam shows nothing terribly awry, then prescribe Cepacol lozenges and saline gargles. If there is a 6-inch gash in the throat and the entire pharynx looks like hamburger helper, get an ENT evaluation.

Session 2

An 18-year-old marine is scheduled for emergency laparotomy for appendicitis. Vital signs are BP 85/50, HR 150, R 28 and shallow. T is 39.7°C.

Preop Questions

1. What do the vital signs indicate?
2. What lab tests are necessary before proceeding?
3. Would you premedicate with sedatives? Antacids? Reglan?
4. How will you determine whether to induce or do an awake intubation?
5. Should you treat his temperature before inducing anesthesia?
6. What effect will his hyperdynamic state have on anesthetic uptake and distribution?
7. What fluid and electrolyte disturbances might you see in such a case?
8. Should an NG be placed preop? If so, should it be removed before induction? What effect does an NG tube have on the GE junction?
9. What would an arterial blood gas likely show? If there is a metabolic acidosis, should you treat with bicarb?
10. How, once the case starts, will you be able to pick up MH if he is already tachycardic?

Answers to Preop Questions

1. All vital signs point to big trouble. Hypotension and tachycardia indicate effective intravascular hypovolemia. The appendix has probably ruptured, causing bacteremia with a drop in SVR plus a tremendous amount of third spacing in the inflamed, infected abdomen. The rapid respirations indicate pain, and the high temperature goes along with a picture of sepsis.

2. None. The longer you wait to go to the OR, the worse for this patient. By history he is young and previously healthy. The only thing that would show up on a test now would be a high white count, as if you need that to make the diagnosis. A urinalysis would show concentrated urine; again, you already know that is the case. So just haul up to the OR pronto.

3. He is in such a bad state now that I would hold off on sedatives. Any sedative given now in effect constitutes part of his anesthetic, and it would be easy to overdo it in a patient already hypotensive, so no sedative. I would give no aspiration prophylaxis either. His inflamed GI tract will not be emptying anything, so giving medications now will not help. An oral antacid may just make him vomit.

4. Examination of the airway, looking for all the usual suspects—receding chin, large teeth, overbite, limited neck or jaw mobility. If the airway looked suspect, then I would prepare the patient for the awake snake, the seeing-eye scope, the cobra of carinal cannulation.

5. No. The temperature is a marker of the intraabdominal process. Treat the cause of the high temperature, not the temperature itself.

6. High cardiac output means that his anesthetic uptake will be slower. The accumulation of anesthetic gas in his alveoli and establishment of the partial pressure in the alveoli are lessened in this high cardiac output state. And can I confess something to you, Dr. Examiner? Ted Eger may understand that, but I just never will. I always thought that with a higher cardiac output, you'd suck that juice into your system just that much faster. Just goes to show you that you've got to be a lot smarter than I am to really understand uptake and distribution.

7. First, the overall intravascular volume will be reduced. That will be the biggest, most dangerous vexation, particularly at the time of induction. From the pain of his appendicitis, the patient has probably been vomiting, resulting in a loss of hydrogen and potassium. So this patient will present with a hypovolemic, hypokalemic metabolic alkalosis.

8. If the patient had an NG placed in the ER, then I would keep it in and place it on suction. If the patient came to me as is, I would not place an NG. NGs hurt and the patient, already in pain, may fight it and suffer more. And the NG is no perfect guardian against aspiration. Large chunks of T-bones, baby back ribs, and triple decker club sandwiches are not sucked out by the little holes of the NG. Also, the NG blocks the GE junction and can act like a wick for aspirate to track upward.

9. Metabolic acidosis. More important than giving a base (bicarb) to treat excess acid, is treating the cause of the acidosis, hypovolemia. So give large amounts of fluids, liters in this case. The man is young and healthy, so you are unlikely to place him in cardiac failure. Do give bicarb if the pH is so low (say, below 7.25) that cellular enzyme systems are unlikely to work properly.

10. Malignant hyperthermia, a metabolic kaboom, can be hard to differentiate from the hypermetabolic state of sepsis as seen here. Tachycardia, an early sign of MH, is already present. Excess CO_2 production is already present. High oxygen consumption is already present. Even the late sign, elevated temperature, is already present. I would look for persistence in these signs in spite of adequate resuscitative measures. For example, after a few liters of fluid, and after the pain relief afforded by anesthesia, this patient's heart rate should start to fall. If the tachycardia persists or worsens, that inclines toward MH.

Intraop Questions

1. What agent will you use to induce? Why? Give one alternative to your agent of choice.
2. You induce and see a pharynx filled with emesis. What do you do?
3. After intubation, wheezing is heard in all lung fields. What are your Dx and Rx?
4. In spite of a "careful induction," the BP goes to caca. How will you raise the pressure? Is Neo a good choice? Ephedrine? Epi?
5. The surgeon sees massive spillage of contaminated material. Will you place invasive monitors?
6. Urine output drops to tumbleweeds and sand dunes blowing through the Foley. What do you do?
7. A Swan shows a cardiac output of 10 and an SVR of 300. BP is still low. How will you treat?
8. At least overnight ventilation is planned. Which relaxant will you use and why?
9. How will you sedate this man overnight? Is a propofol infusion a good option? What problems are associated with propofol?
10. A chest x-ray taken in the room shows a bilateral whiteout of the lungs. What is "shock lung" and how is it treated?

Answers to Intraop Questions

1. After I had poured fluids into this young man, had preoxygenated, and had good cricoid pressure on, I'd do a rapid sequence induction. My agent of choice is ketamine. An alternative is etomidate. Neither of these has cornered the market on the "induction in the unstable patient" market. The fact is, small doses of whatever agent—thiopental, propofol—are also suitable in such a case. And in a similar vein, no agent is without risk. On their very last vesicle of sympathetic tone, any agent can make a patient decompensate.

2. Head down and to the side, suction. Once the airway is cleared, intubate. Then get on your cricoid pressure person, for cricoid pressure, though useless against active vomiting, should protect against passive regurgitation.

3. Most likely the patient aspirated. Keep him on 100% oxygen, suction, use fiberoptic guidance if the original suctioning doesn't do the trick. In case of complete obstruction and an inability to ventilate, remove the ETT and perform rigid bronchoscopy to fish out the offending blocking agent. As the Taco Bell chihuahua would say, "Pull out the chalupa."

4. Volume, feet up, all inhalation agents off, then start with phenylephrine. Use up the whole stick if necessary, this is no time to be shy. Don't bother with ephedrine if there is no response with the phenylephrine; go to the guns. Go to epi and increase the doses geometrically, not arithmetically. That is, give 1 ml, if no response, give 2 ml, then 4 and on up. Don't give 1 ml, then another one, then another one. You want to get an effect.

5. Yes. Even though this man is in baseline good health, his initial vital signs, response early in the case, and now this, make him a setup for all kinds of trouble. He will be septic, could go into ARDS, and will likely need inotropic support. Postop, he will need ventilatory support too. So place an arterial line and a Swan.

6. If you can't answer the oliguria question by now, I'll send you a phone card. Call your mother and tell her that this whole doctor thing just isn't working out for you and that you'll be home soon.

7. Back to the functional definition of SVR. This SVR is what is known in the parlance as too low. He will need intravascular vasoconstriction to counter this low SVR, so I'd start a norepinephrine drip.

8. If his kidneys are still functioning well, I'd use pancuronium. Keep a twitch monitor at the bedside and make sure the ICU staff is familiar with it. More important than the muscle relaxant will be the sedation, for you don't want a patient on a ventilator, paralyzed but not sedated.

9. Propofol is expensive and can support bacterial growth. Sedate with the inexpensive stuff, morphine, for example.

10. "Shock lung" or "Da Nang lung" or a million other names all describe the lung as an insufficient exchange mechanism. Due to shock or fluids or sepsis or aspiration (in this case) or any number of causes, the normal architecture of the lungs is altered and the air spaces fill with fluids and debris, making efficient gas exchange impossible. Large V/Q mismatch occurs and the patient requires ventilatory support and PEEP.

Keep talking. I'm looking at you from the pages of this book and I see you reading a lot, falling into a trap. "I'll just keep reading these answers. Yeah, that's what I would have said." Wrongo. Don't drift into bad habits. Put this book down and go do a practice exam aloud with someone right now.

You heard me.

No one available? Call someone and do one over the phone then.

OK, you're back. Let your own conscience flog you if you didn't do it.

Grab Bag Questions

1. You attempt to induce a child with rectal Brevital but he defecates the Brevital all over you. What will you do next?
2. A nurse anesthetist working with you says that when he checked the circuit this morning he smelled "something funny." New construction is going on in the next wing of the hospital. What do you do?
3. Midway through an ACL reconstruction, someone hears the line isolation monitor going off. What do you do?
4. What special considerations accompany a mediastinal mass?

Answers to Grab Bag Questions

1. Well, evidently plan A didn't work. So go to plan B. Keep in mind that some of that rectal Brevital may have been absorbed, so under no circumstances leave the child unattended. Do an inhalation induction, using pleasant smelling, quick acting Sevoflurane. To calm the patient, tell a nice story or recite a poem to him as he goes off to sleep. (I suggest *The Cremation of Sam McGee*; the OR staff will be amazed when you recite the whole thing.)

2. Let no case begin. Any case that is in progress, convert to oxygen cylinders and ambu-bags, if necessary. Work on pipelines plus anything abnormal could indicate that anything, *ANYTHING* could be in the pipelines. Carbon monoxide (obviously, you wouldn't smell that), exhaust fumes, explosive stuff, corrosive solvents, anything that comes from an industrial site could be making its way into your oxygen supply with potentially hospital-wide catastrophic implications.

3. Check the patient and make sure all is well. Specifically, make sure there is no rhythm disturbance. Then go around the room, unplugging machines one by one until you find the one that has some break in its insulation.

4. The mass may collapse onto the vascular and respiratory structures once anesthesia has been induced, creating vascular compromise and an inability to ventilate even if the trachea is intubated. In its most extreme cases, fem-fem bypass is needed to provide oxygenation.

Pause for the cause. Before we launch into the last practice exam, let's review what these practice exams are meant to do and what they are not meant to do.

These practice exams *do not*:

- Cover *all* material that could be covered. There are an infinite number of other questions and scenarios. The answers provided here just touch on the main points, but they are not in-depth answers by any stretch. (Just look at the last answer, you could write a whole chapter on mediastinal masses.)
- Provide enough of a "cushion" to pass the exam. Just memorizing these answers and thinking you can skate by is folly.

These exams *do:*

- Show you the framework of the exam.
- Give you a sample of what a test *could* be like.

What should you do:

- Tomorrow, say your first case is a hip. Make up your own practice test in the mode of a Session 1.

- Your next case is a retinal detachment. Make up your own practice test in the mode of a Session 2.
- From the ICU and PACU questions you get tomorrow, make up your own grab bag questions.

That is the take home lesson from these practice exams. Use the framework we showed you to make up and answer your own tests.

Now, on to the last sample exam. I wonder if Waldo is in there?

SAMPLE EXAM #10

Session 1

A 75-year-old woman is scheduled for right total hip revision.

HPI: This woman with multiple medical problems has a loose hip prosthesis that was placed 8 years ago. Pain is so severe that she cannot ambulate and she needs a new hip.

PMH: Renal failure on dialysis. Last dialyzed yesterday with a K of 4.6. Her Hct is 28 which is her baseline. Congestive heart failure is under nominal control with the usual litany of meds.

Physical exam: Obese, endentulous, a graft in her left arm.

She is in your OR now with large bore IV access in anticipation of large blood loss, an oximetric Swan, and an A-line.

Intraop Questions

1. How will you induce? Is a combined technique useful? A pure regional technique?
2. What special considerations do you take into account with her renal failure, her arm graft?
3. If the surgeon requests low blood pressure to minimize bleeding, will that adversely affect her graft? Her heart?
4. How will you detect ischemia? Is a TEE useful? Will you place one?
5. How are her hemodynamics affected by the lateral position? Her Swan readings? Say the wedge is 25, what will you do?
6. The surgeon starts losing blood at a brisk pace and you replace cc per cc. What concerns do you have with transfusion? How will you detect a transfusion reaction if she's already oozing from a large surgical wound?
7. A blood gas shows a pO_2 of 65 on 100% O_2. What will you do?
8. The oximetric Swan reads 100%. Is this cause for joy? What affects an oximetric Swan?
9. Your resident tells you, "Oops, I put the A-line in her shunt. I thought it was a hell of a pulse." What do you do?
10. You placed a spinal with Duramorph and Marcaine. How will you tell intraop if it is working?

Answers to Intraop Questions

1. Preoxygenate, intravenous induction with fentanyl, thiopental, and succinylcholine. I would use a combined technique of a spinal with intrathecal morphine plus a general anesthetic. I'm looking for good pain relief after the operation is over, but I don't want to do a hip revision on her side without the airway secured. A revision can take a long time, and it can be uncomfortable to lie on your side that long. Also, if the case goes on and on, the spinal might wear off and then I'd be intubating her on my, and her, side. I would not use an epidural. She is in renal failure and therefore has poor platelet function. The thin spinal needle does not give me pause. The thick Tuohy needle does.

2. Renal failure patients require close fluid management, for if you overdo it, there is no place for the fluid to go. And recent dialysis puts her at risk for having low intravascular volume, a problem if there is the usual bloodletting seen in a hip revision. Renal patients are setups for infection, as their AV grafts allow blood to skip the normal "filtering" effect of the lungs. The graft itself will require special padding to make sure no occlusion occurs. Potassium from blood transfusions places the renal patient at risk. Finally, platelet function and clot formation are impaired.

3. Yes and yes, respectively. The patient already has an impaired ventricle, so reducing the perfusion pressure to her coronaries could place her myocardium at risk. Also, a low blood pressure could result in such low flow through the graft that the graft might be clotted at the end of the case.

4. EKG is not the best detector of ischemia, but it is the most practical as you can observe the EKG throughout the case. The TEE requires a dedicated observer, and you'd have to watch for wall motion abnormalities in the middle of this big thrash of a case. So I would not place a TEE. The other detector I would use is the oximetric Swan. If the mixed venous started to go down, or if the PA pressures started to rise, that would tell me, not precisely that ischemia was occurring, but that "something was awry," and I'd change something. (Transfuse more, raise the perfusion pressure, start nitroglycerin.)

5. When the patient is placed on her side, her diaphragm is compressed, the weight has shifted, and all the axillary rolls and other things are all settled down, the best you can say is that you have a new baseline to work with. If the wedge is now 25, you do look overgenerous on the fluids, but look at all the other numbers (blood pressure, mixed venous, EKG) before you react too quickly. Follow trends based on the "new reality" of the patient on her side.

6. Any transfusion can cause a transfusion reaction (hypotension, oozing, hemolysis), most often from some clerical error or mislabeling. It may be difficult, if you are pouring in gallons of blood, to tell the oozing of a transfusion reaction from the oozing of dilutional thrombocy-topenia (another problem with transfusions.) If oozing is accompanied by hematuria, and the blood pressure starts requiring extensive support (epinephrine) then you have a transfusion reaction. There is no absolute here, as a desperately bleeding patient may also develop hemolysis leading to hematuria, and may also require inotropic support. Other problems with transfusions include hypocalcemia and hypothermia.

7. Go through the oxygen delivery system from the wall, to the connector, to the endotracheal tube, to the proper position of the endotracheal tube (right mainstem is the most likely cause of all) to the lungs themselves. Make sure the patient really is getting 100% oxygen, correct the endotracheal tube position, and treat any bronchospasm that may have occurred.

8. The Swan may have traveled a bit far out and is now in the wedge position. In such a case, it may "see" more richly oxygenated blood. The mixed venous reading tells you of global oxygen delivery, that is, a good cardiac output favors a higher mixed venous. Good oxygenation in the blood and good oxygen carrying capacity all produce a high mixed venous. Some methods "cheat" the accuracy of a mixed venous. A shunt (as in this patient) can yield a more optimistic mixed venous than is the case. And cellular poisoning can rob the cells of the ability to use oxygen, so the cells are starved for oxygen (cyanide poisoning), but the mixed venous hums merrily along at a high number. Oximetric Swans are also affected by correct calibration at the beginning of the case, the mood of the oximetric box and cable, sunspots, gamma rays from outer space, demonic possession, evil genies, and a leprechaun at the back of your machine who makes sure things go wrong right when you need them most.

9. It's not the end of the world. When the technicians do dialysis, they put big needles in the shunt. Just live with the A-line where it is, then slip it out at the end of the case and hope no one notices your embarrassed look. Tell your blushing resident a "real world" hint. In a code with a renal patient, if you can't get a line, go ahead and stick the shunt. Better to get some access and save the patient than to "avoid and protect" the shunt and have the patient die.

10. When the armed and dangerous surgeons make the incision, there should be no change in the vital signs if the spinal is working.

Ischemia, in one form or another, will appear on your test as sure as you are born. Make sure you have that one down.

Postop Questions

1. In the PACU, the patient is breathing inadequately. What is the differential diagnosis? What is recurarization?

2. Her temperature is 33.6°C. What problems are associated with hypothermia?

3. Her AV graft does not have a thrill in it. What do you do?

4. In spite of the intrathecal narcotics, the patient still has pain. What orders will you write for pain relief?

5. How will you monitor the patient for respiratory depression? When can this occur?

6. Your resident, the one who stuck the AV graft, tells you he forgot to give the prophylactic antibiotics. What do you do and what do you tell the surgeon?

7. The patient runs a persistent tachycardia in the PACU. How will you treat this?

8. Forty-five minutes postop and the blood pressure drops to 75/40. How will you evaluate this?

9. As the patient is being transferred, the Swan is pulled out. Can you get by without it now? Do you still need an oximetric Swan?

10. The surgeon is concerned about ongoing bleeding plus the need for dialysis with its attendant heparin. "When should we dialyze next?" he asks you.

Answers to Postop Questions

1. If the patient is not breathing right, systematically go through the breathing mechanism. Is the brain sending out the information to breathe? (Still anesthetized, respiratory depression from intrathecal narcotics?) Are the muscles capable of responding to these signals (muscle weakness—the infamous recurarization, hypothermia potentiating weakness)? Are the heart and lungs overloaded with fluid? (Renal failure plus poor baseline cardiac function plus a big case could easily result in overload.) The most likely cause is fluid overload. Reintubate to assure adequate oxygenation, then treat the overload.

2. Muscle weakness, coagulopathy, and altered consciousness. Plus, as the patient rewarms, she may shiver with its attendant high oxygen consumption.

3. EEK! The darned thing may be clotted. Try to reestablish flow by making sure the patient has adequate fluid volume and a good blood pressure. Make sure there is no undue pressure on that arm. If the thrill is still gone, the patient will need a radiologic study to see if they can declot the graft.

4. Intramuscular narcotics, such as Demerol. The goal is to provide additional pain relief, but not provide a high amount of narcotic at one time (as with intravenous injection) that could further depress respirations. An intramuscular supplement will provide a more gradual rise and fall of narcotic. Nothing is guaranteed, and you will still need to observe for delayed respiratory depression.

5. The best monitor is respiratory rate. Patients tend to gradually slow down their rate, rather than go from 18 breaths a minute right down to 0. Make sure the nurse takes hourly vital signs, paying special attention to the respiratory rate and state of consciousness. Respiratory depression can occur up to 24 hours post placement.

6. Be like George Washington and take a hatchet and chop the resident's head off. No, wait, I mean, go tell the surgeons and be an honest person. Then give the antibiotics right away.

7. Seek the cause of the tachycardia. Pain? Give pain relief. Anemia (a distinct possibility)? Transfuse. Hypoxemia? More oxygen. Make sure the tachycardia is nothing sinister, such as new onset atrial fibrillation or a slow V tach.

8. Hypotension has many causes, but the one I'd look for first here is hypovolemia from ongoing bleeding into that big surgical area. To do a hip revision requires a lot of rending and tearing. Pulling out old cement can even tear something on the other side of the acetabulum, like an iliac artery (it has happened to me). So draw a hematocrit, rule out other causes (cardiac failure, arrhythmia) and go with the percentages—transfuse.

9. Replace the Swan. With her multisystem organ involvement, rocky course in the PACU, and possibility of ongoing bleeding and third spacing, she needs the invasive monitors. Can she get by without an oximetric? Yes, she could. If later on, with all the information at your disposal (cardiac output, lab values, hip drainage evaluation, PA pressures, blood gases), you can't manage her, then replace the oximetric.

10. Dialysis could definitely worsen bleeding, plus the volume shifts could result in more hypotension. Unless the patient needs her potassium reduced, hold off on dialysis for 2 days. And yes, the 2-day figure is arbitrary.

Grab Bag Questions

1. Differ between a placenta previa and a placenta accreta. What are the anesthetic implications of each?

2. An EMT brings in a coding patient with a Combi-tube in place. "Couldn't intubate him, Doc, couldn't see a damn thing." Do you replace the Combi-tube with an ETT?

3. Differ between an anaphylactic and an anaphylactoid reaction. How do you treat each?

4. After a prolonged labor that included an epidural, the woman complains of leg weakness. Evaluate this.

Answers to Grab Bag Questions

1. A placenta previa is a normal placenta that is in an abnormal place, at the exit from the uterus. The baby will have to "tear through" the placenta with attendant blood loss. Placenta accreta means a placenta that has "bored into" the uterus. At birth, rather than separating from the uterus, the placenta accreta may have to be ripped out. Blood loss will be astounding and alarming. The big implication for anesthesia is preparation for massive blood replacement. Some would say a regional technique, with its consequent sympathectomy, is contraindicated in such cases. I say that you must consider all aspects (airway, patient history) before you rule out a regional technique.

2. First make sure you are at least ventilating OK with the Combitube. Then pull it out (you can always put it back in) and look with your laryngoscope. At this point, if you can't place an ETT, go for a surgical airway. While that is going on, mask ventilate.

3. An anaphylactic reaction is mediated by IgE antibodies binding to mast cells or basophils by a specific receptor. An anaphylactoid reaction, in contrast, does not involve a specific antibody. From a clinical standpoint, the difference is moot, because both result in bronchospasm, shock, and edema. Airway obstruction can occur from upper airway swelling. Treatment is fluids and epi, epi, epi. All the disaster stories regarding anaphylactic and anaphylactoid reactions have the same theme—people didn't go to epi fast enough. All the salvation stories have the same theme—people went to epi right away.

4. See the patient and examine her, looking specifically for signs of an epidural hematoma—back pain, motor and sensory loss. If she has these, get neurosurgery and a CT *now*. A more likely possibility is a femoral nerve stretch injury from the baby's head pressing down and/or the patient's legs being in extreme lithotomy position.

As an exercise in reverse psychology, go back through that session, and deliberately answer everything as wrong as you can. Give answers that would automatically flunk any examinee. By now, you should be able to answer so automatically, that it's harder to think of a *wrong* answer than a right one.

Session 2

A 50-year-old woman with multiple sclerosis is scheduled for resection of a gastric carcinoma. Her vital signs are all normal. She can walk with a walker on some days, but at other times needs a wheelchair.

Preop Questions

1. What are the anesthetic implications of multiple sclerosis?
2. Is a preop neuro consult indicated? Why or why not?
3. What preop labs are necessary? Is an EKG necessary if she has no cardiac symptoms?
4. She asks, "Can this operation make my MS worse?" How do you respond?
5. Discuss with the patient the pros and cons of an epidural for postoperative pain relief.
6. Should the OR be heated more than usual before the case? Cooled? Kept the same as usual?
7. She says, "If the cancer has spread, don't wake me up." Your response?
8. How would you premedicate this patient?
9. She asks if she can go to sleep "with a mask, I'm so sick of needles." What can you do in response to this request?
10. Will you give steroids preop or intraop?

Answers to Preop Questions

1. The disease itself has a waxing and waning course. The stress of surgery may exacerbate the symptoms, so discuss that with the patient ahead of time. With muscle wasting, there is the possibility of a hyperkalemic response to succinylcholine. General anesthetics have no specific adverse reaction with MS, and no specific technique is safer than another. Placing any regional block in a patient with preexisting neuro difficulties, especially one whose symptoms may worsen as part of the disease's natural history, is problematic.

2. Yes. Get a preop neuro consult to document the exact state of the current condition. Sometimes steroids are given for treatment. Ask the neuro consult specifically whether steroids should be given perioperatively. And finally, the neurologist can better evaluate and help with the patient's management if the neurologist has seen the patient already. In the best of all worlds, the patient will already have a neurologist that is familiar with her.

3. Hematocrit, creatinine, potassium. This is a big operation and you want to know where you stand regarding blood and renal function. Get a preop EKG. Although the patient has no symptoms, her debilitated state means she does little to stress her system. This operation will be a stress. After the operation, you will be happy you had a preop EKG for comparison. You don't want to be staring at a flipped T wave and wonder, "Gee, was it flipped before?"

4. The short answer is, "No one knows." By making sure her temperature doesn't rise (a possible cause of MS worsening) and minimizing stress to as great a degree as possible, you can tell her that you will do everything to prevent a worsening of symptoms. In other words, be honest but not brutally insensitive. There is always room for cautious optimism and reassurance.

5. An epidural with local anesthetic and a narcotic in it can provide good pain relief. Some doctors hesitate to place an epidural, for fear they will be blamed later for some neurologic loss that was not their fault. Having laid it all out for the patient, and documenting all this, along with a good neuro evaluation, let the patient decide what he or she is comfortable with.

6. Two forces are at work here. An increase in the patient's temperature may exacerbate the MS. The stress of the usual "deep freeze" OR may also worsen MS. I would heat the OR up until the patient is covered and induced, to avoid the "cold slap in the face," then I would cool the OR, watching her temperature like a hawk.

7. In a compassionate way, tell her that you can't do that, but that you can do all in your power to keep her comfortable. Even if the cancer has spread, she will have time for family visits and getting her house in order. Then when you leave the patient, tell the surgeon about the discussion and see what he/she thinks. This patient may need more counseling before the operation.

8. Heavy sedation. IM morphine and midazolam to minimize her stress. Going in for a big cancer resection is an awful thing, so get her as relaxed and forgetful as possible. Given her debilitated state, send her to the OR on supplemental oxygen and make sure someone observes her for signs of respiratory depression.

9. A gastric carcinoma implies a full stomach, so an inhalation induction could pose a problem. With sufficient preoperative sedation, you should be able to get an IV in and perform an intravenous induction.

10. If she has been on steroids in the last 6 months, as is sometimes the case with MS, then I would give a stress-covering dose of steroids to prevent any possibility of adrenal insufficiency.

You're in the home stretch now.

Intraop Questions

1. The patient is thin and the airway looks good. Describe how you could perform an inhalation induction in an adult.
2. Halfway through the inhalation induction the patient goes into laryngospasm. How would you treat this?
3. After induction you attempt a central line. What are the advantages and disadvantages of an upper body line versus a groin central line?
4. Intraop the blood pressure rises to 180/100. Your response?
5. The pulse oximeter stops working. How will you troubleshoot this?
6. You attempt but can't place a radial arterial line on either side. Where will you go next and why?
7. End-tidal CO_2 starts to rise in the middle of the case. How would you tell if rebreathing of CO_2 is occurring and how would you fix it?
8. You have a Bair Hugger on and the temperature has risen to 38.5°C. How will you cool the patient?
9. Your twitch monitor says zero twitches but the surgeon says, "She's tight." What do you do?
10. At extubation you notice blood on the endotracheal tube. How will you evaluate this?

Answers to Intraop Questions

1. For reasons mentioned above, I'd prefer an intravenous induction. But this is how I'd do an inhalation induction: preoxygenate, use sevoflurane, gradually increase the inhaled concentration, monitor the patient's respiration and saturation. When she no longer responded to further commands, put in an oral airway, then give relaxant and intubate. You can also do a single breath technique by having the patient breathe all the way out and take a vital capacity of high concentration of sevo. I would not do this as I have never done it before and am unfamiliar with that technique.

2. Positive pressure, a nondepolarizing relaxant (she may have muscle wasting and I don't want to risk a hyperkalemic response), 100% oxygen, and pressure behind the ramus of the mandible to break the laryngospasm.

3. An upper body central line is less likely to get infected as the groin is hard to keep clean. Also, an upper body line will pose fewer problems when it's time for the patient to sit up and ambulate. A lower body central line has fewer problems if you stick the needle in the wrong place. That is, if by the femoral approach you drop a lung, you may be using too large of a needle.

4. Make sure nothing bad is going on metabolically—hypoxemia, hypercarbia—then treat the most likely cause, inadequate anesthesia. Deepen the anesthetic with IV or inhalational anesthetic.

5. Place the patient on 100% oxygen right away, and listen to the lungs to make sure the physical signs go along with adequate oxygenation and ventilation. Send a blood gas if there is any doubt, because looking at nail beds and the like is not too accurate. Move the pulse oximeter probe around, looking for a better site—another finger, the ear, the nose, the lip as a last resort. If all the probes fail, replace the cable, then replace the machine. All the time, keep looking at the patient; don't be too carried away looking at the machines.

6. Brachial artery. That artery is bigger. Although sometimes described as heresy to place a line in this "has no collateral" artery, the fact is the brachial artery does just fine with lines in it. Sticking an axillary artery is difficult because the artery isn't anchored down too well and you might spear some of the nerves of the brachial plexus while you are fishing around. The next choice would be the femoral artery.

7. Examine the one-way valves and make sure they are opening and closing correctly. Look to the end-tidal trace and see if the CO_2 line does not go back to zero; that would indicate rebreathing. To fix the problem, I'd fix the inspiratory or expiratory valves. Most likely they are sticking from moisture build-up.

8. Turn the Bair Hugger off. Cool the room, and uncover the patient as best you can. Admittedly hard with the surgical drapes on. Stop heating the IV fluids.

9. Change twitch monitors. Believe the surgeon and give a small amount of additional relaxant, but no so much that you will be stuck if the case ends soon.

10. First, make sure there is not a massive amount of blood, so bad that the patient needs reintubation and definitive airway protection. If there was a small amount of trauma with intubation, a little blood on the endotracheal tube won't matter that much.

Grab Bag Questions

1. You induce a 7-year-old child and he develops masseter spasm. What do you do?
2. What are the different fluid requirements for a full-term newborn versus a premature newborn?
3. What are the anesthetic implications of scleroderma?
4. A 350-pound man is scheduled for a carpal tunnel release. Is a Bier block an option? An axillary? What if his airway looks difficult?

Answers to Grab Bag Questions

1. Cancel the case if it is elective. True masseter spasm, a clenching of the teeth that a crowbar couldn't open, may be a precursor to MH. If the case is emergent, proceed with a trigger-free anesthetic, get a clean machine in the room, locate the dantrolene, get help, and at the first sign of MH, start treating with dantrolene.

2. A premature infant has fewer energy stores, so the infant may need some caloric replacement. Also, the newborn has less fluid reserve, and may need more fluids. Keep in mind, a full-term baby is born puffy, bursting with extra fluid to get it through the first few days NPO before the mother's milk is let down. A premature does not have that "storage fluid" on board.

3. Scleroderma affects multiple organs. Intubation may be a beast because TMJ mobility is impaired. Reflux is common, so aspiration is a risk. Restricted lungs can lead to hypoxemia, which then leads to right heart failure. Raynaud's is seen in scleroderma making arterial line placement problematic. Vascular insufficiency can extend to the kidneys. Finally, the patient's overall stiffness can extend to the myocardium, with attendant problems of poor LV function.

4. Exsanguinating and getting a good tourniquet fit on this man's arm will be difficult, so a Bier block is not a good option. A carpal tunnel release can be done under a local only in most cases, so that is a good option. Even if this man's airway looked difficult, I would attempt an axillary block. Even more than usual, I would aspirate frequently to avoid a toxic reaction, and I would use mepivacaine as opposed to bupivacaine. That way, if I did get a toxic reaction, it would be shorter lived. Even if the axillary block were incomplete or started to wear off, I'd ask the surgeon to supplement in the field.

That's it! Did you find Waldo? Yes? A bunch of Waldos? Do you want me to tell you which one it was, or which ones they were?
Never!

24 | Sweet Sorrow

"Good night, good night! Parting is such sweet sorrow."
—William Shakespeare, *Romeo and Juliet*, 1595

Use this book as a guide; don't use it as a text. Practice your exams aloud; the more you do the better.

Dress up nice, show up sober, and stick to the point.

Index